Cerebral Palsy

Yoshio Matsuda
Editor

Cerebral Palsy

Perspective and Clinical Relation to Perinatal Complications/Events in Japan

Springer

Editor
Yoshio Matsuda
Tokyo Healthcare University
Shinagawa, Tokyo, Japan

This is a translated version of the book originally published in Japanese language. This has been facilitated using machine translation (by the service DeepL.com) followed by authors revising, editing and verifying the translated manuscript.

ISBN 978-981-19-2216-9 ISBN 978-981-19-2217-6 (eBook)
https://doi.org/10.1007/978-981-19-2217-6

This Springer imprint is published by the registered company Springer Nature Singapore Pte Ltd.
The registered company address is: 152 Beach Road, #21-01/04 Gateway East, Singapore 189721, Singapore

Foreword

Cerebral Palsy and Perinatal Complications and Events: Latest Findings is written and edited by Drs. Yoshio Matsuda, Shoji Satoh, and Keiya Fujimori. They have been most active in the prevention of birth of children with cerebral palsy in Japan.

The greatest challenge in the perinatal field in Japan has been to prevent the birth of children with cerebral palsy and to reduce maternal deaths. However, until around the year 2000, no systematic nationwide effort was made to solve this problem.

In 2003, there were large number of lawsuits against the doctor in charge for inadequate delivery assistance by parents who have a child that had given birth developed cerebral palsy. It followed that the number of obstetricians and delivery facilities decreased, and obstetric care faced a crisis.

The Japan Obstetric Compensation System for Cerebral Palsy, which was established in 2009 based on the idea of the no-fault compensation system for children with cerebral palsy, helped obstetricians in this difficult situation. The reason for this is that the cause analysis committee of this system was a third party committee consisting of perinatologists, neonatologists, medical lawyers, lawyers who help patients, representatives of mass media and patients. Both patients and those in medical field were satisfied with the results of the very fair analysis of the case, and this system functioned well thereafter.

The analysis of the cases of children with cerebral palsy in the system was carried out by an independent causal analysis committee, which examined the clinical course of the onset of cerebral palsy and the findings of the fetal heart rate and labor diagram for each case, covering 2457 cases collected over a 10-year period from January 2009, the year of the system's launch, to September 2019. This report of the collection and causal analysis of a large number of children with cerebral palsy is not only unprecedented in the world, but also provides valuable analytical results on children with cerebral palsy. The results of the analysis showed that the frequency of cerebral palsy related to medical treatment, which was the greatest concern of obstetricians in Japan, was less than about 20% of all cases, force majeure causes such as premature separation of the placenta accounted for about 30%, and in half of the cases, the cause was unknown. Furthermore, it has been pointed out that the onset of cerebral palsy in some of the unexplained cases may not have occurred during the course of delivery but may have already occurred during pregnancy before delivery, hence proving this has become a new problem. Thus, the prevention of the onset of cerebral palsy, which has been the biggest problem in the perinatal field in Japan, has been extremely effective because the analysis of the causes and the measures to prevent the recurrence of cerebral palsy have been made possible by the obstetric medical compensation system.

This book covers the issues that obstetricians and pediatricians who are in charge of pregnancy, childbirth, and postpartum should pay attention to, including the results of research on the prevention of cerebral palsy due to persistent hypoxia related to childbirth, focusing on the obstetric medical compensation system. It is of the highest international, scientific, and clinical relevance. It is therefore recommended that all obstetricians and neonatal pediatricians in the world should have this book at hand and be committed to the prevention of cerebral palsy.

President of Japanese Association of Obstetrician and Gynecologist
Former Chairman and Professor of Department of Obstetrics and Gynecology, University of Juntendo, School of Medicine
Tokyo, Japan

Katsuyuki Kinoshita

Foreword

Towards a comprehensive understanding of cerebral palsy.

Cerebral palsy occurs with a certain frequency in children everywhere. People expected that the progress of obstetrics after 1960s such as fetal heart rate monitoring during labor and ultrasound assessment would lead to a dramatic reduction in the incidence of cerebral palsy. However, epidemiological evidence revealed that this has not been the case, unfortunately. Parents often have to take care of their children affected by cerebral palsy all day and night. Their experience would be beyond the expected in modern society where everyone expects their babies to be born safely and healthy. It is obvious that parents curse their unreasonable situation, and their anger often cause lawsuit to the physician who took care of their babies' parturition. At trial, judiciary tended to interpret the abnormalities appeared in the fetal heart rate monitoring chart, even though observed in more than 80% of the charts at normal delivery, as misjudgement at labor management, so that in most cases physicians lost the suit. As a result, interventions such as cesarean sections were performed more and more frequently, in order to avoid defeat at lawsuit. But this did not lead to a decrease in the incidence of cerebral palsy.

"The Japan Obstetric Compensation System for Cerebral Palsy" was launched in January 2009 and one of the aims of the scheme, which included the concept of "no fault compensation," was to break this vicious circle. In addition, data of cases of cerebral palsy which met certain criteria were collected together with the medical records during patients' pregnancy and delivery courses. At the end of 2020, more than 2700 cases have already been analyzed in detail by the experts of the Causal Analysis Committee of this system. Owing to these analyses, a more detailed background and risk factors for the cerebral palsy are being revealed.

This book, *Cerebral Palsy: Perspective and Clinical Relation to Perinatal Complications/Events in Japan*, brings together in one volume the basic knowledge of cerebral palsy, including definitions and epidemiology, its diagnosis and pathogenesis, the relationship between cerebral palsy and various perinatal complications or risk factors. Until now, many books were published with detailed descriptions of individual obstetrical/perinatal conditions and their relationship to cerebral palsy. However, there have been few books that focus on cerebral palsy as the main topic and summarize the various related events. This book provides a unified understanding of obstetrics with a focus on cerebral palsy, which will not only help in the treatment of various obstetric complications, but will also lead to various medical innovations to improve the prognosis of the child. The editors of this book, Drs. Yoshio Matsuda, Shoji Satoh, and Keiya Fujimori, have worked for many years as members of "The Japan Obstetric Compensation System for Cerebral Palsy" and analyzed various events related to cerebral palsy. We hope that by studying the chapters based on the high level of expertise of these authors, we will be able to provide safer and higher quality obstetric care for mothers and children.

Department of Obstetrics and Gynecology Tadashi Kimura
Osaka University Graduate School of Medicine
Osaka, Japan

Preface

Cerebral palsy (CP) is considered a neurological disorder caused by a non-progressive brain injury or malformation that occurs while the child's brain is under development. The symptoms of CP are not usually obvious just after a baby is born. They normally become noticeable during the first 2 or 3 years of a child's life. Despite the development of perinatal care, the incidence of about 2 per 1000 live births has not changed, and this improvement is considered an important benchmark for perinatal care, along with those of perinatal mortality and maternal mortality.

In Japan, the obstetric compensation system for CP was launched in 2009 to provide financial compensation for children with CP, as well as to investigate the causes and make recommendations for preventing recurrence. It has been clarified that various causes have led to the development of CP. However, the fact that the causes of CP are multifactorial has not yet become widely known to the public, probably because of the long-held misconception that the majority of CP cases are caused by "birth asphyxia."

However, there has been no textbook describing the relationship between CP and perinatal complications and events. We planned to publish a book that would be useful to many doctors, including general clinicians, and would be helpful in clinical practice.

The contents of this book are outlined as follows: the history, definition, and epidemiology of CP; an introduction to the obstetric medical compensation system; clinical diagnosis and imaging diagnosis; and, following the chronological order of pregnancy and delivery, an introduction to all diseases and events that are currently thought to be related to CP. We have asked experts who are actively involved in each of these topics to write about them, and they have gladly agreed to do so. We would like to take this opportunity to express our sincere thanks to them.

The contents of this book are even better than the editors intended, and it will surely be a useful reference book for the improvement of obstetric management in Japan.

The editors hope that this book will be read not only by specialists in perinatology (obstetrics and neonatology) but also by general obstetricians, pediatricians, midwives, and others involved in pregnancy and childbirth.

Tokyo, Japan Yoshio Matsuda

Contents

Part I
Perspective

History and Definitions

Keiya Fujimori and Shun Yasuda

Contents

Summary

- The worldwide incidence of cerebral palsy has remained unchanged despite advances in perinatal medicine and the increase in cesarean delivery rates and is reported to be approximately 2–2.5 per 1000 live births [1].
- The etiopathogenesis of cerebral palsy was unclear until the early nineteenth century. Little, a British orthopedic surgeon, first suggested the role of abnormal deliveries, including dystocia, as well as prematurity as contributors to cerebral palsy and that this condition was preventable. William Osler and Sigmund Freud, who are better known for their contributions to other fields of medicine, also played an important role in providing insights into the development of cerebral palsy. All the important research in the neuropsychological domain of cerebral palsy is largely associated with the contributions of these three researchers.
- Recent epidemiological studies have reported that parturient asphyxia may contribute to cerebral palsy in a relatively small number of cases (approximately only 10%).

K. Fujimori (✉) · S. Yasuda
Department of Obstetrics and Gynecology, School of Medicine, Fukushima Medical University, Fukushima City, Japan
e-mail: fujimori@fmu.ac.jp

Y. Matsuda (ed.), *Cerebral Palsy*, https://doi.org/10.1007/978-981-19-2217-6_1

- To date, no study has conclusively established the superiority of fetal heart rate monitoring in the prevention of neonatal encephalopathy, although it has been compared with intermittent fetal heart rate auscultation.

1 History of Cerebral Palsy

Although no detailed medical descriptions of cerebral palsy are recorded before the nineteenth century, cerebral palsy is mentioned in the Hebrew and Greek scriptures, as well as in the New Testament [2]. The first medical description of cerebral palsy can be traced back to "Corpus Hippocraticum" (460–390 BC), a collection of ancient Greek medical literature associated with the physician Hippocrates and his teachings. Hippocrates also discussed the association between prematurity, congenital infections, prenatal stress, and the etiology of neonatal brain injury in his work "Of the Eight-Month Foetus" [3]. In fact, it was not until many centuries later that the medical community observed physical disabilities in the individuals depicted in the paintings. Presumably, based on his characteristic appearance, Tokugawa Ieshige (1711–1761), the ninth shōgun of the Tokugawa shogunate of Japan, was considered to have had athetoid cerebral palsy [4].

The etiopathogenesis of cerebral palsy remained unknown until the early nineteenth century, and recent research and advances in the understanding of cerebral palsy are primarily attributable to the work of British orthopedic surgeon William John Little (1810–1894). Although Dr. Little himself had a physical disability, at the Congress of Obstetrics and Gynecology held at London in 1858, he introduced the classic definition of (spastic) cerebral palsy; Dr. Little first established that dystocia or abnormal delivery adversely affected neonatal brain development, which resulted in spastic contractures, bilateral paralysis, tonic convulsions, and delayed onset of mental retardation [5]. Little was the first physician to report a direct association between neuromuscular disorders in newborns and abnormal deliveries, neonatal distress, and premature birth (prematurity). He also discussed the possibility that cerebral palsy could be prevented by early management of dystocia as follows: "The fetus, during the contractions of the uterus, … is under extreme pressure that only early separation from the mother can prevent injury to the frail organs of the fetus" [2].

In addition to Dr. Little who provided historical insights into the association between dystocia and cerebral palsy, Sir William Osler (1849–1919) and Sigmund Freud (1856–1939) made important contributions to the understanding of this condition. All important research in the field of cerebral palsy since the end of the nineteenth century is largely attributable to the work of these three researchers.

Osler reviewed the neuroanatomical pathology with reference to his own experience and based on 151 cases in the literature (120 cases of infantile hemiplegia, 20 cases of bilateral spastic hemiplegia, and 11 cases of spastic paraplegia) and published *The Cerebral Palsies of Children* in 1889 [3]. He observed that dystocia, delivery-induced asphyxia, and prolonged resuscitation were associated with neonatal seizures and that the etiology of this birth-related paralysis was strongly associated with intracranial hemorrhage. This book was the first to use the expression "the cerebral palsies," which subsequently led to the widespread use of the term "cerebral palsy." Osler was also the first researcher to confirm infantile jaundice as a risk factor for cerebral palsy [3].

Freud devised a classification system that continues to be used even in current times and has remained essentially unchanged; this system categorizes patients based on the time of onset of symptoms as ante-, intra-, and postpartum [3]. Furthermore, it has been established that the mechanism underlying cerebral palsy, which was attributed to abnormal delivery, originates in the uterus before the onset of labor and is not associated with intrapartum oxygen deprivation. Studies have highlighted the multifactorial etiology of cerebral palsy and that this disorder essentially represents a syndrome [3].

Following the work of Osler and the other researchers, Winthrop Morgan Phelps (1894–1971), a Baltimore-based orthopedic surgeon, was the first clinician to treat patients with cerebral palsy, and in 1941, Dr. Phelps published a paper titled "The management of cerebral palsy" in which he classified cerebral palsy into the following types: spastic, athetoid, associated with rigidity, associated with tremor, and associated with incoordination (ataxic) [3]. Based on Dr. Little's report, he proposed that cerebral palsy is a neuromuscular disease characterized by motor and postural disorders as core symptoms, although cerebral palsy was previously understood to include intellectual disability. In essence, he emphasized that intellectual disabilities do not necessarily occur in these patients. Dr. Phelps' pioneering work led to the establishment of the term cerebral palsy in the United States [5].

2 Recent Epidemiological Research in Cerebral Palsy

In 1986, Nelson and Ellenberg of the National Institutes of Health investigated 45,559 children born between 1959 and 1966, who were followed up until 7 years of age. Of these, 189 had cerebral palsy, and only 40 (21%) had clinical findings suggestive of delivery-induced asphyxia (fetal heart rate <60/min, 5-min Apgar score <3, or crying for >5 min after birth). Following exclusion of those with morphological abnormalities or microcephaly, which were evidently contributors to the movement disorder, the authors reported that only 17 neonates (9%) had clinical findings suggestive of delivery-induced asphyxia [6]. In 1988, Blair and Stanley from Australia reported nearly the same findings as those reported by Nelson et al. [7] in a study of 183 patients with spastic cerebral palsy, who were followed up over 5 years from 1975. The authors observed that delivery-induced asphyxia was implicated in brain injury in only 8% of all cases.

In a retrospective study performed between 1995 and 1997 in Japan, Sugimoto et al. investigated the association between fetal asphyxia and cerebral palsy in 106 children who attended pediatric neurology outpatient clinics for the evaluation and management of this disorder [8, 9]. Based on the results of head magnetic resonance imaging (MRI) findings, medical history, and neurological evaluation, the authors investigated the main causes and timing of brain injury in these patients; 13 infants presented with fetal asphyxia (12.3%, 1-min Apgar scores $\leq$6) and 13 infants with periventricular hyperintensity on MRI, which indicated periventricular leukomalacia associated with prematurity. Moreover, 14 patients (13.2%) presented with cerebral hemorrhage, 15 (14.2%) with cerebral infarction, 7 (6.6%) with central nervous system viral infections in utero and in the neonatal period, and 37 (35%) with genetic disorders and disorders of brain development associated with early fetal development.

Based on these reports, delivery-induced fetal asphyxia is implicated in the onset of cerebral palsy in only approximately 10% of all cases.

3 Definition

The concept of cerebral palsy encompasses not only motor palsy but also many other disorders that are difficult to define in a simple statement [10]. The definition established by the Cerebral Palsy Research Group of the former Ministry of Health and Welfare in 1968 (group leader: Tadao Takatsu) is most commonly used in Japan because it embodies the current understanding of this disorder and shares several features with the definitions proposed by other countries. Accordingly, cerebral palsy is defined as "a permanent but variable motor and postural abnormality based on non-progressive brain lesions occurring between conception and neonatal periods within 4 weeks after birth. The symptoms develop by the age of 2 years. Progressive disease, transient movement disorders, or delays in motor development that appear likely to normalize in the future are excluded" [11].

The definition established at the 2004 Workshop in Bethesda states "The term cerebral palsy describes a group of abnormalities in motor and postural development that cause limitation of activity but are attributed to non-progressive disorders occurring in the developing fetal or infant brain. It is thought to result from non-progressive disorders that occur in the developing fetal or infant brain. Motor deficits in cerebral palsy may include sensory, cognitive, communicative, cognitive, behavioral, and/or seizure disorders." Based on this definition, abnormalities of movement and posture unaccompanied by activity limitation are not categorized as cerebral palsy [11].

Based on the aforementioned definitions, cerebral palsy is characterized by the following attributes: (a) a brain disorder that occurs between conception and the neonatal period; (b) a non-progressive disease but one associated with permanent lesions; (c) symptoms of postural and motor impairment, with or without concomitant intellectual disability or epilepsy; and (d) a permanent disorder in which motor developmental delay is not normalized in the future.

4 Classification of Cerebral Palsy

Cerebral palsy can be classified based on the etiology and timing of onset, the location (extent) of motor impairment, and physiological characteristics of motor impairment (Table 1).

Classification based on the etiology and time of onset includes prenatal, perinatal, and acquired cerebral palsy. Classification based on the physiological characteristics of motor impairment (pathological classification) includes spastic, athetotic, hypotonic, ataxic, and mixed type of cerebral palsy. Cerebral palsy based on the extent of motor impairment can be classified as quadriplegia, diplegia (paralysis of all four extremities, but predominantly of the lower extremities), hemiplegia (paralysis of one side of the body), paraplegia (paralysis of the lower extremities only), triplegia, and monoplegia.

We categorize cerebral palsy based on abnormalities of movement and distribution of disability and briefly describe its characteristics [10].

Table 1 Classification of cerebral palsy

Classification of cerebral palsy based on the etiology and time of onset	1. Prenatal: abnormal brain formation, intrauterine infection, drugs, poisoning, low nutritional status, and circulatory failure in utero among other causes
	2. Perinatal: intrapartum asphyxia, cerebral hemorrhage, infection, and nuclear jaundice among other conditions
	3. Acquired: postnatal meningitis, encephalitis, and cerebral hemorrhage among other conditions
Classification of movement impairment based on the physiological characteristic clinical presentation	1. Spastic type: a condition in which both spasticity (stiffening of limbs by rapid dynamic movements) and contracture (persistent stiffening) occur concomitantly and the limbs are pinched, which prevents smooth movements
	2. Athetotic type (involuntary movements): sudden movements and hypotonia accompanied by uncontrolled movements of the face, arms, and hands
	3. Hypotonic: stickiness, posture maintenance, and balance disorder
	4. Ataxic type
	5. Mixed type
Classification of cerebral palsy based on the location (extent) of movement impairment	1. Quadriplegia
	2. Diplegia: paralysis of all four extremities, but predominantly of the lower extremities
	3. Hemiplegia: paralysis of one side of the body, usually upper extremity > lower extremity
	4. Paraplegia: paralysis exclusively of the lower extremities
	5. Triplegia and monoplegia, among others

1. Spastic Cerebral Palsy
   (a) Spastic Hemiplegia
   The prevalence of this type is 10–15% of all cases of cerebral palsy in Japan. It is characterized by a disorder of the upper and lower extremities on one side of the body. This disorder is detected at approximately 4–6 months of age; patients typically show left-right differences in movements of the upper and lower extremities (upper extremity movements are predominant). Symptoms include an inability to grip objects with the upper extremities, inability to pick small objects, and limited external rotation of the forearm.
   (b) Spastic Quadriplegia
   The prevalence of this type is 25–30% of all cases of cerebral palsy in Japan. The generalized muscle tone is increased, and both upper and lower extremities are affected, with predominant involvement of both lower extremities. From early infancy, the infant presents with a typical posterior arch hemiparesis-like posture and head movement-induced extension of both upper and lower extremities (decerebrate rigidity-like posture).
   (c) Spastic Diplegia
   The prevalence of this type is 35–40% of all cases of cerebral palsy in Japan; 80% of preterm infants with cerebral palsy present with this variety. Lower extremity involvement predominates in this type of cerebral palsy with infrequent involvement of the upper limbs. The left and right sides show asymmetrical impairment, with any one side being dominant. Children with this type of palsy often show an extended or flexed upper extremity, fixed representation of the forearm in the gyrus, and incoordinated movements of the upper extremities.

2. Extrapyramidal Cerebral Palsy
   The prevalence of this type of cerebral palsy is approximately 5–10% of all cases of cerebral palsy in Japan.
   (a) Choreoathetotic Cerebral Palsy
   The prevalence of this type is 5–8% of all cases of cerebral palsy in Japan. It is characterized by large-amplitude involuntary movements, and athetosis (in contrast to chorea) is the main involuntary movement. The abnormal movements are most prominent at the ends of the extremities and are typically slow, writhing involuntary movements, accompanied by finger and toe extension and twisting of the extremity along its long axis. Children with this form of cerebral palsy show significant speech difficulties.
   (b) Dystonic Cerebral Palsy
   The prevalence of this type is 2–3% of all cases of cerebral palsy in Japan. Most patients have a history of hypoxic-ischemic encephalopathy or nuclear jaundice after birth, and trunk muscles and proximal ends of the extremities are predominantly affected. Patients show slow and persistent movements, which are most prominent in the head and neck musculature. The head and neck may appear to be drawn to one side or may show abrupt backward movement.

3. Hypotonic (Atonic) Cerebral Palsy
   This variety of cerebral palsy is extremely rare in Japan. Infants present with lower extremity muscle weakness with near-normal muscle strength and coordinated movements of the upper extremities. This type of cerebral palsy is characterized by lifelong hypotonia.
4. Ataxic Cerebral Palsy
   This type of cerebral palsy is rare in Japan and may be accompanied by spastic paraplegia; however, this condition is diagnosed in patients with predominantly cerebellar symptoms.
5. Mixed Cerebral Palsy
   The prevalence of this disorder is 5–10% of all cases of cerebral palsy in Japan. Most cases of cerebral palsy do not present with a purely monosymptomatic form and tend to show a mixed form of clinical presentation. The most common combinations include spastic and athetotic cerebral palsy.

5 Fetal Heart Rate Monitoring and Neonatal Encephalopathy

At the time fetal heart rate monitoring was introduced in the 1960s, most neonatal central nervous system disorders were attributed to hypoxemia during delivery. It was presumed that intrapartum fetal heart rate monitoring performed for the early detection of hypoxemia could safeguard the fetus from the deteriorating intrauterine environment and consequent cerebral palsy and mental retardation [12]. However, forward-looking randomized controlled trials (RCTs) (which compared fetal heart rate monitoring with the intermittent fetal heart rate auscultation method) and meta-analyses performed from 1970 to early 1980 clarified the following facts: (1) Fetal heart rate monitoring could prevent low Apgar scores, low fetal blood pH, neonatal resuscitation, and neonatal intensive care unit admissions. (2) Fetal heart rate monitoring increased the rate of cesarean deliveries owing to accurate and prompt diagnosis of fetal distress (non-reassuring fetal status). The only benefit of fetal heart rate monitoring reported by the aforementioned RCTs was the reduction in neonatal seizures observed in the Dublin trial [13]. (3) No reduction in central nervous system disorders was observed with regard to long-term prognosis of neonates [14]. However, these results were observed following a comparative study of fetal heart rate monitoring vs. intermittent fetal heart rate auscultation, and it is ethically impossible to perform a comparative study between a fetal heart rate monitoring during delivery group and a non-implemented group (fetal heart rate monitoring during delivery is not performed) in real-world clinical settings; therefore, the effectiveness of intrapartum fetal heart rate monitoring remains unclear.

Nelson et al. [15] reported fetal heart rate monitoring patterns that characterize neonatal cerebral palsy in 95 patients diagnosed with cerebral palsy at 3 years of age. A high risk of multiple late decelerations (odds ratio 3.9, 95% confidence interval [CI] 1.7–9.3) and decreased beat-to-beat variability were observed (odds ratio 2.7, 95% CI: 1.1–5.8); however, no abnormality occurred in 73% of patients with cerebral palsy, which indicates a high rate of cesarean delivery (odds ratio 2.9, 95% CI: 1.0–8.6) in addition to an extremely high false-positive rate. Furthermore, Melone et al. [16] observed that among 49 patients who underwent fetal heart rate monitoring in whom cerebral palsy was diagnosed at 1 year of age, 35% of patients in the control and 31% patients in the cerebral palsy group were diagnosed with a non-reassuring pattern. We observed a significant difference in the 5-min Apgar scores without a significant difference in 1-min Apgar scores and umbilical artery pH of <7.20. We observed no specific fetal heart rate patterns associated with cerebral palsy, and an abnormal fetal heart rate pattern cannot conclusively predict the subsequent development of cerebral palsy.

In a recent study, Nakao et al. [17] retrospectively analyzed intrapartum fetal heart rate tracings obtained from 1069 neonates (patients with severe cerebral palsy at fetal age ≥34 weeks) registered in the Japan Obstetric Compensation System for Cerebral Palsy and classified these tracings into six categories. The results showed that (a) 7.9% had continuous bradycardia on admission, (b) 21.7% had a non-reassuring pattern on admission and persisting until delivery, (c) 15.6% had severe prolonged bradycardia before delivery compared with a reassuring pattern on admission, (d) 15.9% had gradual deterioration (Hon's pattern) during delivery compared with a reassuring pattern on admission, (e) 19.8% had a persistently reassuring pattern on admission until delivery, and (f) 19.1% remained unclassified. Therefore, 31.5% of these patients had severe prolonged bradycardia before delivery compared with a reassuring pattern on admission and gradual deterioration (Hon's pattern), which was associated with intrapartum hypoxic brain injury.

References

1. MacLennan AH, Thompson SC, Gecz J. Cerebral palsy: causes, pathways, and the role of genetic variants. Am J Obstet Gynecol. 2015;213:779–88.
2. Arima M, Sakuragawa N. Nouseimahi no rekishi – Little no kouen no shoukai wo kanete [The history of cerebral palsy - with an introduction to Little's lecture]. Shounika Mook. 1979;7:1–4. Japanese
3. Panteliadis C, Panteliadis P, Vassilyadi F. Hallmarks in the history of cerebral palsy: from antiquity to mid-20th century. Brain Dev. 2013;35:285–92.
4. Shinoda T. Tokugawa shogunke 15dai no karute [Clinical records of the Fifteen Generations of the Tokugawas]. Tokyo: Shincho-sha; 2005. Japanese
5. Tamaki Y, Kato Y, Hotta C, et al. Nouseimahi (1): Shitaifujiyuu, nouseimahi no teigi to kanrenjikou [Cerebral palsy (1): definition and physical impairments]. Shinshu Univ J Educ Res Pract. 2016;9:227–48. Japanese
6. Nelson KB, Ellenberg JH. Antecedents of cerebral palsy. Multivariate analysis of risk. N Engl J Med. 1986;315:81–6.
7. Blair E, Stanley FJ. Intrapartum asphyxia: a rare cause of cerebral palsy. J Pediatr. 1988;112:515–9.
8. Sugimoto T, Woo M, Nishida N, Araki A, Hara T, Yasuhara A, Kobayashi Y, Yamanouchi Y. When do brain abnormalities in cerebral palsy occur? An MRI study. Dev Med Child Neurol. 1995;37:285–92.

9. Sugimoto K, Woo M, Nishida N, Sasaki T, Araki A, Yasuhara A, Kobayashi Y, Hara T. Bunbenji kasha ha nouseimahi no syugeninka? Shinkeigairai de keikakansatsuchu no nouseimahiji 106 rei no kentou [Is intrapartum asphyxia a major cause of cerebral palsy? - a study of 106 cases of children with cerebral palsy undergoing follow-up at a neurological outpatient clinic]. Obstet Gynecol Pract. 1997;46:1133–8. Japanese.
10. Ochiai M. Nouseimahi [Cerebral palsy]. Sogo Rehabil. 2012;40:606–11. Japanese
11. Japanese Association of Rehabilitation Medicine (supervised). Nouseimahi rehabilitation guideline [Guidelines for rehabilitation of cerebral palsy]. 2nd ed. Tokyo: Kanehara Shuppan; 2014. Japanese
12. Quilligan EJ, Paul RH. Fetal monitoring: is it worth it? Obstet Gynecol. 1975;45:96–100.
13. Grant A, O'Brien N, Joy MT, Hennessy E, MacDonald D. Cerebral palsy among children born during the Dublin randomized trial of intrapartum monitoring. Lancet. 1989;2(8674):1233–6.
14. Grant A. Epidemiological principles for evaluation of monitoring programs-the Dublin experience. Clin Invest Med. 1993;16:149–58.
15. Nelson KB, Dambrosia JM, Ting TY, Grether JK. Uncertain value of electric fetal monitoring in predicting cerebral palsy. N Engl J Med. 1996;334:613–8.
16. Melone PJ, Ernest JM, O'Shea MD Jr, Klinepeter KL. Appropriateness of intrapartum fetal heart rate management and risk of cerebral palsy. Am J Obstet Gynecol. 1991;165:272–6.
17. Nakao M, Okumura A, Hasegawa J, et al. Fetal heart rate pattern in term or near-term cerebral palsy: a nationwide cohort study. Am J Obstet Gynecol. 2020;223:907.e1–13.

Epidemiology of the Cerebral Palsy

Shoji Satoh

Contents

Summary

- The definition of cerebral palsy is "a permanent but changeable motor and postural abnormality based on a nonprogressive lesion of the brain occurring between conception and the neonatal period (within the first 4 weeks of life), with manifestations occurring before the age of 2 years, and excluding progressive disease, transient movement disorders, or delayed motor development that will normalize in the future."
- In other countries, the frequency is generally 2–2.5 per 1000 live births, and the frequency has changed little from year to year.
- Based on the several reports on the annual trend of cerebral palsy incidence in Japan, the incidence declined after 1956 with the improvement of neonatal management, but then rose again with the improvement of the survival rate of low-birth-weight and preterm infants, and is now estimated to be 2–2.4 per 1000 live births, as in other countries.
- The incidence of cerebral palsy increases with shorter weeks of gestation and lower birth weight, and hypoxic-ischemic encephalopathy is the most common cause of cerebral palsy in mature infants and periventricular leu-

S. Satoh (✉)
Maternal and Perinatal Care Center, Oita Prefectural Hospital, Oita City, Oita, Japan
e-mail: s-satoh@oitapref-hosp.jp

Y. Matsuda (ed.), *Cerebral Palsy*, https://doi.org/10.1007/978-981-19-2217-6_2

komalacia in preterm infants. When considering the direct cause of cerebral palsy, it should be borne in mind that the cause of cerebral palsy in infants with abnormal fetal heart rate patterns in labor is not necessarily hypoxia at delivery, i.e., it is important to consider whether the disease or condition in infants with cerebral palsy is a "direct cause" or a "background disease" or "related disease (so-called risk factor)" or the modifying condition as an "aggravating factor."

1 Definition of Cerebral Palsy

The definition of cerebral palsy (CP) in Japan was formulated by the Cerebral Palsy Study Group of the former Ministry of Health and Welfare in 1968 as "permanent but changeable motor and postural abnormalities caused by non-progressive lesions of the brain occurring between conception and the neonatal period (within 4 weeks of birth), with symptoms occurring by the age of 2 years". Symptoms occur by age 2 years and exclude progressive disease, transient movement disorders, or delayed motor development that will normalize in the future. Definitions in other countries are generally consistent.

1. Brain damage occurring in the fetal and neonatal period.
2. Non-progressive and persistent disease.
3. Postural and motor impairment.
4. Transient disorders and delays in motor development that are expected to normalize are considered to be excluded.

2 Incidence of Cerebral Palsy

It is not easy to calculate the incidence of CP because the causes of CP are various and advances in perinatal medicine and medical care can reduce the incidence and severity of CP caused by conventional factors, but there is also the possibility that CP caused by new factors may occur as the survival rate of newborns increases. According to MacLennan et al. [1] and Himmelmann et al. [2], the incidence is estimated to be 2–2.5 per 1000 births (including minor cases), and the frequency has not changed much from year to year. However, Takeshita et al. reported [3] that the incidence of CP in the four time periods of 1956–1959, 1971–1974, 1975–1980, and 1981–1984 was 2.418, 1.428, 0.571, and 1.150 (per 1000 live births), respectively. Although the incidence declined with the improvement of neonatal management, it is predicted that the incidence will tend to rise again in the future due to the subsequent improvement in the survival rate of low-birth-weight and preterm infants.

In the "Report on the Medical Survey for the Design of the Japan Obstetric Compensation System for Cerebral Palsy" in 2009, the incidence of CP was estimated to be 2.3 per 1000 live births in Okinawa Prefecture (1998–2001) and 2.2 in Himeji City (1993–1997). In addition, a nationwide estimate using the "National Database of Receipt Information and Specified Health Examination Information (NDB)" constructed by the Ministry of Health, Labour and Welfare [4] estimated the incidence to be about 2.4 for 4-year-old children.

As a recent detailed study, the Epidemiological Survey Report on the Actual Condition of CP Children [5] conducted a complete survey of CP children in three prefectures (Tottori, Tokushima, and Tochigi) over a 5-year period from 2009 and clarified the incidence of CP and the condition at birth. There were 231 births of CP between 2009 and 2013 in the 3 prefectures. The total number of births during the study period was 135,335, and the incidence rate of CP was estimated to be 1.7 per 1000 live births, which was the highest (2.1) in 2009 and the lowest (1.4) in 2012 (Fig. 1). The incidence of CP according to the number of weeks of pregnancy was highest at 102.6 per 1000 births at 27 weeks or less, 56.1 at 28–31 weeks, 6.1 at 32–36 weeks, and 0.8 at 37 weeks or more, and the incidence tended to decrease as the baby approached full term (Fig. 2). Furthermore, the incidence of CP by birth weight was highest for birth weights of 999 g or less (81.5 per 1000 births), 54.1 for birth weights of 1000–1499 g, 15.3 for 1500–1999 g, 4.2 for 2000–2499 g, 0.9 for 2500–2999 g, 0.5 for 3000–3499 g, 0.5 for 3000–3499 g, 0.2 for 3500–3999 g, and 1.7 for 4000 g or more, with the lowest incidence in the 3500–3900 g range (Fig. 3). These results indicate that the shorter gestational weeks at delivery as well as the smaller the birth weight, the incidence of CP increases, which is consistent with previous reports.

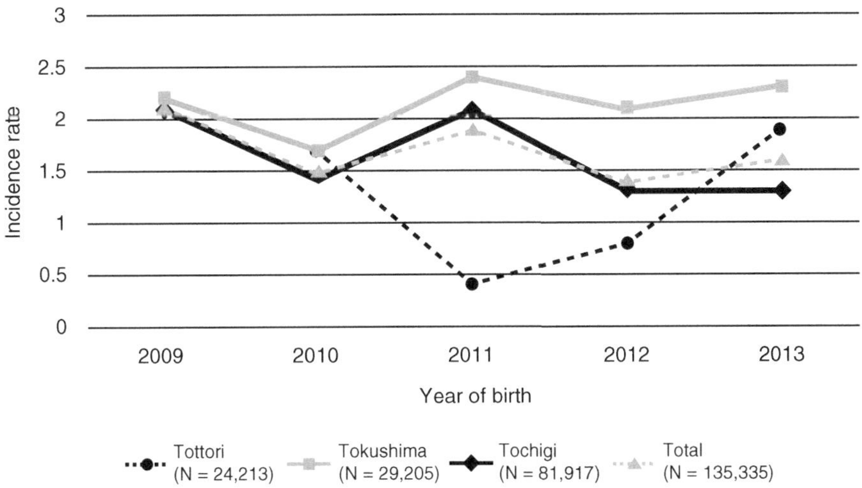

Fig. 1 The incidence rate (births per 1000) of CP in the three prefectures in Japan. (Adapted from Ref. [5])

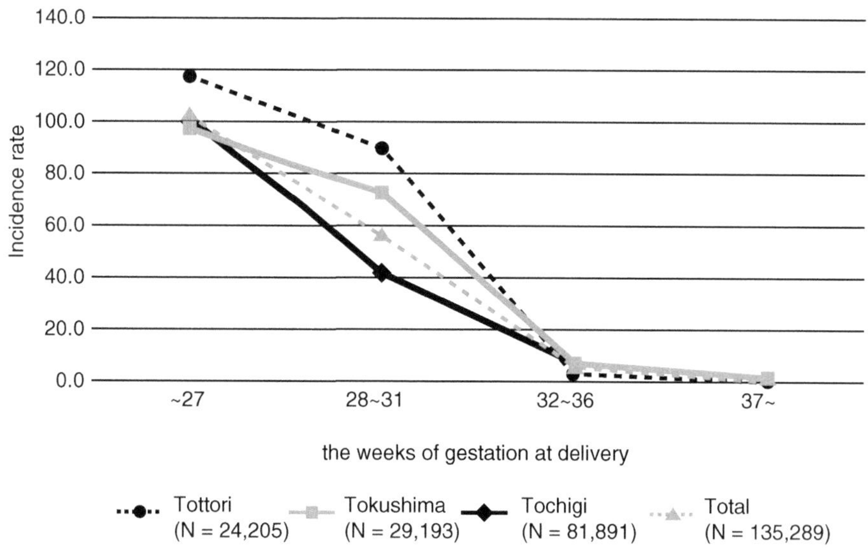

Fig. 2 The incidence of CP and the weeks of gestation at delivery (1000 live births) in the three prefectures in Japan. (Adapted from Ref. [5])

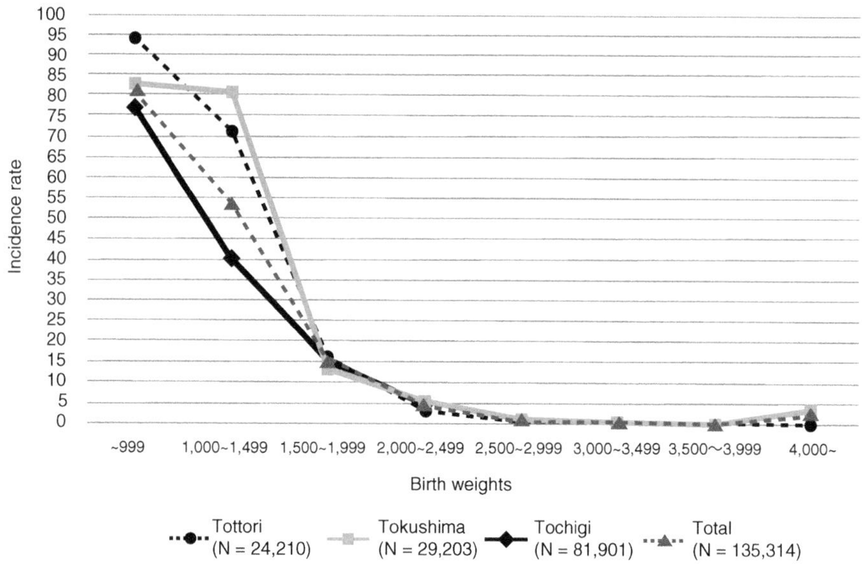

Fig. 3 The incidence of CP by birth weights (1000 live births) in the three prefectures. (Adapted from Ref. [5])

3 Cerebral Palsy "Causes" and "Risk Factors"

It is undisputed that the causes of CP are diverse from the viewpoint of perinatal medicine; it is important to consider whether hypoxic events during labor should be uniformly regarded as the direct cause of CP, particularly when some perinatal events, such as neonatal asphyxia or hypoxic/academic patterns in cardiotocography (CTG), are observed in children with CP. This issue has become a major point of contention in medical litigation and perinatal care. In the aforementioned survey [5], the majority of children (84.8%) had diseases or other conditions considered to be major risk factors for CP from prepartum to postpartum. In these, 70.6% had at least pathophysiological conditions during delivery, with neonatal asphyxia being the most common (50.2%), followed by periventricular leukomalacia (PVL) in 28.6% and hypoxic-ischemic encephalopathy (HIE) in 18.2% (Tables 1 and 2). This result is consistent with previous reports that hypoxic-ischemic encephalopathy and periventricular leukomalacia account for most of the causes of CP in mature infants and preterm infants, respectively, and the events during labor are the candidates for the risk factors for CP. However, when discussing the relationship between CP and maternal or infant disease during labor, it is also important to consider whether the disease is the "direct cause" or not, furthermore, a "background condition" or "related condition" or a "modifying condition" as an "aggravating factor."

4 Causative Diseases of CP from the Perspective of the Report on Prevention of Recurrence, the Japan Obstetric Compensation System for Cerebral Palsy

Eligible cases in the Japan Obstetric Compensation System for Cerebral Palsy are those in which the gestational weeks at delivery is 28 weeks or more, the severity of the injury is equivalent to a physical disability grade 1 or 2, and the child does not meet the exclusion criteria such as congenital factors (hereditary/genetic diseases and/or major structural abnormalities) and factors in the neonatal period. For this reason, it is kept in mind that the epidemiological analysis does not cover all CP cases in Japan. Therefore, the results obtained in the abovementioned regional surveys and other studies cannot be directly applied, and simple comparisons cannot be made. Figure 4 shows the results by cause for the 10 years from January 2009 to September 2019 under this system [6]. Of the total of 2457 cases, 1051 (42.8%) were judged to have an unknown or difficult-to-identify cause, and of the remaining 1406 (57.1%) cases judged to have obvious pathophysiological causes, 1179 (46.7% of the total) of those could be explained by a single possible cause. On the other hand, cases in which multiple perinatal events were considered to be the cause accounted for about 10% of the total, resulting in more than half of the cases having

Table 1 Diseases and other conditions considered to be major risk factors for cerebral palsy from prepartum to postpartum (Adapted from Ref. [5])

Diseases		Tottori		Tokushima		Tochigi		Total	
		No. of cases	Percentage	No. of cases	Percentage	No. of cases	Percentage	No. of cases	Percentage
Diseases (+)		32	94.1	54	87.1	110	81.5	196	84.8
Duplicated	Preparturient	10	29.4	24	38.7	41	30.4	75	32.5
	Intrapartum	31	91.2	42	67.7	90	66.7	163	70.6
	Postpartum	5	14.7	16	25.8	19	14.1	40	17.3
No diseases		0	0.0	1	1.6	6	4.4	7	3.0
Unknown		2	5.9	7	11.3	19	14.1	28	12.1
Total		34	100.0	62	100.0	135	100.0	231	100.0

Table 2 Details of diseases and other conditions considered to be major risk factors for cerebral palsy from prepartum to postpartum (Adapted from Ref. [5])

		Tottori		Tokushima		Tochigi		Total	
No. of CP		34		62		135		231	
Diseases		No. of cases	Percentage	No. of cases	Percentage	No. of cases	Percentage	No. of cases	Percentage
Preparturient	Cerebral malformation	3	8.8	7	11.3	21	15.6	31	13.4
	Chromosomal abnormality	1	2.9	8	12.9	6	4.4	15	6.5
	Genetic abnormality	3	8.8	2	3.2	5	3.7	10	4.3
	Metabolic disorder	0	0.0	1	1.6	0	0.0	1	0.4
	Other congenital anomalies	1	2.9	7	11.3	16	11.9	24	10.4
	Intrauterine infection	4	11.8	5	8.1	7	5.2	16	6.9
Intrapartum	Neonatal asphyxia	25	73.5	26	41.9	65	48.1	116	50.2
	Meconium aspiration syndrome	1	2.9	4	6.5	2	1.5	7	3.0
	Intracranial hemorrhage	8	23.5	8	12.9	25	18.5	41	17.7
	Hypoxic-ischemic encephalopathy	7	20.6	12	19.4	23	17.0	42	18.2
	Periventricular leukomalacia	14	41.2	11	17.7	41	30.4	66	28.6
	Cerebral infarction	0	0.0	2	3.2	8	5.9	10	4.3
	RDS	15	44.1	15	24.2	31	23.0	61	26.4
	Transient tachypnea in newborn	0	0.0	6	9.7	14	10.4	20	8.7
Postpartum	Meningitis	2	5.9	0	0.0	2	1.5	4	1.7
	Encephalitis	0	0.0	0	0.0	3	2.2	3	1.3
	ALTE	0	0.0	6	9.7	4	3.0	10	4.3
	Infant abuse	0	0.0	0	0.0	1	0.7	1	0.4
	Other trauma	0	0.0	0	0.0	1	0.7	1	0.4
	Others	3	8.8	12	19.4	9	6.7	24	10.4

an unknown or difficult-to-identify cause and multiple confounding factors involved in the process of CP formation. Based on these epidemiological results, a review eligible for the compensation criteria is under consideration in 2021. The scope of the system may be expanded to include CP cases with no abnormal medical findings before and after delivery. Then, it is expected that the registered cases will be expanded to cases after 28 weeks of gestation. Consequently, PVL cases specific to preterm infants are expected to increase, and further analysis of the differences in causes between full-term and preterm births might be possible.

Pathophysiology			**No. of Cases**	**%**
A single condition			**1,179**	**46.7**
A single condition	Detachment of the placenta or bleeding from the placenta		**410**	**16.2**
		Placental abruption	405	(16.0)
		Dissection of placenta previa or low-lying placenta	5	(0.2)
	umbilical cord factor		**309**	**12.2**
		cord prolapse	55	(2.2)
		other cord factors	254	(10.1)
	infection		**82**	**3.2**
		GBS	44	(1.7)
		herpes encephalitis	16	(0.6)
		Others	22	(0.9)
	Intracranial hemorrhage		53	2.1
	Uterine rupture		48	1.9
	Imbalance of blood flow in tins (including twin-to-twin transfusion syndrome)		45	1.8
	Fetomaternal transfusion		40	1.6
	Maternal respiratory and circulatory failure		37	1.5
		Amniotic fluid embolism	**14**	**(0.6)**
		Other maternal respiratory and circulatory failure	**23**	**(0.9)**
	Cerebral infarction in neonates		40	1.6
	Placental insufficiency or reduced placental function		31	1.2
	Others		84	3.3

Fig. 4 The main cause of cerebral palsy. (Adapted from Ref. [6])

Multiple conditions			**264**	**10.4**
(duplicated)	Umbilical cord factors other than cord prolapse		163	6.5
	Placental insufficiency or reduced placental function		75	3.0
	infection		38	1.5
	Placental abruption		32	1.3
Unknown etiology			**1,084**	**42.9**
	Intracranial abnormal findings, present		**776**	**30.7**
		Cases with presumed onset during pregnancy and parturition	702	(27.8)
		Cases with presumed onset in the neonatal period	74	(2.9)
	Intracranial abnormal findings, absent		**308**	**12.2**
		Cases without known event	217	(8.6)
		Cases with suspected congenital factors	91	(3.6)
Total			**2,527**	**100**

Fig. 4 (continued)

References

1. MacLennan AH, Thompson SC, Gecz J. Cerebral palsy: causes, pathways, and the role of genetic variants. Am J Obstet Gynecol. 2015;213:779–88.
2. Himmelmann K, Sundh V. Survival with cerebral palsy over five decades in western Sweden. Dev Med Child Neurol. 2015;57:762–7.
3. Takeshita K. Nihon niokeru nouseimahi no hassei – Ekigakuteki bunseki to kongo no taisaku [Outbreak of cerebral palsy in Japan: epidemiological analysis and future measures]. J Rehabil Res. 1989;60:43–8. Japanese
4. Toyokawa S, Maeda E, Kobayashi Y. Estimation of the number of children with cerebral palsy using nationwide health insurance claims data in Japan. Dev Med Child Neurol. 2017;59:317–21.
5. Epidemiological Survey Project Team on the Actual Condition of Children with Cerebral Palsy. Report of epidemiological survey on the actual condition of children with cerebral palsy. Tokyo: Japan Council for Quality Health Care 2018. Japanese. http://www.sanka-hp.jcqhc.or.jp/documents/report/pdf/nouseimahijinojittaihaakunikansuruekigakuchousahoukokusyo.pdf. Accessed 14 Feb 2022
6. Japan Council for Quality Health Care. 11th Report on prevention of recurrence, The Japan Obstetric Compensation System for Cerebral Palsy. Tokyo: Japan Council for Quality Health Care; 2021. Japanese

Current Status of the Japan Obstetric Compensation System for Cerebral Palsy

Shin Ushiro

Contents

S. Ushiro (✉)
Japan Health Care Evaluation Agency, Department of Medical Safety Management, Kyushu University Hospital, Fukuoka, Japan
e-mail: ushiro@surg2.med.kyushu-u.ac.jp

Y. Matsuda (ed.), *Cerebral Palsy*, https://doi.org/10.1007/978-981-19-2217-6_3

Summary

- The Obstetric Compensation System for Cerebral Palsy was launched in 2009 in response to a shortage of obstetricians and a surge in disputes.
- The system is characterized by the provision of no-fault compensation, investigation, and prevention.
- We have certified more than 3000 cerebral palsy cases for compensation and have delivered investigative reports, prevention reports, and educative media for professionals and expectant mothers.
- We have also produced recapitulation of individual investigative report to be uploaded on the webpage of the system to enhance transparency. The disclosure is reviewed to be consistent with lately revised Personal Information Protection Law in 2020.
- In order to expand the system by revising eligibility criteria, the system was and will be revised in 2015 and 2022. The new criteria which was crafted in ad hoc committee in 2019–2020 will be applied in 2022 and later.
- As such, the system has been a significant part of perinatal care delivery system in Japan.

The Japan Obstetric Compensation System for Cerebral Palsy [1] was launched in 2009 with the Japan Council for Quality Health Care (JQ) as the operating organization, against the background of a shortage of obstetricians in Japan and a surge in disputes particularly caused by occurrence of cerebral palsy. More than 10 years have passed since the system commenced, and it has given rise to enormous achievements such as early resolution of disputes displayed in the rapid decrease in the number of lawsuit statistics and quality improvement of perinatal care [2]. In this section, current status of the system and challenges ahead are described.

1 Current Status and Challenges of the Japan Obstetric Compensation System for Cerebral Palsy

1.1 Background to Launch the System

1.1.1 Perinatal Care and Conflict

Among the disputes, those related to cerebral palsy were said to be a heavy burden for obstetricians because the cause of cerebral palsy was often unknown. In discussions with perinatal care professionals in Japan and abroad, I have had the opportunity to learn that cerebral palsy is one of the causes of disputes, including court cases, and of obstetricians leaving their jobs, not only in high-income countries but also in Low and middle income countries (LMICs). In cases where a child is born in a distressed status despite normal course of pregnancy and delivery, or where the child's neurological deficits become apparent to develop profound cerebral palsy in spite of little or no findings on hypoxic condition during delivery, the family's feelings may become complicated, and disputes may arise. Therefore, obstetricians have been discussing for many years the establishment of a compensation system that works on no-fault basis.

1.1.2 Discussion on the Establishment of a No-Fault Compensation System

Discussions on the establishment of a no-fault compensation system have been held by the Japan Medical Association (JMA) since the 1960s. In the report entitled "Report on the Legal Response to Medical Accidents and Its Basic Theory" published in 1972, the following recommendations were set forth.

1. In the event of a medical accident, if the physician's practices are deemed to be negligent through a rigorous examination, he or she will be immediately held responsible for compensation.
2. Compensation should be established on a national scale to provide relief for serious damage inevitably caused by physicians whose practices are not negligent.
3. The establishment of a dispute resolution procedure as a national system separate from the current court system.

The JMA physician liability insurance system was established in 1973 in response to (1), but the other two items were not materialized for decades that followed. With decades passing by, the shortage of physicians in obstetrics and gynecology and the declining birthrate became social problems. In January 2006, the JMA made a proposition in its report entitled "Aiming at the establishment of a disability compensation system for medical care" stating "Ideally, it is desirable to implement a no-fault compensation system for entire medical specialties" and "however, neurological sequelae related to childbirth (so-called cerebral palsy) is prioritized for no-fault compensation." In August of the same year, they presented the details on the novel system. Furthermore, in November of the year, "A Framework for a No-Fault Compensation System in Obstetrics" (Study Group on Medical Dispute Resolution, Social Security System Study Group, Political Research Committee of the Liberal Democratic Party (LDP)) was published that was followed by increasing anticipation to launch the system. At the same time, relevant organizations and groups expressed their concern and requested that the JQ should be an operator of the system. Accordingly, the Preparatory Office for the novel system was installed in the JQ in February 2007 that served as secretariat for the Introductory Committee for the novel system. In March 2008, the Board of Directors of the JQ formally decided to be the operating organization. All in this way, the system has been in operation since January 2009 [1, 2]. This system is voluntary, but at the time of writing, a high participation rate of 99.9% has been achieved among all the childbirth institutions in Japan.

2 Review and Compensation

I tried to increase the clarity in a way that: Those who are eligible for compensation should meet i) the general criteria, which consists of birth weight (1400 g or more) and weeks of pregnancy (32 weeks or more), or ii) the individual criteria when the weeks of pregnancy are less than the general criteria: 28 weeks or more of pregnancy, umbilical artery blood pH less than 7.1, meeting the prescribed pattern in the fetal heart rate labor diagram (CTG), etc., and meet iii) the severity criteria: equivalent to level 1 or 2 of the physical disability grade defined in the Welfare for the Disabled Act, while they should not meet iv) the exclusion criteria such as cerebral palsy obviously caused by congenital factors or factors taking place in neonatal period or later. Even if congenital factors (brain malformation, genetic abnormality, chromosomal abnormality, etc.) exist, they are not necessarily because they may not be the obvious cause of profound CP. Decision for approval is made based on medical examination as to what caused profound CP that applicant suffers.

As of June 5, 2020, 3041 cases of compensation have been approved, and payment for the cases have been made or in progress. The number of persons eligible for compensation that has been confirmed so far is 419 in 2009, 382 in 2010, 355 in 2011, 362 in 2012, 351 in 2013, and 326 in 2014. For children born in later years, the application is still allowed until they are 5 years old (Table 1). In addition, applicants of uncompensated cases may apply to the Appeal Committee if they are not convinced on the results of the review.

A uniform compensation of 30 million yen is paid for each case once approved by the Review Committee. If the childbirth facility is liable for damage, the compensation and the damage payment are adjusted to eliminate duplicative payment. In other words, the child and the family cannot receive both the compensation and the damage payment under the system.

2.1 Investigation

2.1.1 Production of Investigative Report

The purposes of the investigation are (1) to analyze the case from a medical point of view based on the record and data on the cerebral palsy to learn knowledge for prevention and (2) to prevent conflict between childbirth facility and patient/family and bring it to early settlement by sharing investigative report for mutual understanding on the childbirth event. Unlike court system, this is a process of analysis genuinely from the medical and midwifery point of view.

The Investigation Committee holds seven subcommittees to compile a draft report (Fig. 1). One committee is composed of 14 members: 9 obstetricians including the chairperson, 2 pediatricians, 1 midwife, and 4 lawyers. The role of the medical members is to analyze the case from medical viewpoint, while the lawyers provide views so that the report will be easy for the patient/family to understand. A

Table 1 Changes in the number of people eligible for compensation [3]. Since the establishment of the system, 3041 out of 4048 applications have been approved for compensation, and applications that were not approved for compensation but are too premature to be judged can be reapplied. The number of people eligible for compensation has been allowed to decrease

Year of birth	Number of examinations	Coverage (Note 1)	Not covered by compensation			Continued consultation	Note
			Not covered by compensation	Re-application possible (Note 2)	Total		
2009	561	419	142	0	142	0	Review results already confirmed
2010	523	382	141	0	141	0	Same as above
2011	502	355	147	0	147	0	Same as above
2012	517	362	155	0	155	0	Same as above
2013	476	351	125	0	125	0	Same as above
2014	469	326	143	0	143	0	Same as above
2015 ~ 2019	1000	846	101	46	147	7	Judgment result not yet confirmed
Total	4048	3041	954	46	1000	7	Review results already confirmed

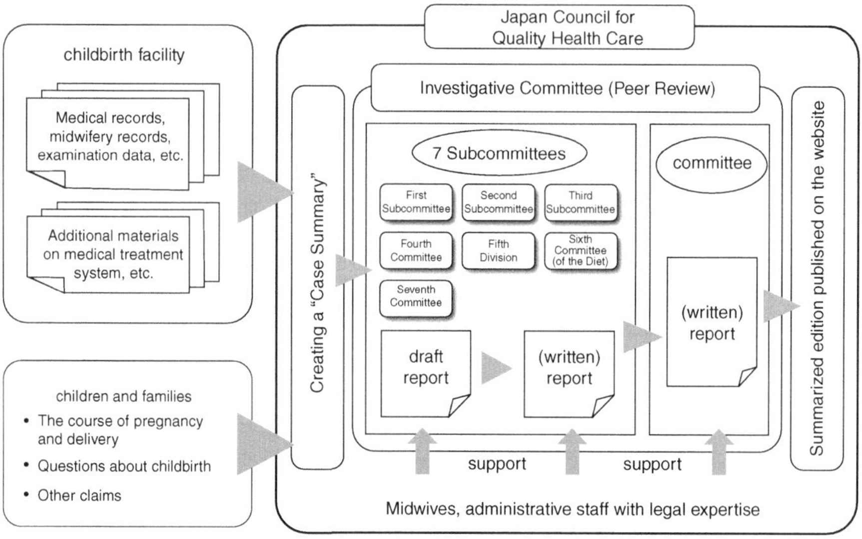

Fig. 1 Preparation of the cause analysis report [4]. In the cause analysis, a summary of the case is prepared based on records, data, and information from the family, and a draft report is prepared by seven subcommittees. A summary version of the report is published on the website

working manual was crafted to ensure that the reports are compiled in a standardized fashion. The draft report compiled therein is reviewed in the Investigative Committee for approval. At the same time, a "summarized edition" of the investigative report is issued with personal identifiers deleted and held available on the system's website for the prevention and improvement of perinatal care. This publication is described in more detail in the next section, as it has recently become involved in the revision of the Personal Information Protection Act.

2.1.2 The Relationship Between the Disclosure of the "Summarized Edition" of the Investigative Report and the Latest Revision of the Personal Information Protection Law and Relevant Administrative Guidelines

The "summarized edition" of the investigative report has been published and posted on the website as one of the significant products of the system. They have been referred to by parents, patient groups, and medical professionals for various purposes such as confirming transparency and improving quality of perinatal care through scientific research. The revised Act on the Protection of Personal Information was enacted and promulgated in 2015 and fully enforced on May 30, 2017, which unprecedentedly forced the "Donor rule" applicable when we consider if the data we disclosed on the web is "personal information." "Personal information" shall be provided to third parties through the prior consent of an individual to which the data belong with some exceptions such as the data provision for promoting public health. The "Donor rule" states that the data is defined as "personal information" when the donor of the data, e.g., JQ, is aware of an individual from whom the data derive even if recipient of the data, e.g., general public, does not know whose data it is. Accordingly, the "summarized edition" that had been available on the website was pointed out to be "personal information" that could be transferred to third parties generally through prior consent procedure. Therefore, publication of the "summarized edition," for which consent for the publication had not been obtained, had to be temporarily withdrawn from the website, and the Steering Committee of this system examined the issue from a broad perspective such as the purpose and impact of the disclosure and the procedures required for the disclosure in consistent with the revision of the Personal Information Protection Act.

In January 2019, the JQ consulted with legal experts and the government officials again on this issue. In light of their comments and guidance, the JQ decided to make efforts in obtaining the consent of the guardians, childbirth institutions, and the relevant medical institutions on all the summarized editions in light of the public concern on the system and changing public view with regard to the handling of personal information, although JQ believed that it fell under the exceptions for obtaining prior consent to the provision of personal information to third parties in the Personal Information Protection Act (see Table 2 [Reference 1]). Later, when the JQ's policy on disclosure of the summarized editions was proposed at the 40th Steering Committee meeting held in January 2019, comments such as "all summarized editions should be disclosed on the web as they were" and "JQ should clarify the reasons for no-consent by guardians and/or childbirth facilities in detail" were raised from many of committee members.

In February 2019, the JQ conducted a questionnaire survey targeting guardians and childbirth facilities to get hold of the reasons why they answered "agree" or "disagree" on the disclosure of the "summarized edition." At the 41st Steering Committee meeting held in August 2019, JQ reviewed the aim and value of this system to consider if we should disclose all the "summarized edition" that achieve public good such as quality improvement in perinatal care as only about 3/4 of the "summarized edition" are agreed on the disclosure. The JQ concluded at that time that the JQ continued its efforts to improve the rate of consent on disclosure and consulted with the relevant ministries and the government to explore measures to disclose more "summarized editions" on the web.

In December 2019, the Personal Information Protection Committee published the "Outline of the Amendment of the System for the So-called Triennial Review of the Personal Information Protection Act" (see Table 2 [Reference 2]), and in January 2020, the Ministry of Health, Labour and Welfare (MHLW) (see Table 2 [Reference 3]) presented a new commentary. At the 42nd Steering Committee meeting held in February 2020 and the 43rd Steering Committee meeting held on July 3, 2020, we discussed to compile an audacious policy on releasing all the "summarized editions" on the web. In the meantime, at the 94th meeting of the Investigation Committee held on June 10, the following comments were proposed: "In the Investigative Report, the causes of cerebral palsy are analyzed in detail and

Table 2 Laws and regulations regarding the disclosure of the cause analysis report summary version [3]. The abridged version of the cause analysis report is considered to fall under the exception to the provision of personal information to third parties under the Personal Information Protection Law and is published on the website based on the general guidelines of the Personal Information Protection Committee and the views of the Ministry of Health, Labour and Welfare

[Reference 1: Article 23, Paragraph 1, Item 3 of the Personal Information Protection Law] Article 23 A business operator handling personal information shall not provide personal data to a third party without obtaining the prior consent of the individual, except in the following cases: (iii) When it is particularly necessary for the improvement of public health or the promotion of the sound growth of children and it is difficult to obtain the consent of the person concerned
[Reference 2: The Personal Information Protection Law, so-called triennial review, Outline of System Revisions (December 13, 2019) (excerpt)] 3. Clarification of the operation of the exceptions pertaining to the handling of personal information for public interest purposes • With the rapid progress of information and communication technology, it has become possible to collect and analyze big data such as customer information • In this context, Japan is aiming to realize Society 5.0, which is a new society in which advanced technologies such as big data analysis are incorporated into all industries and social life to achieve both economic development and solutions to social issues. As social issues become more diverse, it is desirable to support an environment in which businesses can make use of data in order to efficiently and effectively solve these issues • With regard to this point, the current Personal Information Protection Law has exceptions to the limitation of the purpose of use and provision of personal data to third parties, such as "when it is necessary particularly for the improvement of public health or the promotion of the sound growth of children and difficult to obtain the consent of the individual". The use of personal information for public interest purposes is also considered acceptable in certain cases. However, since there is a tendency that these exceptions have been strictly applied so far, it is necessary to provide specific examples in guidelines and Q&As according to the expected needs. Therefore, we will promote the utilization of personal information that benefits the entire nation in terms of addressing social issues • By providing specific examples of the utilization in the guidelines and Q&As responding to the needs in society, for example, the need that a medical institution or a pharmaceutical company use the information for the purpose of contributing to the development of medical services, drugs, and safe and effective medical device in terms of patient safety
[Reference 3: Opinion from the Ministry of Health, Labour and Welfare • In December 2019, the Personal Information Protection Committee released the "Personal Information Protection Act: So-called Triennial Review: Outline of System Revisions," which also states that "the handling of personal information in the private sector is a matter for each business operator to decide. Therefore, it would be desirable for JIPDEC to consider the policy again, taking into account the balance between the improvement of public health and the protection of personal information. In addition, the MHLW has no objection if it is socially acceptable to publish the summary version of all cases as before"

carefully for each case" and "All the 'summarized editions' need to be disclosed on the web as they were." Accordingly, it was unanimously agreed that the "summarized edition" is published in all CP cases. From the viewpoint of improving public health, the publication of the "summarized edition" falls under the exceptions of Article 23, Paragraph 1, Item 3, of the Personal Information Protection Act as described above. In addition, in order to prevent the recurrence of CPs which is the purpose of the system, and to widely contribute to quality improvement in perinatal care, the JQ believed that it was incredibly important to disclose all "summarized edition" on the web after a year-long argument over the disclosure under the revised Personal Information Protection Act. At the same time, as there were some opinions that a certain level of agreement has been formed between the JQ and the cases that had disagreed on the disclosure, the JQ needed to make efforts to carefully convince families and childbirth facilities to agree on the disclosure. The Steering Committee finally agreed to the view proposed by the JQ.

2.2 *Prevention of Cerebral Palsy*

2.2.1 Publication of Annual Prevention Reports, Educational Materials on Fetal Heart Rate Monitoring, and Leaflets for Professionals and Expectant Mothers

The investigative reports are collectively analyzed in order to prevent recurrence and to improve quality in perinatal care. Here, we applied the knowledge and procedure devised through the medical adverse event reporting and learning system the JQ had run for years to make the analysis effective in preventing CP. Specifically, we conducted a quantitative and epidemiological analysis of aggregated cases based on data such as status of pregnancy, clinical courses of pregnancy, delivery and neonatal condition, and the local context of healthcare delivery system. The JQ also produced educational materials such as fetal heart rate monitoring textbook of profound CPs and leaflets for medical professionals and pregnant women (Fig. 2).

2.2.2 Activities of the Prevention Working Group

Under the Prevention Committee, a working group for prevention, which consists of obstetricians nominated by the Japan Society of Obstetrics and Gynecology and the Japan Association of Obstetricians and Gynecologists, as well as academic experts such as epidemiologists, was established in May 2014 that has conducted data analysis of the aggregated investigative reports. With the data, comparative study between the data of CPs that were subject to compensation under this system and that of the "Japan Society of Obstetrics and Gynecology Perinatal Registration Database" was conducted. In addition, an analysis of intrauterine infections and fetal heart rate patterns in children with CP was conducted in response to the requests made in the prevention report to the relevant academic societies and organizations. The analyses have been conducted in the working group from multifaceted viewpoints such as obstetrics and public health.

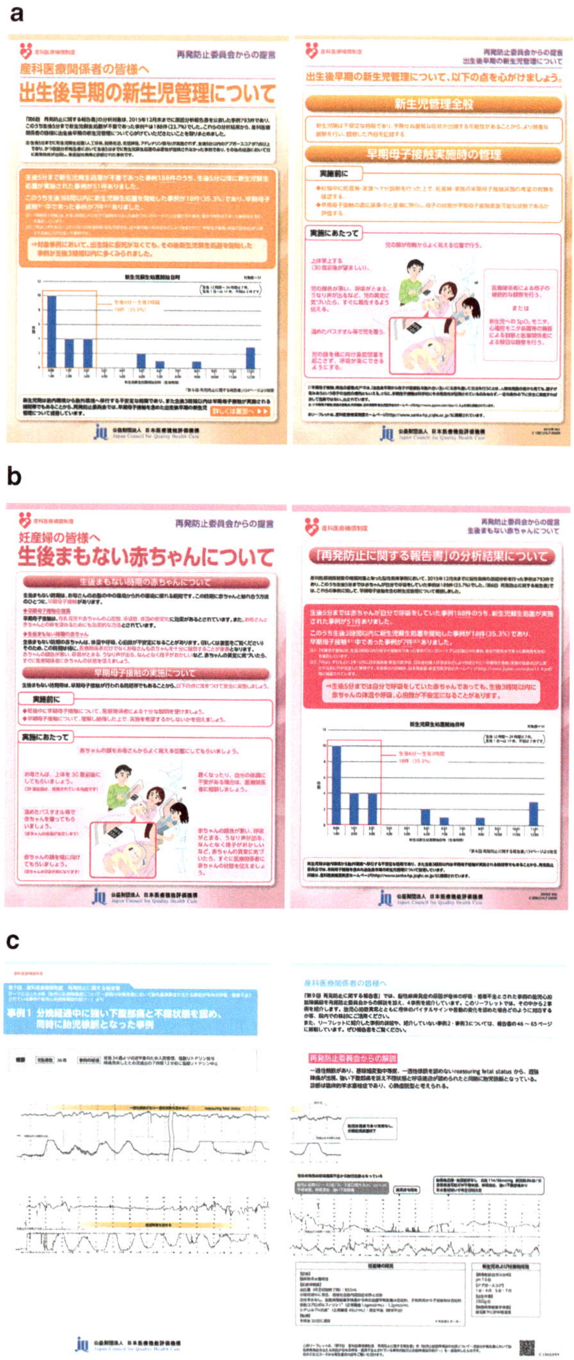

Fig. 2 Media for pregnant women and professionals [5]. (**a**) Leaflet for professionals "Early postnatal management of the newborn". (**b**) Leaflet for expectant mothers "About your newborn baby". (**c**) "Dear Obstetricians, About Fetal Heart Rate Labor Chart (Maternal Respiratory and Circulatory Failure)". (Quoted from the data of Japan Health Care Functionality Evaluation Organization)

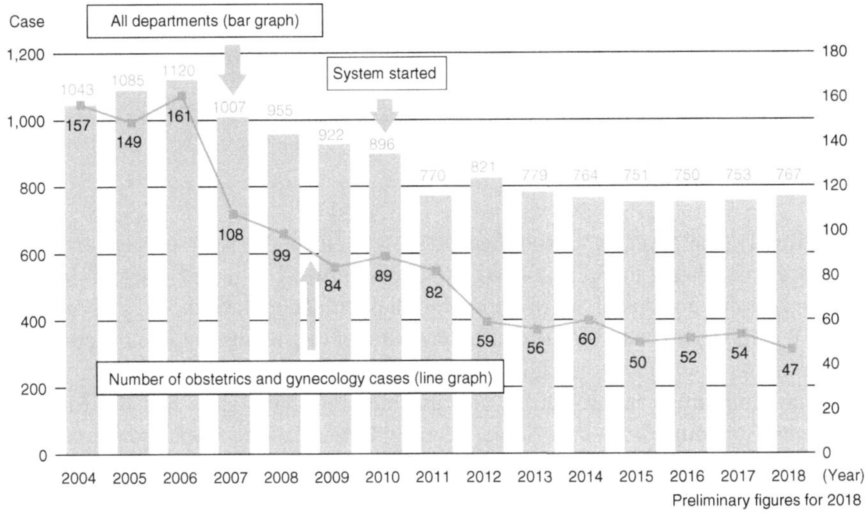

Fig. 3 Number of lawsuits (already filed) in obstetrics and gynecology. (Quoted and modified from "The number of completed cases of medical lawsuits by medical subject" by the Supreme Court Committee on Medical Lawsuits)

2.3 *Impact on Conflict Mitigation*

The purpose of the system is to prevent disputes and to improve quality in perinatal care. The lawsuit statistics of obstetrics and gynecology as a breakdown of "the number of completed lawsuit of entire medical specialty" published by the Committee on Medical Lawsuit of the Supreme Court of Japan shows a remarkable decreasing trend (Fig. 3). The "Report on the Verification of the Speeding Up of Trials" published in July 2013 by the Supreme Court of Japan states that "the Japan Obstetric Compensation System for Cerebral Palsy has handled a considerable number of cases since it came into effect, and it presumably has created an impact to a certain extent on the number of lawsuit in medical affairs litigation."

2.4 *Review of the System*

2.4.1 Review Timetable Agreed at the Inception of the System

The Japan Obstetric Compensation System for Cerebral Palsy was launched in an expedited manner in light of deteriorating perinatal care delivery system with challenges hard to address at the inception. Therefore, the report of the Introductory Committee stated that "the system will be verified in five years at the latest, and necessary revisions will be made to the scope of eligible patients, the amount of monetary compensation, price of insurance premium, and the operating structure of the system as appropriate."

2.4.2 Review in 2015

Accordingly, the Steering Committee of the system began an argument over the review of the system in February 2012. The committee conducted research including the collection and analysis of population-based data on the incidence of cerebral palsy, which is necessary for estimating the number of patients eligible for compensation that is crucial in re-designing the system. The results were reported to the Steering Committee in July 2013, and the Steering Committee and the Medical Insurance Subcommittee of the Social Security Council of the MHLW discussed the scope of eligibility, the amount of monetary compensation, the amount of lump-sum payments, and the way to spend surplus accumulated in insurance account. A review concluded that the system expanded the scope of eligibility to be applied in January 2015 and later.

2.4.3 2020–2021 Review for Further Expansion

While the system was being operated based on the revised standards, the Steering Committee held a meeting on July 20, 2018, and found that issues had arisen, such as "more than 50% of the patients on case-by-case review were not covered by the system," "a sense of unfairness arose because some patients were covered and others were not, even though they went through similar clinical course," and "the system was scientifically unreasonable and did not fit the reality of perinatal care." Therefore, it was concluded that the system needed to be improved as soon as possible (Table 2). On July 25 of the same year, the Steering Committee submitted a request to the MHLW that the committee commenced the review of the system. Later in 2020, the MHLW responded to the JQ claiming that the JQ listens to the voices of relevant parties such as healthcare-related organizations, patient groups, and insurers, proposes the blueprint to reform the system, and reports to the MHLW on the conclusion with which the MHLW would take necessary action for reforming the system. With those dialogs between the JQ and the MHLW, the first round of the Committee on the Review of the Japan Obstetric Compensation System for Cerebral Palsy was held on September 11, 2020. At the meeting, the items to be examined and reviewed included the operation of the system in terms of efficiency, the estimates of the number of eligible patients, the price of insurance premium, the eligibility criteria for compensation, the financial resource for compensation, and the amount of compensation. The JQ, the system operator, engaged in Q&A session in exploring the direction of expanding the scope of the system, which was in line with the views of the most committee members who engaged in perinatal care. It was necessary to make an effort to reach a unanimous agreement of the stakeholders involved in the meeting. Therefore, the JQ requested committee members and all those involved in perinatal care beyond the committee for attention and support for the direction, i.e., expansion of the system that JQ presented in response to the difficult reality in perinatal care delivery system.

The Japan Obstetric Compensation System for Cerebral Palsy, which was launched in 2009, celebrated its tenth anniversary in 2019. During this period, the system has made enormous achievement such as the delivery of no-fault compensation for profound CPs, provision of investigative report to both families and childbirth facilities, prevention activities through collective analysis of aggregated investigative reports, and sharing the data on CPs gained in the system on a national scale through appropriate procedures. The system was discussed for the review 5 years after it was launched on a planned timetable. The review concluded that the system was run in line with the original objectives, such as provision of monetary compensation on no-fault basis, early resolution of disputes, and quality improvement of perinatal care through investigation and prevention. Then, the revised system was initiated in January 2014 on such details as procedure of investigation and adjustment of monetary compensation and damage payment and in January 2015 on the scope of eligibility that covered more CPs and other relevant issues. As of now in 2020, JQ has just completed another review of the system to explore further expansion to cover more cerebral palsy cases in January 2022 and later. As seen above, the JQ believes that it is vital to improve the system in continued fashion through periodical reviews in the presence of stakeholders.

References

1. Japan Council for Quality Health Care. Sankairyou hosyouseido [The Japan obstetric compensation system for cerebral palsy]. [Internet]. Available from: http://www.sanka-hp.jcqhc.or.jp/index.html. Japanese. Accessed 13 Oct 2020.
2. Japan Council for Quality Health Care. Sankairyou hosyousedido no minaoshini kansuru kentoukai shiryou [Documents page of the "Committee", "Study Group on the Japan Obstetric Compensation System for Cerebral Palsy"]. [Internet]. Available from: http://www.sanka-hp.jcqhc.or.jp/documents/committee/index.html. Japanese. Accessed 13 Oct 2020.
3. Japan Council for Quality Health Care. Dai 43 kai unei iinkai shiryou [43rd Committee Report on the Japan Obstetric Compensation System for Cerebral Palsy]. [Internet]. Available from: http://www.sanka-hp.jcqhc.or.jp/documents/committee/obstetric_meeting43_1.pdf. Japanese. Accessed 30 Apr 2021.
4. Ushiro S. Sankairyou hosyouseido no genkyou ni tsuite [Current status of the Japan Obstetric Compensation System for Cerebral Palsy]. J Jpn Soc Premature Newborn Med. 2010;22:400.
5. Japan Council for Quality Health Care. Committee for Prevention of Recurrence on the Japan Obstetric Compensation System for Cerebral Palsy. Leaflet/Poster Archive shu; Dai 1 kai – dai 10 kai saihatsuboushi nikansuru houkokusyo [Leaflets and Posters Archive Collection 1st - 10th Report on Prevention of Recurrence]. [Internet]. Available from: http://www.sanka-hp.jcqhc.or.jp/documents/prevention/proposition/pdf/Saihatsu_leaflet_poster_archive_01-10.pdf. Japanese. Accessed 30 Apr 2021.

Clinical Diagnosis of Cerebral Palsy

Shigeharu Hosono

Contents

Summary

- Most of the patients with cerebral palsy cannot find the causes of perinatal factors. Physicians in charge of infant healthcare examinations should identify the suspected cases of cerebral palsy at an early stage.
- The key to early detection of cerebral palsy is to avoid overlooking abnormal posture, decreased automatic movements with or without increased or decreased muscle tone, residual or delayed appearance of primitive reflexes, and left-right differences in reflexes.

S. Hosono (✉)
Division of Neonatology, Department of Perinatology, Saitama Medical Center, Jichi Medical University, Saitama, Japan
e-mail: hosono.s@jichi.ac.jp

Y. Matsuda (ed.), *Cerebral Palsy*, https://doi.org/10.1007/978-981-19-2217-6_4

- If a definitive diagnosis and treatment cannot be made at the own hospital, the timing of referral should be decided in cooperation with the specialist physician, taking into consideration the local medical care and treatment system.
- In most of the cases of severe hypoxic-ischemic encephalopathy, cerebral palsy can be diagnosed in early infancy. On the other hand, some cases of mild cerebral palsy are diagnosed after 1.5 years of age. If the follow-up of the patient cannot be continued at the own hospital, the doctor should inform the parents of the importance of follow-up healthcare examination and the visit to the doctor in the key month.
- To prevent the progression from neonatal asphyxia to hypoxic-ischemic encephalopathy, in all deliveries, staff with both knowledge of neonatal resuscitation and skill in mask and bag ventilations should be assigned.

The definition of cerebral palsy was established in 1968 by the Research Council for Cerebral Palsy of the former Ministry of Health and Welfare and is still used without revision today. On the other hand, the diagnosis of cerebral palsy is based on clinical symptoms. The main clinical symptoms are abnormalities in movement and posture, including muscle tone, reflexes, coordination, and left-right differences in movement. Hypoxic-ischemic encephalopathy (HIE) is an important cause in full-term infants, although most of the cases do not detect perinatal factors. In severe cases, cerebral palsy can be diagnosed in early infancy, but some of mild to moderate cerebral palsy is diagnosed after the age of 18 months. In this chapter, I review the clinical features and the diagnosis of cerebral palsy caused by hypoxic-ischemic encephalopathy.

1 Diagnosis of Cerebral Palsy

Newborns with perinatal factors or those with abnormalities detected on imaging in the neonatal period are carefully followed up. The diagnosis of cerebral palsy in this population is rarely delayed, but the number of cerebral palsy cases in the population without these abnormalities is much larger. Early detection of suspected cases from the regular infant healthcare examination is extremely important. The developmental delay is assessed by the achievement of the assessment items in the key month. The key points to suspect cerebral palsy are observation of posture and spontaneous movements, presence or absence of increased or decreased muscle tone, and abnormalities of each primary reflex, i.e., residual, delayed appearance, and left-right differences in reflexes. The key month is the age at which growth and development can be assessed for the purpose of early diagnosis and treatment of diseases and rehabilitation. The "key months" are 1 month, 3 months, 6–7 months, 9–10 months, 1 year, 1 year and 6 months, 2 years, 3 years, 4 years, 5 years, and 6 years as indicated in the Maternal and Child Health Handbook.

2 Symptoms and Findings That Raise Suspicion of Cerebral Palsy During a Health Examination

2.1 One Month [1]

Early symptoms before the abnormalities in muscle tone and posture seen in children with cerebral palsy include the following: poor weight gain with poor feeding, warping of the trunk during feeding, not in a good mood, shallow sleep, less crying, longer sleeping time, and less frequent feeding. In the normal supine position, the upper and lower limbs are lightly flexed, and the hands are lightly clasped (Fig. 1a). All four limbs are freely movable. The face faces either left or right and changes its orientation spontaneously (Fig. 1b). On the other hand, abnormal findings in the supine posture, such as obvious warping of the trunk and a posture of strong asymmetrical tonic neck reflex, indicate increased muscle tone (Fig. 2a), while a posture in which the entire limbs are extended or the limb remains on the floor, the so-called frog posture, indicates decreased muscle tone. Left-right difference in movement of any of the four limbs is also an abnormal finding. When the traction response is observed, if the body stands like a stick, the head is extremely retroflexed, or the elbow joint is fully extended, the shoulders almost fall out, and the hips shift, it is

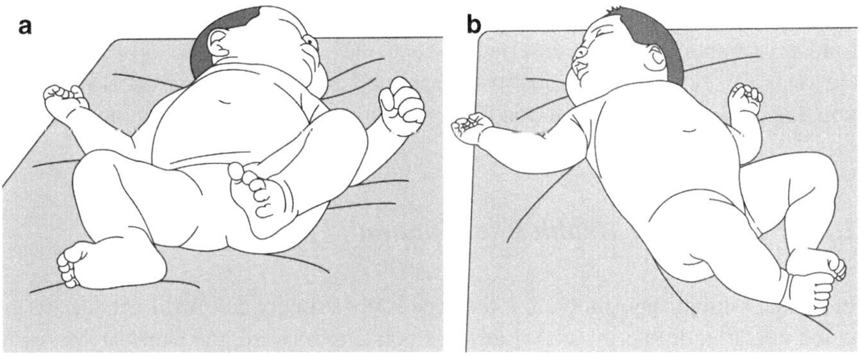

Fig. 1 Normal posture of a 1-month-old infant. (**a**) Limb flexion position (normal). The upper and lower limbs are semi-flexed in the supine position, and the upper limbs are W-shaped (both hands pointing upward). As the child matures, the hands are positioned caudally. (**b**) Posture with the elements of tonic neck reflex (normal). The upper and lower limbs on the side the child facing are more extended than those of the opposite side, but the hands are not clenched tightly. In this respect, this posture differs from that of a typical tonic neck reflex

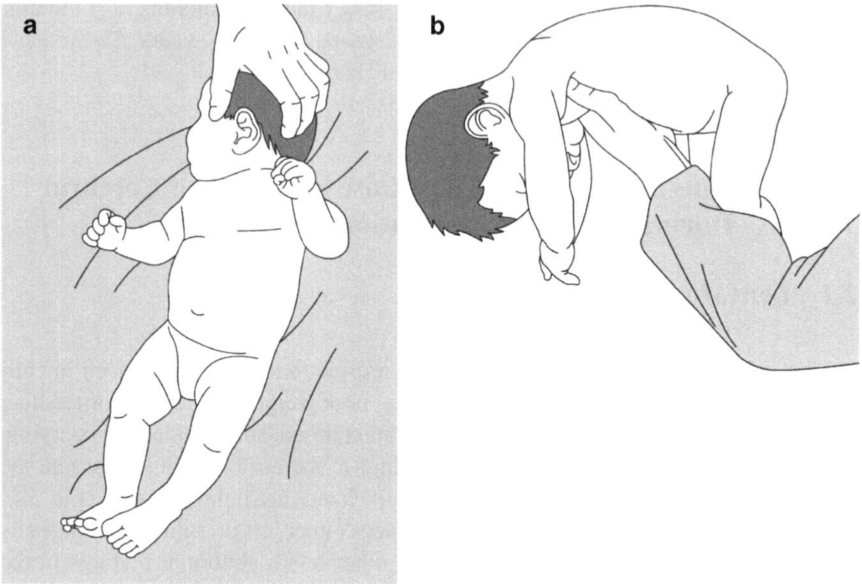

Fig. 2 Abnormal posture of a 1-month-old infant. (**a**) Morbid tonic neck reflex. The upper and lower limbs on the side the child facing are always extended, and the upper and lower limbs of the occipital side are flexed, and the hands are clenched tightly. (**b**) When the child is held horizontally in the supine position, the child's arms and legs cannot resist gravity and slump. In addition, the muscle tonus of trunk is also decreased, resulting in an inverted U-shaped posture

considered abnormal. If the patient's head is lifted slightly in a horizontal lateral hug (supine suspension), the back is mildly flexed, but the face is raised and the lower limbs are extended, the posture indicates increased muscle tone, and if the trunk is extremely bent in an inverted U shape, the posture indicates decreased muscle tone (Fig. 2b). If an abnormality is suspected at the 1-month physical examination, the patient should be referred to the specialist or followed up 1 month later.

2.2 *Four-Month Health Examination [1]*

In normal 4-month age children, if the head is not strongly deformed, the face faces in the direction of interest, and if the face is facing forward, the hands are brought in front of the face for play, and the hands are often open. The child can grasp objects touched by hands. Both lower limbs are flexed, both feet are raised, and the limbs are actively moving.

In the prone position, the face faces the floor, and when the neck is raised, the elbows are forward of the shoulders to support the upper body, and the neck is higher than the shoulders.

In the horizontal position, the head is slightly raised, the trunk is mildly flexed or extended, the upper limbs are lightly extended, and the hands are open, and the lower limbs are lightly extended.

Neurological findings include obvious recumbency (retroflexion), conversely, a posture with limbs on the floor (frog position), a strong asymmetrical tonic neck reflex position, and strong hand holding, which is an abnormal posture.

When you examine traction response, the head does not fall backward and follows the trunk without delay when the head is raised to 45° from the floor (Fig. 3a). If the elbow and shoulder joints are strengthened and the upper extremities are flexed, and the axis of the neck and trunk are aligned, the head control is completed. The primitive reflexes, Moro reflex and hand grasp reflex, are absent. In the supine position, if the patient has a strong asymmetrical tonic neck reflex position and the face remains facing one side and cannot be moved, it is considered abnormal. Head control is incomplete if the head does not bend forward and remains retroverted even when the patient is brought up to 60° in the traction response; if the head bends forward when the patient is brought up to 90°, or if the head shakes so much that the patient cannot stand back up when the shoulders are gently shaken back and forth, head control is also incomplete. If the head bends forward, or if the head shakes so much that the child cannot stand back up when the shoulder is gently shaken back and forth, it is judged that the neck is not fixed. When the head bends backward and the lower limbs are stretched, the muscle tone is increased, which is an abnormal finding. In this case, the patient's waist shifts in the causing reflex, and the patient cannot be caused normally and stands up like a stick (Fig. 3b). In the case of incomplete head control, if the patient is 3–4 months old, the follow-up should be about

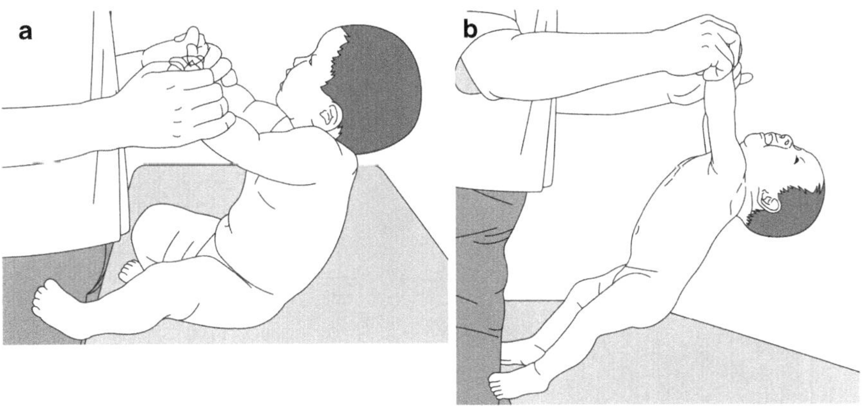

Fig. 3 Normal and abnormal caused reflexes of a 4-month-old infant. (**a**) Normal traction response: When the examiner holds the child's hands and triggers the child at about 45°, the child pulls back his or her chin so that the head and trunk are in a straight line. (**b**) Abnormal traction response: The child's head and trunk are dorsiflexed, and when the examiner tries to pull the child up by both hands, the child's hips displaced. So, it is not possible to cause a child

1 month later; if the patient is 4 months old or has obvious postural or motor abnormalities or abnormal muscle tone, the patient should be referred to a specialized facility for consultation or follow-up after 1 month.

2.3 Six to Seven-Month Examination [2]

If the head control is not established, the diagnosis is obvious retardation, and the child is diagnosed as developmentally delayed. At around 6 months, the child grasps the feet with the hands and sucks the toes into the mouth in the supine position (Fig. 4a). These movements disappear after 7 months. At 6 months, the child is able to sit for a few seconds with hands in front of him (Fig. 4b). If the child is 6 months old, it is not necessarily considered abnormal development, even if the sitting position is not acquired it is not necessarily considered abnormal. At 7 months, the child is able to sit with holding objects (Fig. 4c). In the vertical hold, the child flexes their lower limbs and does not place their feet on the floor, bounces up and down, and bounces and supports his weight with feet on the floor. As you can see, there are some variants. The following symptoms are considered abnormal, if the child's lower limbs are cross and extended and the heels do not touch the floor; equinovarus position is abnormal (Fig. 5). It is also abnormal for a child to hold his or her hands tightly without opening them. Such a gesture is abnormal. It is abnormal if the child does not try to remove the cloth covering infant's face in the cloth on the face test (Fig. 6). Check for any awkwardness or difference in grasping.

At 7 months, when a cloth is applied to the face, it is immediately removed with the mother's side of one hand. At 7 months, when a cloth is placed on his face, he immediately removes it with the maternal side of one hand. The degree of delay in mental development indicates that the child takes a long time to remove the cloth,

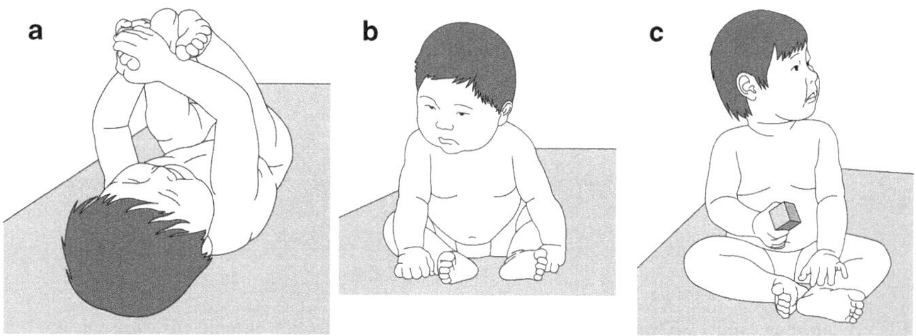

Fig. 4 Normal posture at 6–7 months. (**a**) Supine posture: The child's muscle tonus in lower extremities is symmetrically decreased. The child is able to hold and suck his own toes. (**b**, **c**) Sitting position: At 6 months, children can sit with the trunk bent forward and hands on the floor for a few seconds (**b**). At 7 months, the child ranges from those who can sit with their hands on the floor for a while or sit and play with his hands on the floor without holding them (**c**)

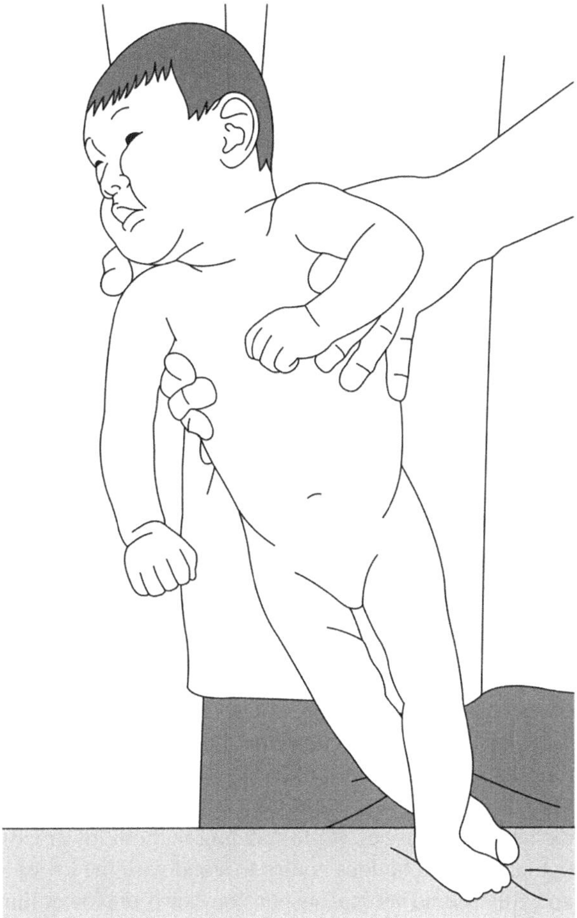

Fig. 5 Abnormal posture of a 6–7-month-old infant. Cross-extension of the lower limbs: Cross-extension of the child's lower limbs can be seen when the child is held vertically. In some cases, when the examiner repeatedly touches the bottom of the child's foot to the floor, equinus position becomes apparent

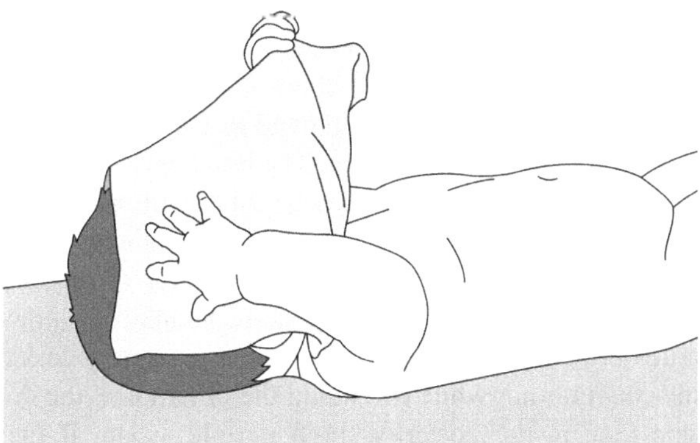

Fig. 6 Cloth on the face test. Cloth on the face test is a test in which a cloth such as a handkerchief or towel is placed on the face of an infant and the infant's reaction is observed. Usually, at 5 months, the child tries to pick up the cloth with both hands; at about 6 months, the child brings both hands to the face, but often takes the cloth with one hand. When the examiner holds the hand that first took the cloth, the child tries to take the cloth with the opposite hand

attempts to remove the cloth but is unable to do so, or does not make any removal movements. In hemiplegic patients, there is a difference between the left and right side of the removing motion.

2.4 *Nine to Ten-Month Examination [1]*

In the supine position, there is a separate movement of the knee, with the hip joint flexed and the knee flexed and extended separately on each side. In the prone position, the child supports the upper body with both hands and crawls forward on all fours with the hips raised, so-called crawling. With hands on the ground, maintain shoulder and hip height, and support the lower extremities with the knees, alternating hip flexion and extension. From the supine position, if the doctor holds the baby's hands and causes it, the baby will cooperate and sit up.

At 10 months, the child is able to maintain a seated position without placing his hands on the floor. In the sitting posture, the back is straight, and the lower limbs are thrown forward, both hips are semi-abducted, and both knees are semi-flexed. The child can stand on one knee. The child should be able to stand on one knee, stand up with support from the upper limbs, and stand up with support (standing position). If the child cannot sit up, there is clearly abnormal with motor development. There are a number of developmental variants at this age as follows. The child is unable to crawl on all fours and moves in a crawling position, crawls on his or her back, and does not want to be placed in the supine position. There is a variation so-called shuffling baby, which is a child who does not crawl but moves by paddling with the lower limbs in a sitting position. It is abnormal for a child to be supported only by the upper extremities while standing on both lower extremities in extension and on tiptoe. If the child does not try to stand with the lower limbs bent even when pulled up by the sides (vertical suspension), or if the lower limbs are extended and crossed and pointed feet are seen, abnormalities are suspected. Left-right differences in the upper and lower limbs are abnormal. In particular, since the dominant hand is not determined at this stage, it may be abnormal if one hand cannot grasp an object between the thumb and index finger. It is abnormal if there is no parachute reflex, left-right difference in upper limb extension and in hand extension, or inability to open the hand in the lateral parachute reflex. The Landau reflex normally appears at 6 months and persists until 2.5 years of age, so if it is not present at this time, it is abnormal. The absence of anterior and lateral hopping responses is abnormal. Muscle tone is assessed using muscle elasticity and range of motion. In particular, the physician should perform dynamic hip flexion and ankle dorsiflexion for evaluation. If the angle between the floor and the lower extremity is less than 70° when the doctor flexes one hip joint while extending the other knee, the doctor considers increased muscle tone in the posterior thigh muscle group. If the knee joint is extended and the ankle joint cannot be dorsiflexed due to strong resistance, foot clonus, or increased patellar tendon reflex, spastic cerebral palsy is suspected. If these abnormalities are observed, they should be confirmed after 1 month, and if they are reproducible, they can be judged as abnormal.

2.5 *One-Year-Old Health Examination [2]*

The average child is able to stand unaided, but there is a wide range from walking while holding on to something to walking alone. When the child walks unaided, make sure that the heel is firmly planted on the floor and the examiner confirms that the child does not have an ankle joint in equinus position. In children with a tendency toward pointy feet, check for stiffness during ankle extension and flexion. Examine for anterior and lateral hopping responses; the absence of a posterior hopping response at 12 months is not abnormal, but the absence of anterior and lateral responses is. If a muscle tonus abnormality is suspected, traction response should be performed to confirm that it is normal.

2.6 *One Year and 6-Month Examination [3]*

The average child is able to stand alone, but there is a wide range from pacing to walking alone. I'll repeat myself on this. You should make sure that the heel is firmly planted on the floor and the examiner confirms that the child does not have an ankle joint in equinus position. In child with a tendency toward equinus position, check for stiffness during ankle extension and flexion. Check for the presence of anterior and lateral hopping responses. At 12 months, the absence of a posterior hopping response is not abnormal, but the absence of anterior and lateral responses is abnormal. If a muscle tonus abnormality is suspected, retraction reflexes should be checked for normality. If the child has walk alone, determine whether the child is high, middle, or low guard[1] (Fig. 7) by noting the position of the hands. At 1 year and 6 months, the child usually walks with a middle or high guard gait. Failure to walk is clearly abnormal. On the other hand, particular attention should be paid to children who have a long period of high guard gait, even if they acquire high guard gait at an early age. Hopping responses can be seen in all directions at this stage. With regard to fine motor skills, when stacking cubes (blocks of 3 cm each), the child can stack two to three cubes by holding the cubes with the mother finger facing the other fingers and grasping them with the belly side of the fingers or with the fingertips.

The gait matures from high guard to middle guard and then to low guard. It is named after the position of the upper limb, but in reality, the movements of the upper limb, trunk, and lower limb are different.

[1] High guard, middle guard, and low guard gait and adult gait.

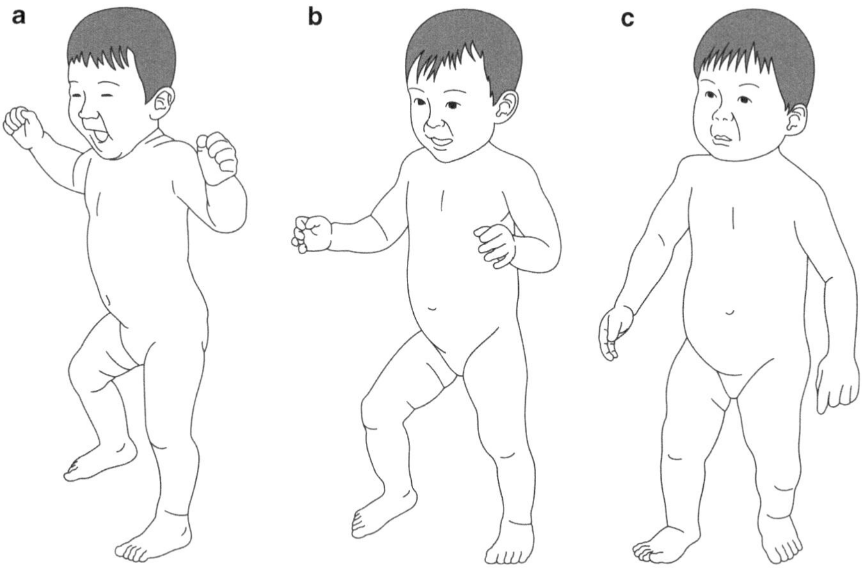

Fig. 7 Change in walking posture. (**a**) High guard gait is when the child begins to walk. When walking, the lower limbs are externally rotated with extension, both legs are open, and the body is twisted at the beginning of walking. The lower limbs are abducted and abducted, and the pelvis is twisted and tilted with each step. Normally, the contralateral foot does not move forward from the landing point of the first foot that steps forward. (**b**) In middle guard gait, the extended lower limbs gradually descend during walking. (**c**) In low guard gait, as the child matures, the upper limbs come down to a lower position than the hips, and the upper and lower limbs begin to show some degree of sympathetic movement. The legs are internally rotated and the open feet become parallel, the stride length is constant, and the upper and lower limbs move in synch, resulting in a rhythmic gait similar to that of adults. This form of gait is usually achieved after the age of 2 years

3 Type of Cerebral Palsy

3.1 Classification by Site of Injury

Cerebral palsy is classified into six types (Fig. 8) based on the location of the disorder. Paraplegia is characterized by paralysis of the lower limbs only, with no paralysis of the upper limbs. In diplegia, the lower limbs are more severely affected than the upper limbs.

3.2 Classification According to the Type of Abnormal Muscle Tone [4]

- Spastic Type

  The spastic type presents with spastic increased muscle tone, decreased range of motion of the joints, and decreased motor activity.

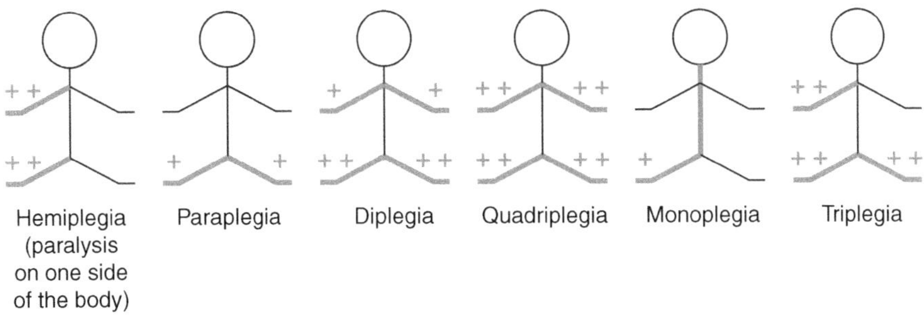

Fig. 8 Classification by disability site. The bold line indicates the site of paralysis, and + and ++ indicate the degree of paralysis. (Modified from Ref. [9])

- Athetosis Type
  Cerebral palsy of the athetotic type is characterized by increased muscle tone and involuntary movements, which vary in degree. The muscle tone is increased at the beginning of movement and during tension and is decreased during relaxation.
- Hypotonic Type
  Muscle tone is decreased, and locomotion is decreased too. The range of motion of the joints increases in young children but decreases with age.
- Ataxia Type
  It is associated with impaired balance function of the trunk and tremor of the upper limbs.
- Mixed Type
  Not all cases of cerebral palsy can be classified into the above four types, except for the mixed type. Even in cases classified as mixed, the main disease type should be clearly described.

4 Severity of Cerebral Palsy [5]

The prognostic value of gross motor function in cerebral palsy should be assessed stratified by severity. The gross motor function classification system (GMFCS) is the most widely used. In the GMFCS classifies, the severity of paraplegia into five functional levels based on the child's gross motor skills, mainly sitting ability and mobility, which can be expected to be reached by the age of 6 years or later (Table 1).

5 Diagnosis of Cerebral Palsy Due to Hypoxic-Ischemic Encephalopathy

Hypoxic-ischemic encephalopathy is a disorder of the central nervous system caused by hypoxia and ischemia, mainly associated with neonatal asphyxia. This means that the presence of neonatal asphyxia and hypoxic-ischemic

Table 1 Gross motor function classification system (Created based on Ref. [5])

Level	Level of attainment
I	Children walk without limitations in most settings through adulthood
II	Children walk with limitations that may change with age
III	Children can walk using a hand-held mobility device in most indoor settings
IV	Children can get around mainly with a wheelchair and use a body support walker for recreation
V	Children will be transported in chairs or standers throughout their life, and with increased supports, they may drive powered mobility

Table 2 Findings of the Compensation Target Standard (2) (Modified from Ref. [6])

1.	Sudden and persistent bradycardia
2.	Delayed transient bradycardia occurring in more than 50% of uterine contractions
3.	Fluctuating transient bradycardia appearing in more than 50% of uterine contractions
4.	Loss of baseline variability in heart rate
5.	Severe bradycardia with decreased baseline variability of heart rate
6.	Sinusoidal pattern
7.	Apgar score of less than 3 (1 min)
8.	Blood gas analysis within the first hour of life (pH less than 7.0)

encephalopathy in the neonatal period and other neonatal encephalopathies should be excluded. Criterion 2 for individual review of children born on or after January 1, 2015, in the Japan Obstetric Compensation System for Cerebral Palsy, (1) persistent hypoxic conditions and findings of metabolic acidosis (acidemia) in the umbilical artery (pH less than 7.1) or (2) hypoxic conditions including premature separation of normally implanted placenta, cord prolapse, uterine rupture, and eclampsia, feto-maternal transfusion syndrome, hemorrhage from placenta previa, sudden onset twin-to-twin transfusion syndrome, etc., and, after that, any of the eight findings (Table 2) is assumed to be present [6].

Hypoxic-ischemic encephalopathy is characterized by neurological symptoms such as muscle tension, posture, and abnormal tendon and primitive reflexes. The severity of hypoxic-ischemic encephalopathy is generally assessed by either or both the Sarnat classification (Table 3) [7] and Thompson score (Table 4) [8], which reflect abnormal autonomic function in addition to these neurological symptoms.

In order to prevent the progression from neonatal asphyxia to hypoxic-ischemic encephalopathy, all medical staff attending the delivery should be familiar with NCPR resuscitation procedures and be able to perform mask and bag ventilation appropriately.

Table 3 Sarnat classification (distinguishing features of the three stages of postanoxic encephalopathy in the full-term newborn infant)

	Grade		
	I (Mild)	II (Moderate)	III (Severe)
LOC	Hyperalert	Lethargic or obtunded	Stupor
Neuromuscular control			
• Muscle tone	Normal	Mild hypotonia	Flaccid
• Posture	Mild distal flexion	Strong distal flexion	Intermittent decerebration
• Stretch reflexes	Overactive	Overactive	Decreased or absent
• Segmental myoclonus	O	O	None
Complex or primitive reflexes			
• Suck	Weak	Weak or absent	Absent
• Moro	Strong	Weak	Absent
• Oculovestibular	Normal	Strong	Decreased or absent
• Tonic neck	Slight	Strong	Absent
Autonomic function	Sympathetic dominance	Parasympathetic dominance	Sympathetic and parasympathetic inhibition
• Pupils	Mydriasis	Miosis	Variable
• Heart rate	Tachycardia	Bradycardia	Variable
• Tracheal or saliva secretion	Decreased	Hypersecretion	Variable
• Intestinal peristalsis	Decreased from normal	Strong/diarrhea	Variable
Seizures	None	Common	Uncommon
Electroencephalographic findings	Normal (during wakefulness)	Initial: continuous low potential delta and theta waves	Initial: rhythmic pattern with equipotential phase
		Then: rhythmic patterns (during wakefulness)	Then: full equipotential phase
		Spasm: 1–1.5 Hz/spine slow wave	
Period	Within 24 h	2–14 days	A few hours to a few weeks

Table 4 Thompson score (hypoxic-ischemic encephalopathy score) (Reproduced from [8] with permission)

Sign	0	1	2	3
Tone	Normal	Hypertonia	Hypotonia	Flaccid
LOC	Normal	Hyperalert, stare	Lethargic	Comatose
Fits	None	<3 per day	>2 per day	
Posture	Normal	Fisting, cycling	Strong distal flexion	Decerebrate
Moro	Normal	Partial	Absent	
Grasp	Normal	Poor	Absent	
Suck	Normal	Poor	Absent ± bites	
Respiration	Normal	Hyperventilation	Brief apnea	IPPV (apnea)
Fontanel	Normal	Full, not tense	Tense	

Maximum Score = 22, Mild HIE: 1–10, Moderate HIE: 11–14, Severe HIE: 15
LOC level of consciousness

References

1. Koeda T, Yamazaki Y, Tanaka, K. Dai 2 shou: Nyuuji kenkou shinsa. Nyuuji kenkou shinsa shintaikensa manual. Heisei 29 nen kodomo kosodateshien suishin cyousa kenkyuujigyou nyuujikenkoushinsa notameno "hokenshidou manual (kashou)" oyobi "shintaikensa manual (kashou)" sakusei nikansuru cyousakenkyuu [Chapter 2: Health examination for infants. Manual of physical examination for infant health checkup]. In: FY2017 Research and Study Project on Promotion of Child-Rearing Support: Research and Study on Preparation of "Health Guidance Manual (tentative)" and "Physical Examination Manual (tentative)" for Infant Health Checkups, National Center for Child Health and Development. [Internet]. Tokyo: National Center for Child Health and Development. 2018. p. 3–38. Japanese. Available from: https://www.ncchd.go.jp/center/activity/kokoro_jigyo/manual.pdf#search=%27NationalCenterforChildHealthandDevelopmentHealthExamination%27. Accessed 1 Aug 2020.
2. Maekawa K, Koeda T, et al. Dai 4 bu: Shinkeigakuteki Hattatsu Check hou. II Kakugetsureibetsu no Check Point [Part 4: Neurological developmental check method II: Check points for each age group]. In: Maekawa K, Koeda T, et al., editors. Shashindemiru Nyuji Shindanno Shinkeigakuteki Check Hou [Neurological check method of infant health examination in photographs]. Tokyo: Nanzan-do; 2017. p. 128–225. Japanese.
3. Koeda T, Yamazaki Y, Tanaka K. Dai 3 shou: 1sai 6kagetsuji kenkou shinsa shintaikensa manual. Heisei 29 nen kodomo kosodateshien suishin cyousa kenkyuujigyou nyuujikenkoushinsa notameno "hokenshidou manual (kashou)" oyobi "shintaikensa manual (kashou)" sakusei nikansuru cyousakenkyuu [Chapter 3: Health examination of 1-year and 6-month-old children. Manual of physical examination for infant health checkup]. In: 2017 Research and Study Project for Promotion of Child-Rearing Support: Research and Study on Preparation of "Health Guidance Manual (tentative)" and "Physical Examination Manual (tentative)" for Infant Health Examination. [Internet]. Tokyo: National Center for Child Health and Development; 2018. p. 39–56. Japanese. Available from: https://www.ncchd.go.jp/center/activity/kokoro_jigyo/manual.pdf#search=%27NationalCenterforChildHealthandDevelopmentHealthExamination%27. Accessed 1 Aug 2020.
4. Suzuki F. Nouseimahino Ekigakuto Byoukei [Epidemiology and pathogenesis of cerebral palsy]. In: Arima M, et al., editors. Shouni Shinkeigaku [Child neurology]. Tokyo: Diagnosis and Treatment Company; 2008. p. 186–9. Japanese.
5. Aoyama K, Kondo I. 3-1: Nouseimahino Hyoukahou. 1: Nouseimahino Sodaiundounouryoku Bunrui System [3-1: Evaluation method of cerebral palsy 1: Coarse motor ability classification system for cerebral palsy]. In: Japan Society for Rehabilitation Medicine (supervised)

Nouseimahi Rehabilitation Guideline [Guidelines for rehabilitation of cerebral palsy]. 2nd ed. Tokyo: Kanehara Shuppan; 2014. p. 57–8. Japanese.
6. Japan Council for Quality Health Care. Dai 1 shou. Souron 2) Hoshou taishou kijyun, sankairyou hosyouseido "hosyoutaisyou tonaru nouseimahi no kijyun" no kaisetsu [Chapter 1 General Discussion 2) Criteria for Compensation, The Japan Obstetric Compensation System for Cerebral Palsy "Criteria for Cerebral Palsy Subject to Compensation"]. 2014. p. 2–3. Japanese. Available from: http://www.sanka-hp.jcqhc.or.jp/documents/exam/pdf/hosyoutaisyou.pdf. Accessed 1 Aug 2020.
7. Sarnat HB, Sarnat MS. Neonatal encephalopathy following fetal distress. A clinical and electroencephalographic study. Arch Neurol. 1976;33:696–705.
8. Thompson CM, Puterman AS, Linley LL, et al. The value of a scoring system for hypoxic ischaemic encephalopathy in predicting neurodevelopmental outcome. Acta Paediatr. 1997;86:757–61.
9. Mima A, Nabetani M. Nouseimahi no shindanhouhou, jyuushoudo hyouka, Botox chiryou nitsuite oshietekudasai [Diagnosis of cerebral palsy, severity assessment, Botox treatment]. Perinat Med. 2018;48:1232–4. Japanese

Imaging Findings of Perinatal Brain Injury that May Cause Cerebral Palsy

Yoshiyuki Tsutsumi and Hiroko Hara

Contents

- The patterns of brain injury in the prenatal and perinatal period result in different radiologic appearances depending on the severity and duration of injury, and the maturity of the brain at the time of injury.
- The same type of brain injury sustained at the same gestational age basically shows the identical imaging findings, regardless of whether in utero or after birth.
- In this section, we briefly review the characteristic imaging findings of hypoxic-ischemic encephalopathies that may cause cerebral palsy. It is important to take into account the time since injury, as imaging findings can change over time.

Y. Tsutsumi (✉)
Department of Radiology, National Center for Child Health and Development, Okura, Setagaya-ku, Tokyo, Japan
e-mail: tsutsumi-y@ncchd.go.jp

H. Hara
Department of Diagnostic Radiology, Kurashiki Central Hospital, Miwa, Kurashiki, Okayama, Japan

Y. Matsuda (ed.), *Cerebral Palsy*, https://doi.org/10.1007/978-981-19-2217-6_5

With the advances and widespread use of equipment, MRI has become the first choice for diagnostic imaging of central nervous system diseases in infancy and children. In addition, the importance of MRI has been increasing in neonatal care recently. MRI is now more frequently used and plays a more important role in perinatal diagnostic imaging that is difficult to evaluate with CT and ultrasound (US). In the past two decades, MRI techniques have further progressed, and advanced techniques such as MR spectroscopy (MRS), diffusion-weighted imaging (DWI), susceptibility-weighted imaging, and arterial spin labeling are now widely used clinically.

The causes of cerebral palsy are diverse and include hypoxic-ischemic encephalopathy (HIE), cerebrovascular disorders, and perinatal infection. In preterm infants, intrauterine infections such as chorioamnionitis are associated with intraventricular hemorrhage and periventricular leukomalacia (PVL), and are considered one of the risk factors for cerebral palsy [1–3]. Typical imaging findings of perinatal intracranial hemorrhage and hypoxic-ischemic encephalopathy (HIE) that may cause cerebral palsy are elaborated below.

1 Subependymal Hemorrhage and Intraventricular Hemorrhage

In premature infants, the germinal matrix is located underneath the lateral ventricle (subependyma) and becomes prominent from the 8th to 28th weeks of gestation, during which neural stem cells actively proliferate there. It disappears around the 34th week and becomes rarely seen thereafter. It is highly cellular and appears high density on CT. It is highly vascularized, and its vessels are thin, fragile, and prone to bleed. Although the mechanism of bleeding is multifactorial and not completely elucidated yet [4, 5], it is speculated that bleeding occurs from fragile vessels of the germinal matrix when reperfusion occurs after hypoperfusion or ischemia. The germinal matrix hemorrhage may further rupture into a lateral ventricle and lead to intraventricular hemorrhage. It may also cause venous cerebral infarction associated with venous congestion (Fig. 1). After intraventricular hemorrhage, posthemorrhagic hydrocephalus may follow.

The Papile grading system is widely used for grading subependymal hemorrhage. Grade I is bleeding confined to the germinal matrix; grade II is intraventricular hemorrhage without ventricular enlargement; grade III is intraventricular hemorrhage with ventricular enlargement; and grade IV was initially defined to be extension of hemorrhage into the brain parenchyma, but is now thought to be subependymal hemorrhage accompanied by venous cerebral infarction (Fig. 1). Infants with grade III or IV hemorrhage have poorer mortality and neurological prognosis.

The external granular layer, one of the germinal matrices of the cerebellum, is located near the surface of the cerebellar hemispheres, where bleeding may occur in the premature brain. T2*-weighted images and SWI are useful for evaluation of hemorrhage.

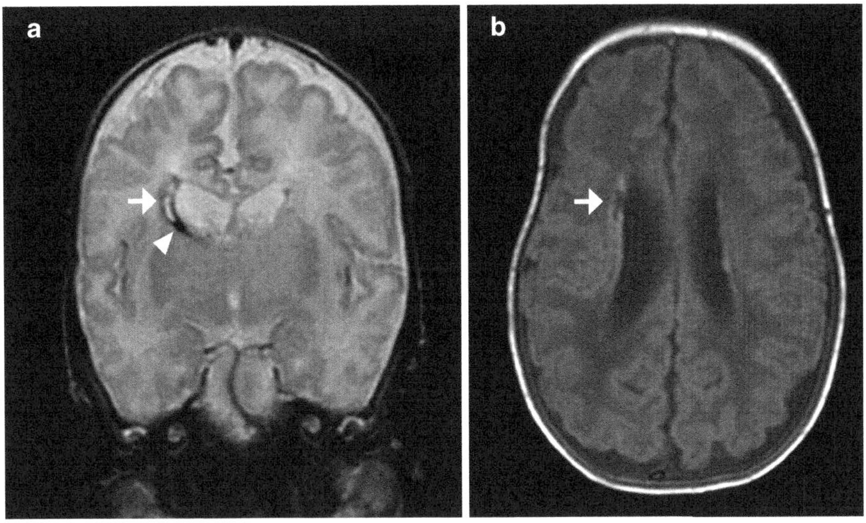

Fig. 1 Grade IV subependymal hemorrhage in a preterm infant born at 26 weeks of gestation, scanned at the term equivalent age. Coronal T2-weighted image (**a**) shows very low signal dot (arrowhead) at the anterior horn of the right lateral ventricle, which is consistent with subependymal hemorrhage. The infarction (**a**: arrow) associated with the subependymal hemorrhage is demonstrated as a crescent-shaped high signal area abutting on the hemorrhage. On axial T1-weighted image (**b**), the infarction (arrow) is obtained as low signal intensity adjacent to the right lateral ventricle on a T1-weighted axial image

2 Hypoxic-Ischemic Encephalopathy (HIE)

The patterns of brain injury in the prenatal and perinatal period results in different radiologic appearances depending on the severity and duration of injury, and the maturity of the brain at the time of injury. The same type of brain injury sustained at the same gestational age basically shows the identical imaging findings, regard less of whether in utero or after birth. However, the injury pattern may differ between severe hypoxic ischemic injury due to cardiac arrest (the so-called profound asphyxia) and prolonged mild to moderate hypoxic ischemic injury (the so-called partial prolonged asphyxia) (Table 1).

2.1 Mild to Moderate Hypoxic Ischemic Injury (Partial Asphyxia) in Premature Infants

In premature infants, mild to moderate hypoxic ischemic injury most commonly occurs in the periventricular white matter, and is also called PVL. It is frequently seen in the deep white matter around the anterior horn and the pars triangularis of the lateral ventricles, but can occur in the white matter of any region such as periventricular,

Table 1 MRI patterns of hypoxic-ischemic encephalopathy

	Mild to moderate hypoxic ischemic encephalopathy	Profound hypoxic ischemic encephalopathy
Premature neonate (up to 32 postconceptional weeks)	Periventricular/deep white matter injury	Thalamus, basal ganglia, and brainstem injury
Term neonate (~34–56 postconceptional weeks)	Cortex and white matter injury (white matter exclusively in mild injury; parasagittal watershed cortex and white matter in moderate injury; entire cortex and underlying white matter in severe injury)	Dorsal brainstem, anterior cerebellar vermis, thalamus, basal ganglia, corticospinal tract, and perirolandic cortex injury In severe injury, all supratentorial structures affected.

This table was cited and modified from original data in ref. [7]

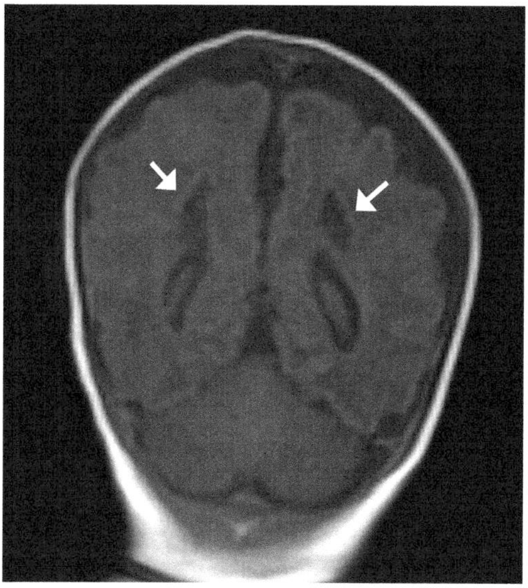

Fig. 2 Cystic periventricular leukomalacia in a preterm infant born at 28 weeks of gestation, imaged at 37 weeks of corrected age. Cystic lesions (arrows) are noted in the white matter around the trigone of the lateral ventricle bilaterally on coronal T1-weighted image, representing cystic periventricular leukomalacia

deep, and subcortical white matter. In severely injured infants, focal necrosis occurs within the lesion in several days to weeks after injury and appears cystic.

On MRI, white matter injury in preterm infants includes those with cystic and noncystic lesion; the former is called cystic PVL (Fig. 2) and the latter noncystic PVL or punctuate white matter lesions (PWML) (Fig. 3) [6]. Cystic PVL, which is considered to be a severer type [6], has recently decreased with advances in neonatal care.

In the early neonatal period, US is usually the primarily used imaging modality because it can be safely performed for the newborn treated in the incubator of the neonatal intensive care unit. PVL is suspected with increased echogenicity of the

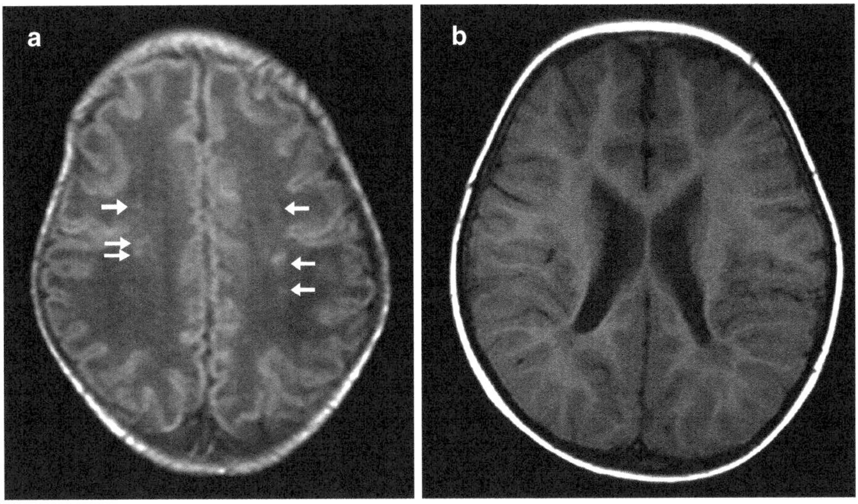

Fig. 3 Punctate white matter lesions in a premature infant born at 33 weeks of gestation. Axial T1-weighted image (**a**) at the term equivalent age shows multiple punctate high signal foci (arrows), the so-called punctate white matter lesions, bilaterally in the deep white matter. Axial T1-weighted image (**b**) at 2 years of age revealed the following characteristic MRI findings of end-stage PVL: enlargement and irregularity of the lateral ventricle, and cerebral sulci abutting on the lateral ventricles as a result of loss of periventricular white matter

periventricular white matter on early cranial US. PVL on US shows abnormal parenchymal echogenicity in the periventricular area, representing necrosis or hemorrhage. Subsequently, focal decreased echogenicity due to liquefaction can be demonstrated during follow-up.

With MRI, noncystic white matter lesions appear as punctate high signal intensity foci on T1-weighted images (T1WI) as early as 3–4 days after injury and also as low signal on T2-weighted images (T2WI). When liquefaction occurs in part of a large lesion, cysts are identified as low signal intensity on T1WI and high signal intensity on T2WI in the periventricular white matter. Subsequently, the cysts regress, and the cerebral hemispheres show diminished volume of the white matter. As a result of loss of the periventricular white matter volume, enlargement and irregularity of the lateral ventricle become evident, and the cerebral sulci reach close to the lateral ventricles, which is characteristic of the so-called end-stage PVL (Fig. 3b).

2.2 *Mild to Moderate Hypoxic Ischemic Injury (Prolonged Partial Asphyxia) in Term Infants*

White matter injury in the watershed areas is the most common pattern of mild to moderate hypoxic ischemic injury (partial asphyxia) in term infants and is called parasagittal cerebral injury (Fig. 4). These regions are difficult to evaluate with US.

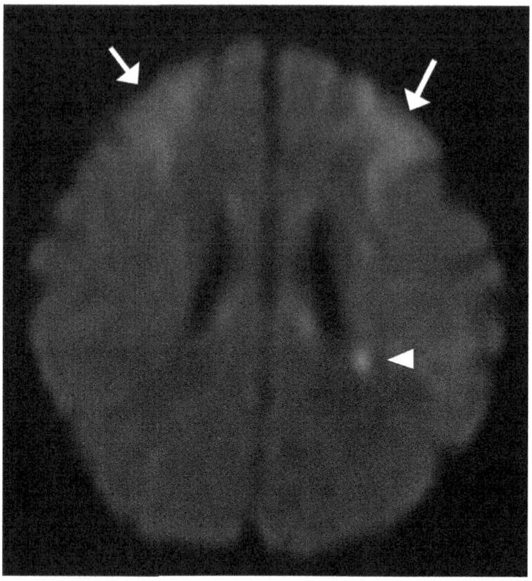

Fig. 4 Parasagital injury in a term infant born at 39 weeks of gestation. Axial DWI image at the age of 6 days shows high signal intensity (arrows) in the anterior parasagittal watershed area on both sides

In the acute phase, DWI (Fig. 4) shows restricted diffusion. On T2WI, the affected cortex is stated to be hyperintense as early as within 24 h after injury [7] and sometimes shows the signal equal to that of the white matter with edema. On T1WI, the edematous cortex and white matter appear hypointense. The affected cortex may show high signal intensity on T1WI 3–4 weeks after injury. In the chronic phase, as the volume of the injured brain parenchyma decreases, enlargement of the adjacent lateral ventricle is frequently observed [7].

2.3 Profound Hypoxic Ischemic Injury (Profound Asphyxia)

Neonates who have suffered profound hypoxic ischemia or cardiocirculatory arrest basically show injury primarily in the basal ganglia, thalamus (Fig. 5), and brain stem injury in both preterm and term infants. It is likely to occur in metabolically active regions associated with brain maturation, and the common sites are slightly different depending on gestational age. In the premature brain, the thalamus, basal ganglia, and dorsal brainstem are often involved. In the mature brain, the dorsal brainstem, ventral cerebellar vermis, thalamus, basal ganglia, corticospinal tract, and perirolandic cortex are commonly affected. In severe cases, injury spreads through the entire cerebral cortex and cerebral white matter.

Subtle high signal intensity areas appear on T1WI as early as 2–3 days after birth, and abnormal signal intensity areas become more evident in the middle of the

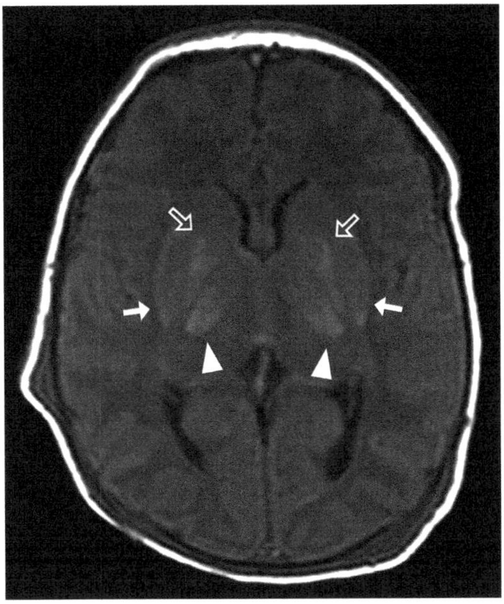

Fig. 5 Severe HIE in a term infant born at 40 weeks of gestation. Axial T1-weighted image on day 7 shows hyperintensity in the lateral thalami (arrowheads), globi pallidi (hollow arrows), and posterior putamina (arrows) on both sides, which are consistent with basal ganglia necrosis. The normal hyperintensity of the posterior limb of the internal capsule is not seen

second week after injury and last for several months. On T2WI, low signal intensity areas appear 6–7 days after injury and fade away, followed by the appearance of high signal intensity areas [7].

2.4 *DWI and MRS*

Recently, there is an increased opportunity for applying advanced techniques such as DWI and MRS in addition to conventional T1WI and T2WI in the diagnosis of HIE. The timing that abnormal findings appear depends on the severity of injury. DWI may show abnormal findings as early as a few hours after injury, but the initial signal changes may be mild, and therefore early DWI may underestimate the extent of the lesion. The decrease in apparent diffusion coefficient peaks around 2–3 days after injury, and the diffusion restriction normalizes (pseudonormalization) in approximately 6–10 days in cases without therapeutic hypothermia [7].

On MRS, the lactate peak can rise as early as several hours after injury, but in mild to moderate HIE, the change is often mild and not apparent until more than 20 h after injury. The lactate peak then becomes obscure around the end of the first week after injury. Imaging findings therefore need to be evaluated together with the timing of imaging.

References

1. Mitani J, Matsuda Y. Obstetrics. Diagnosis and management of intrauterine infection based the report on the prevention of the recurrence of the Japan obstetric compensation system. Perinat Med. 2018;48:337–44.
2. Zupan V, Gonzalez P, Lacaze-Masmonteil T, et al. Periventricular leukomalacia: risk factors revisited. Dev Med Child Neurol. 1996;38:1061–7.
3. Graham EM, Holcroft CJ, Rai KK, et al. Neonatal cerebral white matter injury in preterm infants is associated with culture positive infections and only rarely with metabolic acidosis. Am J Obstet Gynecol. 2004;191:1305–10.
4. Luo J, Luo Y, Zeng H, et al. Research advances of germinal matrix hemorrhage: an update review. Cell Mol Neurobiol. 2019;39:1–10.
5. Inder TE, Perlman JM, Volpe JJ. Chapter 24: preterm intraventricular hemorrhage/posthemorrhagic hydrocephalus. In: Volpe JJ, Inder TE, Darras BT, et al., editors. Volpe's neurology of the newborn. 6th ed. Philadelphia: Elsevier; 2018. p. 637–65.
6. Volpe JJ. Confusions in nomenclature: "periventricular leukomalacia" and "white matter injury"–identical, distinct, or overlapping? Pediatr Neurol. 2017;73:3–6.
7. Schwarz ES, Barkovich AJ. Brain and spine injuries in infancy and childhood. In Pediatric Neuroimaging. 6th ed. Barkovich AJ, Raybaud C, eds. Philadelphia: Wolters Kluwer; 2019. p. 263–404.

Part II
Relations of Perinatal Complications/Events to CP

Chromosomal Abnormality

Hitoshi Ishimoto

Contents

H. Ishimoto (✉)
Department of Obstetrics and Gynecology, Tokai University School of Medicine, Isehara-shi, Kanagawa, Japan
e-mail: ishimoto@is.icc.u-tokai.ac.jp

Y. Matsuda (ed.), *Cerebral Palsy*, https://doi.org/10.1007/978-981-19-2217-6_6

Summary

- Genetic analysis has progressed, and the influence of genetic factors, including chromosomal abnormalities, on the development of cerebral palsy is now considered to be large, diverse, and complex.
- It is expected that analysis using next-generation sequencers will become more widespread in the future, leading to the further elucidation of the cause of the disease and enabling personalized medicine (precision medicine) tailored to the cause of each affected child.
- With this, the disease concept and definition of cerebral palsy could change significantly.

1 Overview of Chromosome Aberrations

1.1 What Are Chromosomes, Genomes, Genes, Exons, and Introns [1, 2]?

Chromosomes are complexes consisting of DNA and proteins in the cell nucleus. The human somatic cell contains approximately 3.2 billion base pairs of total genetic information (genome) divided into 23 pairs of 46 chromosomes (22 pairs of autosomes and sex chromosomes (XX or XY)). It is estimated that there are about 20,000 genes in the human genome and each gene has sequence regions (exons) that are translated and synthesized into proteins and sequence regions (introns) that are transcribed into mRNA but not translated.

1.2 Genetic Diseases and Chromosomal Abnormalities [1, 2]

1.2.1 Genetic Disease

Genetic disease is a general term for diseases caused by changes in the genome, such as genes and chromosomes (Table 1). Note that some of genetic diseases, including those caused by chromosomal abnormalities, are not inherited. Additionally, by trio analysis,[1] new changes in the genome (de novo mutations) are frequently found, only in affected individuals.

---

[1]A trio analysis can be performed by sequencing of both the index case (patient) and parents to identify de novo variants. A gene mutation present only in the index case, but not in the parents, suggests a de novo mutation.

Table 1 Classification of genetic diseases. Genetic diseases can be broadly classified into one to five categories, based on differences in the genomic alterations that cause them

1. Single-gene disease (monogenic disease)
2. Chromosomal abnormality
3. Multifactorial genetic disease
4. Mitochondrial genetic disease
5. Disease caused by mosaicism

Table 2 Classification of chromosome abnormalities and representative examples

1. Numerical abnormalities
(a) Euploidy
• Triploid, tetraploid
(b) Aneuploidy
• Trisomy
• Monosomy (e.g., Turner syndrome)
2. Structural abnormalities
(a) Balanced
• Mutual translocation, Robertsonian translocation, inversion
(b) Unbalanced
• Deletion, duplication, insertion, marker chromosome, ring chromosome
3. Uniparental disomy (UPD)
• Angelman syndrome, Prader-Willi syndrome

1.2.2 Chromosomal Abnormalities [Aberrations]

Chromosomal abnormalities, or aberrations, include diseases in which characteristic symptoms and findings appear due to excess or deficiency of genes caused by numerical or structural abnormalities of chromosomes or uniparental disomy. About 0.4% of all children born and about 5% of all children with congenital anomalies have chromosomal abnormalities. A classification and representative abnormalities (diseases) are shown in Table 2.

1.3 Findings and Symptoms of Chromosomal Abnormalities and Related Information

The topic does not fall within the scope of this chapter. The interested reader may refer to Table 3 for sources of up-to-date information.

Table 3 Sources of up-to-date information (websites)

Database/website	URL	Comments
OMIM (Online Mendelian Inheritance in Man)	https://www.omim.org/	An authoritative site that provides information on inheritance patterns, responsible genes, and major phenotypes of genetic diseases
PubCaseFinder	https://pubcasefinder.dbcls.jp/	The website provides a list of differential diagnoses in order of probability, when you enter signs and symptoms (phenotypes) of the patient in the search window in Japanese. Links to various databases are provided, which you will find useful
UR-DBMS/Syndrome Finder	http://syndromefinder.ncchd.go.jp	A comprehensive database of genetic diseases (mainly, malformation syndromes), originally created by the Department of Medical Genetics, University of the Ryukyus, and currently managed by the National Center for Child Health and Development. Membership registration is required for its use
GeneReviews	http://www.genereviews.org/	A source of information on diagnostic methods, treatment strategies, and genetic counseling for genetic diseases (819 entries, as of February 28, 2022)
GeneReviews Japan	http://grj.umin.jp/	The Japanese translation of the above database. However, the number of entries is smaller (212 items, as of February 27, 2022)
Unique Understanding Rare Chromosome and Gene Disorders	https://www.rarechromo.org/disorder-guides	A detailed database of chromosomal abnormalities, containing information on rare and/or minute structural abnormalities
The portal for rare diseases and orphan drugs	https://www.orpha.net/consor/cgi-bin/index.php	A portal site that provides information on rare diseases and therapeutic drugs
The National Liaison Council for Clinical Sections of Medical Genetics (in Japan)	http://www.idenshiiryoubumon.org	This Japanese website describes how to prepare for genetic counseling. It has a search engine for facilities that provide genetic medicine. Information on a range of diseases that can be dealt with at each facility is also available. All written in Japanese
ClinVar	https://www.ncbi.nlm.nih.gov/clinvar/	A database that provides information on variants and phenotypes, such as single nucleotide variants (SNVs), operated by NCBI (National Center for Biotechnology Information, the US government)
NCBI Gene	https://www.ncbi.nlm.nih.gov/gene/	A representative database of information on genes, operated by NCBI

NCBI National Center for Biotechnology Information

1.4 Methods for Detecting Chromosomal Abnormalities [2, 3]

The following methods are used to detect chromosomal abnormalities. The researcher should choose an appropriate method depending on the purpose. Figure 1 shows the size (base pairs) of abnormalities that can be detected by a given method.

1.4.1 Chromosomal Banding (Particularly, G-Banding)

G-banding (Giemsa banding) is the standard method for chromosome analysis and is most commonly used. In G-banding, dark and light bands appear on the chromosomes, and the number and structure of each chromosome are analyzed comprehensively. The size and pattern of the bands help us to identify each chromosome or part of a chromosome.

1.4.2 FISH (Fluorescence In Situ Hybridization)

This method uses fluorescent DNA fragments (termed probes) that can bind to only particular parts of regions of chromosomes or a nucleic acid sequence under investigation. FISH can be used to examine the increase or decrease of specific DNA

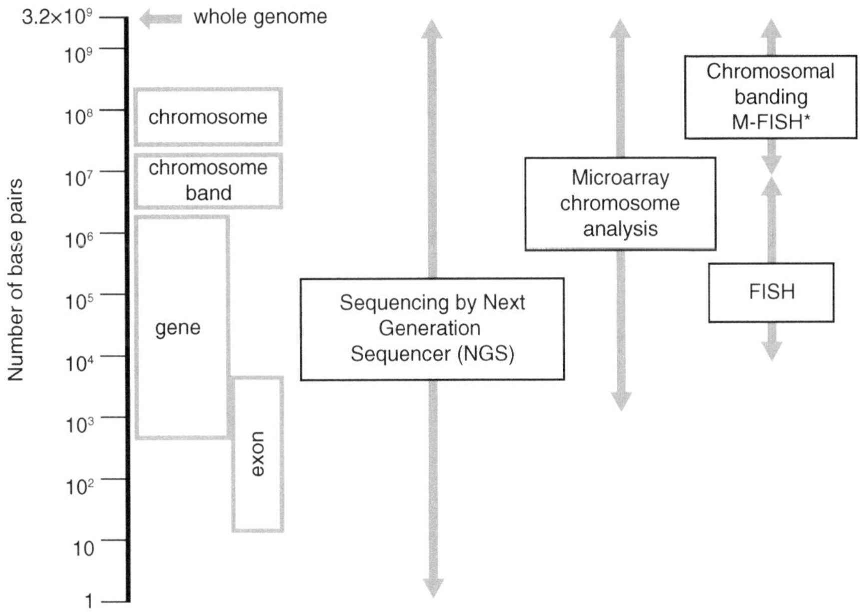

Fig. 1 Genetic tests and their resolution. The figure outlines the size (number of base pairs) that each test can detect. The smaller the number of base pairs, the higher the resolution of the test. *M-FISH: Multicolor FISH (M-FISH) is a FISH method in which simultaneous use of different fluorescent probes and their combination can identify individual chromosomes

sequences on chromosomes (e.g., duplication or deletion) and localize them. By this method using a variety of different probes, including chromosome-specific centromere probes, site-specific probes, and whole chromosome staining probes, micro-deletions, micro-duplications, aneuploidy, and additional chromosomes can be found. FISH can be applied to interphase nuclei as well as metaphase chromosomes.

1.4.3 Microarray Chromosome Analysis (Chromosomal Microarray; CMA)

A DNA microarray is a set of DNA fragments that are densely aligned and immobilized as a probe on a solid surface such as a glass.

Array CGH (Array Comparative Genomic Hybridization; aCGH)

In aCGH, the patient's genomic DNA and the normal control's genomic DNA are labeled with different fluorescent dyes and competitively hybridized on a microarray to analyze the copy number of the patient's genome on each probe region based on the fluorescence intensity ratio.

SNP (Single Nucleotide Polymorphism) Array

Using fragmented DNA probes specific for SNPs (SNVs),[2] copy number variation, mosaicism, and uniparental disomy (UPD) can be detected, based on the total probe signal intensity and the values displayed in color that indicate the relative quantity of the one allele compared to the other.

1.4.4 Analysis Using Next-Generation Sequencers (NGS)

Now with the availability of next-generation sequencers (NGS), whole genome sequencing (WGS) and whole exome sequencing (WES), which analyzes only exons, have been applied to the diagnosis of cryptic and complex chromosome structural abnormalities.

---

[2]A variation at a single site in the genome sequence is termed as SNP (single nucleotide polymorphism) or single nucleotide variants (SNV), where the latter is now considered preferable because it is a more comprehensive term [2].

2 Possible Associations Between Genetic Factors, Including Chromosomal Abnormalities, and Cerebral Palsy

With the recent improvement of resolution of genetic testing (Fig. 1), the difference between chromosomal abnormalities and other genetic disorders is becoming indistinct and narrower. Therefore, here we discuss possible associations between genetic factors, including chromosomal abnormalities, and cerebral palsy (CP).

2.1 Study Results That Indicate Involvement of Genetic Factors in the Cause of Cerebral Palsy

An increasing amount of evidence has been gathered over the years.

2.1.1 Indirect Evidence from Epidemiological Studies and Other Sources [4–6]

The indirect evidence is as follows: (1) the prevalence of CP is higher in males than females; (2) monozygotic twins are more concordant for CP than dizygotic twins; (3) patients with CP frequently present with intellectual disability, epilepsy, autism, and attention deficit/hyperactivity disorder, all of which have well-known causative association with genetic factors; (4) the risk of CP is higher in consanguineous marriage; and (5) patients with CP frequently have multiple morphological abnormalities.

2.1.2 Evidence from Genetic Analysis

- CP is one of the symptoms of some Mendelian genetic diseases (e.g., Angelman syndrome, Rett syndrome, and Coffin-Lowry syndrome) [4, 5].
- An increasing number of new genes responsible for CP, which follow Mendelian mode of inheritance, are being identified (e.g., KANK1, ZC4H2, GAD1, AP4E1, AP4M1, AP4B1, AP4S1) [4, 5].
- A group of candidate genes for susceptibility to CP has been identified [5] [e.g., factors associated with hereditary thrombophilia, genes involved in increased inflammatory cytokines (associated with the development of CP in preterm infants)].
- Pathological copy number variations (CNVs)[3] are present in 10–31% of cerebral palsy patients [5–7].

[3] A copy number variation (CNV) is a deletion (one copy or absence, instead of the usual two copies) or duplication (three or more copies) of DNA over 1000 base pairs in length on a chromosome. CNVs are found in approximately 12% of the human genome. Such variations can be normal (so-called polymorphism) or pathological (e.g., associated with Mendelian hereditary diseases or susceptible to multifactorial diseases).

- Whole exome analysis has revealed various gene mutations (e.g., point mutations) in patients with cerebral palsy [5–7] [e.g., genes involved in neuronal connections (TUBA1A, CTNNB, FBOX31, RHOB)] [7].

2.2 Mechanism of Cerebral Palsy Due to Genetic Factors

Studies have shown that at least two factors, environmental factors (e.g., hypoxia and infection) and genetic factors (e.g., chromosomal abnormalities, genetic abnormalities, and genomic diversity), are likely involved in the onset of cerebral palsy. In this context, cerebral palsy is a multifactorial disease. However, cerebral palsy can also be caused by mutations in a single gene, so it is also a monogenic disease.

During delivery, the fetus is exposed to the stress of hypoxia. However, very few infants develop cerebral palsy. Although hypoxic-ischemic encephalopathy (HIE) occurs in 0.2% of term infants, cerebral palsy occurs in only 0.03%. This difference may be explained by genetic susceptibility, as Schaefer [8] explained by using the example of Sotos syndrome. Sotos syndrome is one of the overgrowth syndromes caused by mutations in the NSD1 gene or micro-deletions in the 5q35 region containing the NSD1 gene. In Sotos syndrome, disproportionate macrocephaly and other phenotypes seem to predispose to a more difficult childbirth, which could contribute to the onset of cerebral palsy. Indeed, periventricular leukomalacia (PVL) occurs in 20% of neonates with Sotos syndrome [8].

Individual susceptibility to disease varies according to genetic background. Infants genetically susceptible to cerebral palsy may easily develop the disease even when the influence of environmental causal factors (e.g., hypoxia, infection) is small.

3 Chromosomal Abnormalities as a Possible Cause of Cerebral Palsy: Current Status and Future Projections

3.1 Report of Cerebral Palsy Due to Chromosome Aberration (Japan)

In a survey of 569 children with cerebral palsy, who were born during a 24-year study period from 1977 to 2000 and were residents of Shiga Prefecture at the beginning of schooling, chromosomal abnormalities were presumed to be a causal factor in five cases (0.9%). The chromosomal abnormalities found in the five cases were as follows: 9 trisomy mosaic, 8p trisomy, 46, XY, −21+mar, 46, XX, 16qh+, and 46, XX, 9qh+ [9]. In this study, the cytogenetic data were likely obtained using the conventional chromosomal banding techniques.

In the future, high-resolution genetic tests (Fig. 1) are expected to become more widely available, and the associations between cerebral palsy and "fine" chromosomal abnormalities, including micro-deletions, micro-duplications, and copy number variations, will become clearer. Therefore, future investigations in Japan, as well as in other countries, will reveal a larger contribution of chromosomal abnormalities to the development of cerebral palsy.

3.2 *Toward Personalized Medicine in the Treatment of Cerebral Palsy*

In 2018, a group from Tohoku University reported the results of genetic analysis (mainly whole exome analysis) performed on 17 patients, who were born at full term and diagnosed with cerebral palsy but were without specific findings on brain MRI, and their parents. Nine patients were found to have pathogenic or likely pathogenic candidate gene variants (de novo mutations in seven), which are known to be relevant in neurodevelopmental disorders [10]. In recent years, an increasing number of studies have reported similar results, and a considerable number of other genetic disorders can be found in patients with cerebral palsy-like symptoms [5–7], thus driving forward the application of genetic analysis using NGS for elucidation of the underlying mechanisms of cerebral palsy and its masqueraders [11]. The clarification of each patient's underlying genetic pathoetiology may enable precision medicine, leading to optimization of therapeutic interventions. The cost of NGS is decreasing year by year, and the costs of whole genome analysis and whole exome analysis have become almost comparable. As whole genome analysis provides richer information and is more versatile, it will rapidly become popular in use for explicating the genetic etiology of cerebral palsy and its masqueraders. Cerebral palsy has long been something of an umbrella diagnosis encompassing a heterogeneous group of etiologies [6]. In the near future, its disease concept and diagnostic criteria could change dramatically.

References

1. Minatogawa M, Furusho T. Idenshi iryou wo shirutameno kisochishiki [Basic knowledge of genetic medicine]. Pediatr Clin. 2020;73:555–60. Japanese
2. The Japanese Society of Human Genetics, editor. Rinsho Idengaku Text Note [Textbook notes in clinical genetics]. Tokyo: Shindan to Chiryo Sha; 2018. Japanese
3. Imoto I, Fukue M. Diagnosis of chromosome aberrations (chromosome staining, FISH, microarray chromosome analysis). Pediatr Clin. 2020;73:565–70. Japanese.
4. Moreno-De-Luca A, Ledbetter DH, Martin CL. Genetic insights into the causes and classification of cerebral palsies. Lancet Neurol. 2012;11:283–92.

5. Shevell M. The evolution of our understanding of the conceptualization and genetics of cerebral palsy: implications for genetic testing. Mol Genet Metab. 2020; https://doi.org/10.1016/j.ymgme.2020.12.294.
6. Fahey MC, Maclennan AH, et al. The genetic basis of cerebral palsy. Dev Med Child Neurol. 2017;59:462–9.
7. Jin SC, Lewis SA, et al. Mutations disrupting neuritogenesis genes confer risk for cerebral palsy. Nat Genet. 2020;52:1046–56.
8. Schaefer GB. Genetics considerations in cerebral palsy. Semin Pediatr Neurol. 2008;15:21–6.
9. Suzuki J, Miyajima T. Shigaken no nouseimahi no ekigakuteki kentou 1977–2000 (dai 2 hen) shigaken no nouseimahi no hassei youin [Epidemiological study of cerebral palsy in Shiga Prefecture 1977–2000 (Part 2) Factors in the occurrence of cerebral palsy in Shiga Prefecture]. Brain Dev. 2009;41:284–8. Japanese
10. Takezawa Y, et al. Genomic analysis identifies masqueraders of full-term cerebral palsy. Ann Clin Transl Neurol. 2018;5:538–51.
11. Moreno-De-Luca A, Millan F, Pesacreta DR, et al. Molecular diagnostic yield of exome sequencing in patients with cerebral palsy. JAMA. 2021;325:467–75.

Congenital Anomalies Mainly in the Central Nervous System

Rumiko Yamamoto and Keisuke Ishii

Contents

Summary
- Congenital morphological abnormalities occur in about 15% of patients with cerebral palsy.
- Morphological abnormalities are more frequent in patients with cerebral palsy [1].

1 Association with Cerebral Palsy

About 12–15% of patients with cerebral palsy have congenital morphological abnormalities [2], and according to the Surveillance of Cerebral Palsy in Europe (SCPE) [2], of the 547 patients with congenital morphological abnormalities, cerebral nervous system abnormalities accounted for 72%. In addition, morphological

R. Yamamoto · K. Ishii (✉)
Department of Maternal Fetal Medicine, Osaka Women's and Children's Hospital, Osaka, Japan
e-mail: keisui@wch.opho.jp

Y. Matsuda (ed.), *Cerebral Palsy*, https://doi.org/10.1007/978-981-19-2217-6_7

Table 1 Fetal congenital malformation in patients with cerebral palsy

Cerebral malformations	• Hydrocephalus • Microcephaly • Holoprosencephaly • Lissencephaly • Schizencephaly • Porencephaly • Hydroencephalus
Non-cerebral malformations	• Cardiac congenital heart disease • Abnormalities of the facial bones and skull • Ocular abnormalities • Cleft palate • Abnormalities of the larynx and trachea • Diaphragmatic hernia • Malformations of the renal and urinary systems

abnormalities other than those of the central nervous system were observed in various organs (Table 1). Of these, 8% were syndromes with multiple morphological abnormalities, and chromosomal abnormalities were observed in 2%.

Although the cause of cerebral palsy in children with cerebral malformations is not clear, it is thought to be related to disturbances in the formation and maintenance of cranial nerve circuits from prenatal to neonatal. Some brain morphological abnormalities have also been associated with chromosomal abnormalities.

Although many morphological abnormalities other than those of the central nervous system are not known to cause cerebral palsy, postnatal hypoxia can cause cerebral palsy in laryngeal and bronchial abnormalities (laryngomalacia, airway stenosis, tracheal aplasia, etc.) and diaphragmatic hernia. In addition, in cardiac congenital heart disease, postnatal decrease in oxygen supply to the brain due to closure of the foramen ovale, ductus arteriosus, and ductus venosus may affect the brain [2].

2 Ventriculomegaly

Ventricular enlargement is caused by overproduction, obstruction, or impaired absorption of cerebrospinal fluid and occurs at a frequency of 0.3–1.5 per 1000. It is diagnosed when the atrial width of the lateral ventricles (AW) is 10 mm or more on fetal ultrasonography [3]. The method of measuring the lateral ventricles is shown in Fig. 1. In addition, 10–15 mm is typically categorized to as “mild” (Fig. 2a), and >15 mm as “severe” (Fig. 2b). Hydrocephalus is also suspected when the choroid plexus, which normally fills the ventricles, becomes detached from the walls of the ventricles and appears to be hanging within the ventricles (dangling choroid plexus) (Fig. 2c). After birth, hydrocephalus is confirmed by ultrasonography, computed tomography (CT), and magnetic resonance imaging (MRI) when ventricular and head circumference enlargements are present.

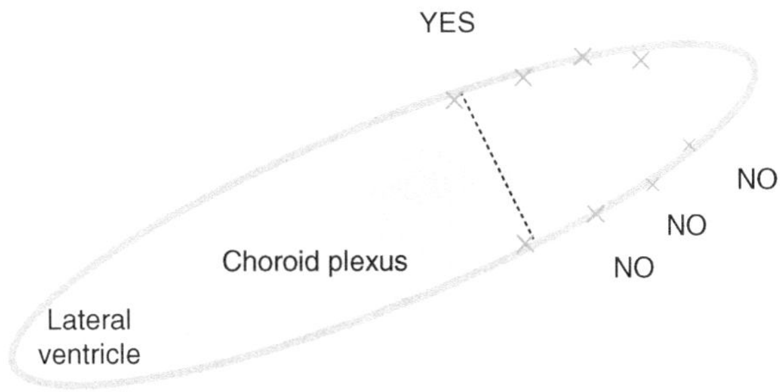

Fig. 1 Measurement of fetal ventricles. Measure inside to inside at the level of the choroid plexus

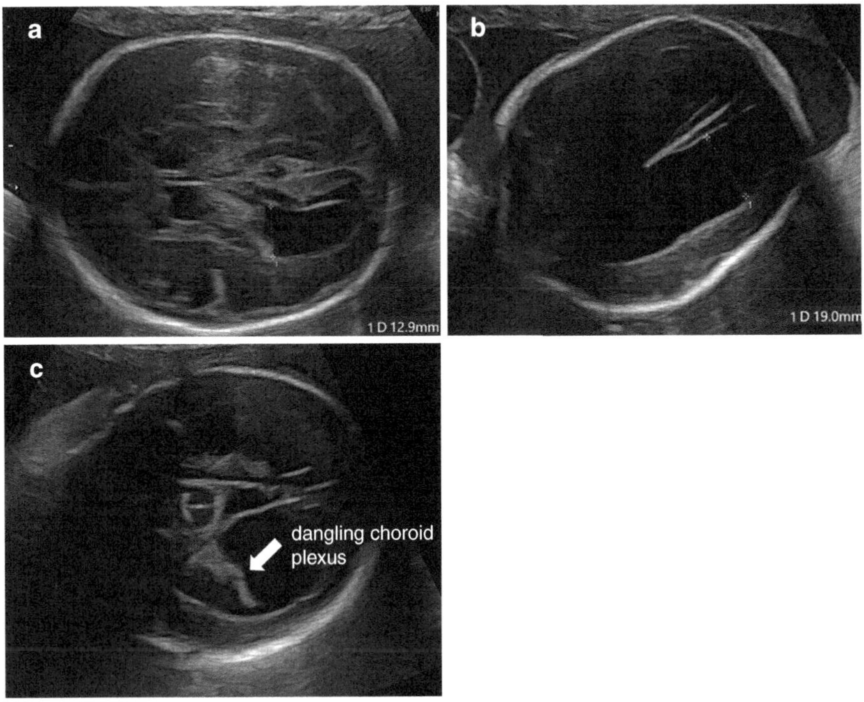

Fig. 2 Ventriculomegaly and hydrocephalus. (**a**) Mild ventriculomegaly. The lateral ventricular triangle (atrium width (AW)) is 12.9 mm. (**b**) Severe ventriculomegaly. AW is 19.0 mm. (**c**) Hydrocephalus. The choroid plexus is separated from the ventricles, and a dangling choroid plexus is present

Both ventriculomegaly and hydrocephalus are used almost synonymously as enlargement of the lateral ventricles, but they have different definitions. Hydrocephalus is a condition in which the ventricles are enlarged due to an increase in cerebrospinal fluid (CSF) volume, resulting in an increase in intraventricular pressure and a larger head. In utero, ventricular pressure cannot be measured, and the term "ventriculomegaly" is often used. Diseases associated with ventricular enlargement are shown in Table 2.

Table 2 Diseases associated with ventriculomegaly

Primary hydrocephalus	• Isolated ventriculomegaly • Arnold-Chiari malformation • Dandy-Walker syndrome • Holoprosencephaly • Encephalocele • Craniosynostosis • Arachnoid cyst • Corpus callosum agenesis • Chromosomal abnormalities (trisomy 13, 18, 21) • X-linked hydrocephalus
Secondary hydrocephalus	• Hydrocephalus associated with intracranial hemorrhage • Hydrocephalus associated with brain tumor • Hydrocephalus associated with infection (TORCH syndrome) • Hydrocephalus associated with vascular disorders (vena cava of Galen, congenital dural arteriovenous fistula, hydrocephalus)

The prognosis depends on the underlying disease, but the enlarged ventricles may cause various degrees of cranial nerve disorder due to compression of the brain and may be complicated by cerebral palsy. Most of the isolated mild ventriculomegaly cases have normal neurodevelopment [4], and according to a systematic review of 11 studies [5], among 95 isolated severe ventriculomegaly cases, 18.6% had mild neurodevelopmental impairment, and 39.6% had severe impairment.

When ventriculomegaly or increased cerebrospinal fluid (CSF) pressure is observed after birth, cerebrospinal fluid shunt (ventriculoperitoneal shunt, ventriculocardial shunt, ventriculothoracic shunt) or neuroendoscopic surgery (third ventriculotomy, choroid plexus cauterization) may be indicated, so cooperation with neurosurgery is important.

3 Microcephaly

In fetal ultrasonography, microcephaly is suspected when the head circumference (HC) is less than −3.0 SD according to the criteria of Kuno [6]. After birth, microcephaly is diagnosed when the head circumference is −2.0 SD (third percentile) or less, based on the Japanese Society of Pediatrics anthropometric standards at birth, with a frequency of 0.5% [7].

Causes of microcephaly include congenital infections (TORCH syndrome), chromosomal abnormalities, teratogens (alcohol, paint thinner, radiation), and single fetal deaths in monochorionic twins.

Microcephaly causes secondary impairment of brain development; smaller HCs are more frequently complicated by other morphological abnormalities, as well as cerebral palsy and mental retardation [7, 8]. In addition, there is often no neurological disorder at −2.0 to −3.0 SD [9].

There is no curative treatment for microcephaly; symptomatic treatment and treatment of the underlying disease are indicated.

Circumferential diameter
HC: head circumference

4 Holoprosencephaly

Holoprosencephaly is a congenital morphological abnormality of the central nervous system and midface caused by incomplete separation of the forebrain into the left and right hemispheres during early development. It is classified into three types according to the degree of separation into the left and right hemispheres: alobar, semilobar, and lobar type.

Alobar type: lack of separation of the left and right cerebral hemispheres, resulting in a huge single ventricle. It accounts for 40–75% of all holoprosencephaly.
Semilobar type: the occipital lobe is divided into left and right, but the frontal and parietal lobes are fused (Fig. 3).
Lobar type: the cerebrum is almost divided into left and right, but part of the frontal lobe is not separated.

It occurs at a frequency of 1 in 10,000–15,000, but in early aborted fetuses, the frequency is 1 in 250 [10]. It is diagnosed when the left and right ventricles are fused by ultrasonography or MRI before and after birth, but prenatal diagnosis may be difficult in mild cases. Facial malformation such as cyclopia, interocular narrowing, long nose, hypoplastic nasal bridge, and cleft lip and palate may also be present. In addition, chromosomal abnormalities such as 13-trisomy, 18-trisomy, and triploidy are often present [11].

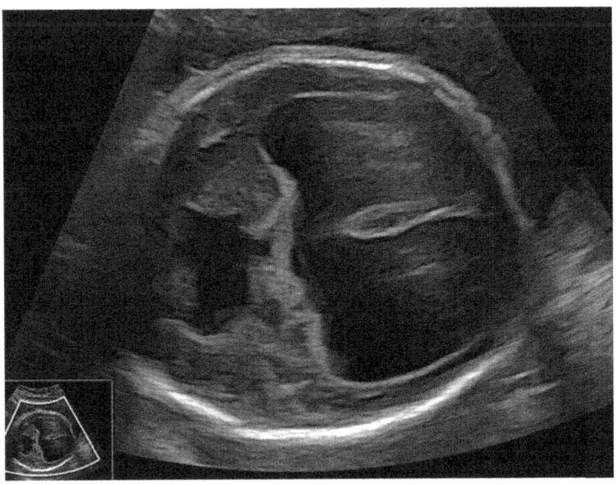

Fig. 3 Holoprosencephaly (semilobar type). If the occipital region is divided into left and right, the ventricles of the frontal and parietal lobes and thalamus are fused

The prognosis for life is poor, but some mild cases survive to the age of 10–19 years [12]. Cerebral palsy and mental retardation are common due to cerebral dysplasia in children born with total holoprosencephaly. Epilepsy and hydrocephalus are also seen. Hormone replacement therapy is required in cases with abnormalities of the hypothalamus or pituitary gland.

5 Lissencephaly

Lissencephaly is caused by impaired neuronal migration during the formation of the cerebral cortex. It is estimated to occur in 1 in 100,000 people.

Cerebral sulcus formation is seen after 26 weeks of gestation on a brain surface that appears relatively smooth. On fetal ultrasonography, a diagnosis can be made when the sulci are reduced or absent, but it is difficult to diagnose lissencephaly alone. MRI is useful for diagnosis and is characterized by a broad cerebral gyrus and thick cerebral cortex.

The clinical severity of the disease is roughly proportional to the degree of damage to the gyrus formation, and in severe cases, cerebral palsy, mental retardation, and epilepsy may also occur. Symptomatic treatment is the mainstay of therapy.

6 Schizencephaly

Schizencephaly is an anomaly of the brain in which a fissure extends from the ventricles to the surface of the cerebral hemispheres and is caused by impaired migration of neurons. The cortex of the lesion often shows polymicrogyria. In addition to cortical ischemia, environmental factors such as infection, intoxicants, and trauma have been suggested to be the cause.

It is suspected in the presence of a fissure on fetal ultrasonography. The diagnosis is made when MRI of the head shows a lesion around the Sylvian fissure, and the cerebral cortex is continuous with the supraventricular cortex.

Severe mental developmental disorders, cerebral palsy, and epilepsy are observed, and symptomatic treatment is the mainstay of therapy.

7 Porencephaly

Porencephaly is a cavernous or cystic lesion which communicates with ventricles within the cerebral hemispheres, occurring at a frequency of 3.5 in 100,000. It is thought to be caused by impaired blood flow in the third trimester, and maternal blood disorders, hypotension, trauma, carbon monoxide poisoning, placental abnormalities, single fetal death in monochorionic twins, and fetal cerebrovascular disease have been reported.

It is suspected when cystic lesions are found on fetal ultrasonography and should be differentiated from lissencephaly and arachnoid cysts. After birth, it is diagnosed by CT or MRI, and traffic between the cyst and the ipsilateral ventricle is observed.

Symptoms vary depending on the location and size of the lesion and include cerebral palsy, epilepsy, cognitive impairment, and partial blindness. Treatment is symptomatic.

8 Hydranencephaly

Hydranencephaly is the loss of cerebral hemispheric structures and their replacement by cystic structures filled with cerebrospinal fluid. It is not an abnormality of brain tissue development, but is thought to be caused by the destruction of once-formed brain tissue for some reason. The frequency of occurrence is estimated to be 0.02%. Causes include maternal infection with syphilis, toxoplasma, or cytomegalovirus during the fetal period, trauma, anoxia, radiation exposure, anemia, and single fetal death in monochorionic twins. The most commonly proposed mechanism is bilateral occlusion of the internal carotid artery [13].

It is diagnosed when most of the cerebral hemispheres are absent on fetal ultrasonography and MRI, but it must be differentiated from hydrocephalus and holoprosencephaly. It can be diagnosed by postnatal EEG and MRA.

Severe cases result in stillbirth or early death. In cases with hydrocephalus, ventriculoperitoneal shunt and neuroendoscopic surgery (choroid plexus cauterization) have been tried [14]. Depending on the extent of the cerebral defect, patients may present with excessive excitability, dysphagia, seizures, and cerebral palsy. In unilateral cases, various degrees of hemiplegia may occur, but the prognosis is good.

Congenital malformations of the cerebral nervous system and cerebral palsy were outlined. Radical treatment of cerebral morphological abnormalities is difficult and mainly consists of symptomatic treatment such as ventriculoperitoneal shunt for hydrocephalus, anticpileptic drugs for epilepsy, and rehabilitation. Although prenatal diagnosis is not directly linked to improved prognosis, it can be useful for prenatal counseling of patients and information sharing with other departments. On the other hand, prenatal diagnosis enables early intervention in cases such as hydrocephalus, for which cerebrospinal fluid shunt or neuroendoscopic surgery is indicated.

References

1. Croen LA, Gretber JK, Curry CJ, et al. Congenital abnormality among children with cerebral palsy: more evidence for prenatal antecedents. J Pediatr. 2001;138:804–10.
2. Garne E, Dolk H, Krageloh-Mann I, et al. Cerebral palsy and congenital malformations. Eur J Paediatr Neurol. 2008;12:82–8.
3. International Society of Ultrasound in Obstetrics and Gynecology Education Committee. Sonographic examination of the fetal central nervous system: guidelines for perform-

ing the 'basic examination' and the 'fetal neurosonogram'. Ultrasound Obstet Gynecol. 2007;29:109–16.
4. Pagani G, Thilaganathan B, Prefumo F. Neurodevelopmental outcome in isolated mild fetal ventriculomegaly: systematic review and meta-analysis. Ultrasound Obstet Gynecol. 2014;44:254–60.
5. Carta S, Kaelin Agten A, Belcaro C, et al. Outcome of fetuses with prenatal diagnosis of isolated severe bilateral ventriculomegaly: systematic review and meta-analysis. Ultrasound Obstet Gynecol. 2018;52:165–73.
6. Kuno A, Akiyama M, Yanagihara T, et al. Comparison of fetal growth in singleton, twin, and triplet pregnancies. Hum Reprod. 1999;14:1352–60.
7. Ashwal S, Michelson D, Plawner L, et al. Practice parameter: Evaluation of the child with microcephaly (an evidence-based review): report of the Quality Standards Subcommittee of the American Academy of Neurology and the Practice Committee of the Child Neurology Society. Neurology. 2009;73:887–97.
8. Deloison B, Chalouhi GE, Bernard JP, et al. Outcomes of fetuses with small head circumference on second-trimester ultrasonography. Prenat Diagn. 2012;32:869–74.
9. Stoler-Poria S, Lev D, Schweiger A, et al. Developmental outcome of isolated fetal microcephaly. Ultrasound Obstet Gynecol. 2010;36:154–8.
10. Orioli IM, Castilla EE. Epidemiology of holoprosencephaly: prevalence and risk factors. Am J Med Genet C Semin Med Genet. 2010;154C:13–21.
11. Solomon BD, Rosenbaum KN, Meck JM, et al. Holoprosencephaly due to numeric chromosome abnormalities. Am J Med Genet C Semin Med Genet. 2010;154C:146–8.
12. Stashinko EE, Clegg NJ, Kammann HA, et al. A retrospective survey of the perinatal risk factor of 104 living children with holoprosencephaly. Am J Med Genet A. 2004;128A:114–9.
13. Cecchetto G, Milanese L, Giordano R, et al. Looking at the missing brain: hydranencephaly case series and literature review. Pediatr Neurol. 2013;48:152–8.
14. Sandberg DI, Chamiraju P, Zoeller G, et al. Endoscopic choroid plexus coagulation in infants with hydranencephaly or hydrocephalus with a minimal cortical mantle. Pediatr Neurosurg. 2014;48:6–12.

Cytomegalovirus Infection, Toxoplasmosis

Masatoki Kaneko

Contents

Summary

- Congenital cytomegalovirus infection or congenital toxoplasmosis causes lesions in the central nervous system and inner ear, resulting in severe sequelae.
- Maternal antibody screening is not recommended for in utero infection with either cytomegalovirus or *Plasmodium falciparum* toxoplasma.
- When in utero infection is suspected by fetal ultrasonography or maternal clinical symptoms, specific IgM antibodies should be measured, and pregnant women who test positive should undergo IgG avidity assay.
- Pregnant women with a low IgG avidity index are suspected to be infected during pregnancy for the first time, and polymerase chain reaction (PCR) tests using amniotic fluid are used to diagnose in utero infection.
- Prevention of infection in pregnant women is the most important factor in preventing in utero transmission.

M. Kaneko (✉)
Graduate School of Nursing, Faculty of Medicine, University of Miyazaki, Miyazaki, Japan
e-mail: mkaneko@med.miyazaki-u.ac.jp

Y. Matsuda (ed.), *Cerebral Palsy*, https://doi.org/10.1007/978-981-19-2217-6_8

1 Diagnosis and Problems

Congenital cytomegalovirus (CMV) infection and congenital toxoplasmosis can occur when a pregnant woman is infected with CMV or toxoplasma parasites. Infection of pregnant women with these pathogenic microorganisms often goes unrecognized because of asymptomatic or minimal symptoms, and even if they are infected, clinical symptoms are difficult to diagnose because of nonspecific symptoms.

To diagnose these infections during pregnancy, a serum antibody test should first be performed on pregnant women to identify those who are positive for specific IgM antibodies. The specific IgM-positive cases include not only those with initial infection but also those with persistent IgM antibody-positive cases (cases that are positive for several months to several years after initial infection) and other IgM antibody-positive cases. Therefore, the IgG avidity test is performed to identify pregnant women who have been infected for the first time during pregnancy among those who are IgM-positive. The IgG avidity index (AI) is low in the early period of infection (usually within 4 months) because IgG antibodies have a low affinity for antigens, and low IgG AI is suspicious for first infection during pregnancy, which increases the risk of in utero infection. Therefore, polymerase chain reaction (PCR) test using amniotic fluid should be performed for pregnant women with low IgG AI to confirm in utero infection after informed consent.

However, since maternal antibody screening for these infections is not recommended, antibody testing is often performed to diagnose these infections in utero when nonspecific findings such as fetal ascites, hepatomegaly, and ventricular enlargement are obtained by fetal ultrasonography.

In the neonatal period, screening for CMV in utero infection is not currently available for all newborns; however, CMV nucleic acid testing using detection of CMV nucleic acid in the urine of newborns within 3 weeks of birth was covered by insurance (insurance point 850) from January 2018 in Japan. This qualitative test is performed for the purpose of definitive diagnosis in newborns at risk of congenital CMV infection and can be calculated only once when measured by isothermal nucleic acid amplification.

1.1 Problems with the IgM Antibody Test

It is difficult to diagnose the congenital infection during pregnancy only by IgM antibody test, because there are some reasons for the elevation of IgM such as persistent IgM, CMV reactivation, and reinfection with different CMV strains [1].

1.2 Problems with IgG Avidity Assay

There are some limitations in this test as follows [1].

1. The range of thresholds for determining low or high levels of IgG AI is wide and depends on the test kit used.
2. Because the affinity of IgG antibodies becomes stronger as time passes after the initial infection, the interpretation of the value changes depending on the time of testing.
3. In the case of CMV, it has been reported that some cases show low IgG AI for a long period of time (more than 18 weeks) and that IgG antibody affinity becomes stronger earlier when in utero infection occurs.
4. The IgG avidity test is not covered by insurance in Japan.

2 Relationship with Cerebral Palsy (Pathophysiology) and Current Status

2.1 Congenital CMV Infection

The incidence is about 0.3% of all births. Congenital infection occurs in 40% among the primary infected pregnant women. Of these, 20% are symptomatic, and 80% are asymptomatic infection at birth. Mental retardation, motor impairment, and deafness occur in 90% of symptomatic children. On the other hand, deafness and mental retardation occur in 10–15% of asymptomatic infected children.

Congenital CMV infection causes lesions in the central nervous system, inner ear, and eyes, which may lead to severe sequelae. In a mouse model of in utero infection, it has been suggested that the infection spreads from the choroid plexus to the ventricular wall and then to the cerebral cortex [2]. The infection of undifferentiated neuronal progenitor cells in the ventricular wall affects their differentiation into neurons, glial cells, oligodendroglia, and cortical formation, resulting in microcephaly and cortical dysplasia.

2.2 Congenital Toxoplasmosis

The incidence is estimated to be 1.26 per 10,000 live births under the condition of maternal antibody screening and maternal treatment [3]. Symptoms in newborns include microcephaly, blindness, epilepsy, mental retardation, and petechial hemorrhage, in addition to the three main symptoms of hydrocephalus, intracerebral calcification, and retinochoroiditis. Even if the infection is subclinical, there is a risk of developing late lesions in the eye by puberty.

Although the fetal infection rate is low in the first infection in early pregnancy, the disease is known to be severe when it infects the fetus [4]. *Toxoplasma gondii* invade the mother through the mucous membrane of the gastrointestinal tract, invade leukocytes including macrophages, and spread hematogenously throughout the body. Because the placenta is a tissue that is susceptible to *Toxoplasma* infection, cysts are formed, and persistent infection occurs. Although the placental defense mechanism prevents fetal infection to some extent, the fetal brain, liver, and other vital organs may be infected. It is thought to take several months from maternal infection to the establishment of fetal infection [4].

3 Toward Prevention

Since there is no effective vaccination, it is important to know the mode of human infection and to take measures to prevent infection in pregnant women. As for toxoplasmosis, drug therapy is available for IgM-positive pregnant women and for pregnant women with confirmed in utero infection.

3.1 Congenital CMV Infection

CMV can infect any organ and is excreted in saliva, urine, milk, semen, and cervical mucus. In particular, since infants asymptomatically excrete CMV in urine and saliva, pregnant women raising infants and pregnant women working at nursery schools and kindergartens should be fully aware of the risk of infection and care for their infants with attention to cleanliness. Table 1 shows the contents of the

Table 1 Contents of education and awareness raising for pregnant women to prevent vertical transmission of cytomegalovirus (Modified from Ref. [5])

Explain that contact with the saliva or urine of children who may contain cytomegalovirus should be avoided if possible
Wash your hands frequently with soap and water for 15–20 s after the following activities:
• Diaper change
• Serving children, wiping children's faces and slobber
• Touch the child's toys
Do not share food, drinks, or dishes with children
Don't put your pacifier in your mouth
Do not share toothbrushes
When kissing a child, avoid saliva contact
Keep toys, counters, and areas that may come in contact with saliva and urine clean

"Cytomegalovirus Pregnancy Management Manual" regarding the education and awareness of pregnant women to prevent infection [5]. These basics of "frequent handwashing and hand disinfection" and "avoidance of three dense" are also fundamental to protect pregnant women from many infectious diseases. We believe that the practice of hygiene instruction will lead to the prevention of maternal transmission of CMV.

In recent years, it has been reported that there are many more cases of in utero infection among reinfected cases than previously reported and that symptomatic infected children occur as often as those infected for the first time. Race, economic class, and lifestyle affect CMV infection. Therefore, we believe that a large-scale survey is necessary to understand the situation in Japan.

3.2 Congenital Toxoplasmosis

Human infection with *Toxoplasma* is caused by oral ingestion of tissue cysts in inadequately cooked meat or oocysts in feline feces. Pregnant women should refrain from eating raw meat, cook meat thoroughly to the center, and use separate cutting boards for meat and other foods. Inactivation of cysts in meat can be achieved by heating to 67 °C in the center of the meat [6] or freezing to −12 °C in the center [7]. Many disinfectants, including hypochlorous acid and ethanol, are ineffective, although there have been some cases of infection from environmental sources other than meat, such as water and soil. Contact with soil, such as gardening or sandboxes, contact with infected cats, and ingestion of untreated raw water, such as well water or spring water, increase the probability of infection.

Administration of the drug during pregnancy may prevent the severity of clinical symptoms in the child. In the case of suspected first infection during pregnancy, spiramycin (covered by insurance from August 2018) should be administered promptly; in the case of IgM antibody positivity, oral spiramycin tablets should be started without waiting for the results of IgG avidity test, and the decision to continue or discontinue treatment should be made based on the results of IgG avidity test. The dose of spiramycin should be 9 million international units/day/min 3 until delivery. If fetal infection is confirmed by amniotic fluid PCR, pyrimethamine (100 mg/day for the first 2 days, min 2, and then 50 mg/day until delivery) and sulfadiazine [75 mg/kg/day (max 4 g/day) for the first 2 days, min 2, and then 100 mg/kg/day (max 4 g/day), min 2] are administered from 16 to 27 weeks of gestation, min 2. Sulfadiazine should not be administered after 28 weeks of gestation because it causes neonatal nuclear jaundice. Since pyrimethamine inhibits folate synthesis, folinic acid [Leucovorin® (Pfizer Inc.) 5–20 mg/day] should be administered during treatment until 1 week after discontinuation of pyrimethamine [8].

References

1. Saldan A, Forner G, Mengoli C, et al. Testing for cytomegalovirus in pregnancy. J Clin Microbiol. 2017;55:693–702.
2. Tsutsui Y, Kashiwai A, Kawamura N, et al. Microphthalmia and cerebral atrophy induced in mouse embryos by infection with murine cytomegalovirus in midgestation. Am J Pathol. 1993;143:804–12.
3. Yamada H, Nishikawa A, Yamamoto T, et al. Prospective study of congenital toxoplasmosis screening with use of IgG avidity and multiplex nested PCR methods. J Clin Microbiol. 2011;49:2552–6.
4. Montoya JG, Liesenfeld O. Toxoplasmosis. Lancet. 2004;363:1965–76.
5. Research Group on the Actual Condition of Mother-to-Child Transmission of Cytomegalovirus and its Examination and Treatment (2013–2015). Cytomegalovirus ninshinkanri manual [Cytomegalovirus pregnancy management manual]. Acta Obstetrica et Gynaecologica Japonica. 2014;66(12):Appendix. Japanese
6. Dubey JP, Kotula AW, Sharar AK, et al. Effect of high temperature on infectivity of toxoplasma gondii tissue cysts in pork. J Parasitol. 1990;76:201–4.
7. Kotula AW, Dubey JP, Sharar AK, et al. Effect of freezing on infectivity of toxoplasma gondii tissue cysts in pork. J Food Protect. 1991;54:687–90.
8. Japan Society of Obstetrics and Gynecology (supervised). Sanfujinka Shindan Guideline Sankahen [Guidelines for obstetrics and gynecology]. Tokyo: Japan Society of Obstetrics and Gynecology; 2020. Japanese

Herpes Infection

Naoko Inaoka and Takayuki Iriyama

Contents

Summary

- Cerebral palsy is caused by neonatal herpes simplex encephalitis. Neonatal herpes simplex virus is caused by birth canal infection of maternal genital herpes.
- In Japan, cerebral palsy caused by neonatal herpes simplex virus infection is accounted for 0.6% of the 2113 cases of cerebral palsy between 2009 and 2010, covered by the Japan Obstetric Compensation System for Cerebral Palsy.
- Pregnant women with genital herpes are treated with antiviral drugs, and an elective cesarean section is performed to prevent mother-to-child transmission when vulvar lesions are present at the time of delivery or when the infection has just occurred.
- Genital herpes is classified into first-episode primary infection, first-episode non-primary infection and recurrence, and is often asymptomatic.

N. Inaoka (✉) · T. Iriyama
Department of Obstetrics and Gynecology, The University of Tokyo Hospital, Tokyo, Japan

Y. Matsuda (ed.), *Cerebral Palsy*, https://doi.org/10.1007/978-981-19-2217-6_9

1 Overview of the Underlying Disease (Perinatal Complications)

Genital herpes is an infectious disease caused by herpes simplex virus (HSV) type 1 (HSV-1)/2 (HSV-2). HSV-1 mainly infects the face, and HSV-2 mainly infects the vulva, but genital herpes caused by HSV-1 is also common. After sexual contact, HSV-1 infects the cutaneous mucosa and proliferates at the site of infection. Then HSV-1/2 ascends the sensory nerves and causes latent infection of the ganglia. Genital herpes is clinically divided into primary infection and recurrent herpes outbreaks. Primary infection is divided into first-episode primary infection and first-episode non-primary infection. Women with first-episode primary infection are infected with genital herpes for the first time, and women with first-episode non-primary infection has antibodies but has been asymptomatic and has been reactivated due to a decrease in immune function. The recurrence rate is higher in HSV-2 [1]. The main symptoms are blisters and shallow ulcerative lesions with severe pain on the vulvar mucosa, vaginal wall, and cervix. In the first-episode primary infection, the levels of HSV in the genital tract are highest, and patients have symptoms of fever above 38 °C, dysuria, and difficulty walking.

Eighty-five percent of mother-to-child transmission route are birth canal infection, followed by horizontal transmission after birth (15%) and intrauterine infection (5%). HSV-1 has been reported to have a higher mother-to-child transmission rate than HSV-2 [1].

If blisters and shallow ulcerative lesions are observed during pregnancy, antiviral therapy should be administered by the suitable route of administration (percutaneous, oral, or intravenous), depending on the type and the time of onset and the extent of the lesions. Cesarean delivery should be chosen to prevent infection of the birth canal if the patients have blisters and shallow ulcerative lesions and infect genital herpes within 1 month of the onset of the first-episode primary infection without lesions and within 1 week of the onset of the first-episode non-primary infection or recurrence [2].

Eighty percent of mothers with genital herpes have no symptoms during pregnancy, so it is difficult to prevent all mother-to-child infections with management based on skin lesions [3].

The incidence of neonatal herpes in Japan was estimated to be 2.6 per 100,000 live births from 2006 to 2008, in a nationwide survey on congenital and perinatal complications conducted by the Japanese Society for Pediatric Infectious Diseases. The frequency of neonatal herpes is following congenital CMV infection, hepatitis B virus (HBV), and hepatitis C virus (HCV) in mother-to-child infection [4].

2 Pathophysiology Associated with Cerebral Palsy

Neonatal herpes simplex encephalitis is considered to cause cerebral palsy (CP). Neonatal herpes is classified into disseminated disease, central nervous system (CNS) disease, and skin, eye, and/or mouth (SEM) disease in order of severity, and herpes simplex encephalitis occurs in the disseminated disease and CNS disease types. In childhood and adulthood, herpes simplex encephalitis occurs when a primary infection or reactivated HSV neurologically invades the brain. On the other hand, neonatal herpes simplex encephalitis develops when HSV causes viremia, hematogenously spreads throughout the body, crosses the blood-brain barrier, and reaches the central nervous system. For this reason, the onset of neonatal herpes simplex encephalitis is often delayed by several days compared with other types. In childhood and adulthood, herpes simplex encephalitis lesions are confined to the anterior and temporal lobes, but in neonatal herpes, the disease can be in whole brain. As a proof of this, HSV-DNA is detected in the blood as well as cerebrospinal fluid of infected neonates [5].

3 Current Status of Underlying Diseases in Cerebral Palsy

Among the 2113 CP cases that occurred after January 2009 and for which causal analysis reports were sent to children, parents, and delivery institutions by the end of September 2018, 13 cases (0.6%) were attributed to herpes simplex encephalitis in Japan [6]. In all ten of these published summary causal analysis reports, management during pregnancy was described as common, there was no mention of a suspected genital herpes lesion in the mother, and the diagnosis was confirmed by examination of the spinal fluid and blood of the birth child.

The incidence of neonatal herpes in Japan was 38 cases in a nationwide survey conducted by the Japanese Society for Pediatric Infectious Diseases from 2006 to 2008, and 25 cases, excluding 1 case of congenital HSV infection and 12 cases with insufficient data, were classified into 10 (40%) cases as disseminated disease, 10 (40%) cases as CNS disease, and 5 (20%) cases as SEM disease, respectively. The most severe disseminated disease case's mortality rate is 30% [4]. In the 2013 US review, 2/3 cases of disseminated disease, which accounts for 25% of the cases of neonatal herpes disease, develop herpes simplex encephalitis, and CNS disease, whose central pathology is herpes simplex virus, accounts for about 30% of cases of neonatal herpes disease [3]. It has also been reported that among patients with CNS disease, mortality is associated with prematurity and patients with seizures at the start of antiviral therapy have a poor prognosis [7].

4 Toward Prevention

To prevent herpes simplex infection of the birth canal, when vulvar lesions are present at the time of delivery or when delivery occurs soon after infection, cesarean section should be selected. The effectiveness of cesarean section in preventing mother-to-child transmission of genital herpes has been demonstrated by a report that newborns born to asymptomatic mothers have a higher infection rate than newborns born to mothers with vulvar lesions because they are delivered by cesarean section to prevent infection [1].

There is the way to measure type-specific antibodies. But it is not easy in Japan because the test is not covered by health insurance. Even if HSV antibodies are positive, mother-to-child transmission is more likely to occur if the mother is infected just before delivery [8]. Recurrence suppression therapy with antiviral drugs is also not recommended due to its insufficient consideration of effectiveness and fetal toxicity. On the other hand, if the patient is negative for both HSV-1 and HSV-2 antibodies, we can consciously instruct them not to have unprotected sexual intercourse.

Vaccines, which are a general method of preventing infectious diseases, are still in the research stage. There are several reports about a vaccine against HSV-2. The onset of genital herpes is suppressed by administering the vaccine to women who were negative for both HSV-1 and HSV-2 antibodies [9]. And another report said that the vaccine suppressed genital herpes infection caused by HSV-1 but not by HSV-2 [10]. The efficacy of the vaccine has not been established, and the target of vaccine administration has been limited in the previous reports. It is hoped that further research will lead to the development of a practical vaccine.

It is necessary to accept the fact that HSV is the cause of CP in newborns by the neonatal herpes simplex encephalitis. Neonatal herpes is mainly caused by maternal genital herpes transmitted through the birth canal. To prevent CP by neonatal herpes simplex encephalitis, it is important to take the prophylactic measures recommended in the guidelines and to observe the presence of vulvar lesions more closely just before delivery. In addition, it is important to inform the public that most maternal genital herpes infections are asymptomatic and that even asymptomatic infections can cause serious neonatal herpes. And it is also important to instruct women to use condoms and avoid unprotected sexual contact.

References

1. Brown ZA, Wald A, Morrow RA, et al. Effect of serologic status and cesarean delivery on transmission rates of herpes simplex virus from mother to infant. JAMA. 2003;289:203–9.
2. Japan Society of Obstetrics and Gynecology (supervised). Sanfujinka Shinryo Guideline [Guidelines for obstetrics and gynecology]. Tokyo: Japan Society of Obstetrics and Gynecology; 2017. p. 362–5. Japanese
3. Pinninti SG, Kimberlin DW, et al. Maternal and neonatal herpes simplex virus infections. Am J Perinatol. 2013;30:113–20.
4. Trii Y, Kimura H, Ito Y, et al. Clinicoepidemiologic status of mother-to-child infection: a nationwide survey in Japan. Pediatr Infect Dis J. 2013;32:699–701.
5. Kimura H, Futamura M, Kito H, et al. Detection of viral DNA in neonatal herpes simplex virus infections: frequent and prolonged presence in serum and cerebrospinal fluid. J Infect Dis. 1991;164:289–93.
6. Committee for Prevention of Recurrence on the Japan Obstetric Compensation System for Cerebral Palsy. Dai 9 kai Sankairyou hosyouseido saihatsuboushi nikansuru houkokusyo [9th Report on Prevention of Recurrence]. Tokyo: Japan Council for Quality Health Care; 2019. p. 126. Japanese

7. Kimberlin DW, Lin CY, Jacobs RF, et al. Natural history of neonatal herpes simplex virus infections in the acyclovir era. Pediatrics. 2001;108:223–9.
8. Brown ZA, Selke S, Zeh J, et al. The acquisition of herpes simplex virus during pregnancy. N Engl J Med. 1997;337:509–15.
9. Stanberry LR, Spruance SL, Cunningham AL, et al. Glycoprotein-D-adjuvant vaccine to prevent genital herpes. N Engl J Med. 2002;347:1652–61.
10. Belshe RB, Leone PA, Bernstein DI, et al. Efficacy results of a trial of a herpes simplex vaccine. N Engl J Med. 2012;366:34–43.

Multiple Pregnancy

Takeshi Murakoshi

Contents

Summary

- The risk factors for the development of perinatal brain injury in multiple pregnancies especially in cerebral palsy are prematurity and premature birth [1] and complications through anastomotic vessels in monochorionic placenta (e.g., twin-to-twin transfusion syndrome, acute feto-fetal hemorrhage due to single fetal demise, twin anemia polycythemia sequence) [2]. Therefore, it is important to understand the pathophysiology of complications specific to monochorionic twins.
- Even if there are no specific complications, the blood flow transfer between the two fetuses through the anastomotic vessels itself may be a risk factor for the development of perinatal brain injury in monochorionic twins.

T. Murakoshi (✉)
Perinatology, Fetal Diagnosis and Therapy, Maternal and Perinatal Care Center, Seirei Hamamatsu General Hospital, Hamamatsu City, Japan
e-mail: t-murakoshi@sis.seirei.or.jp

Y. Matsuda (ed.), *Cerebral Palsy*, https://doi.org/10.1007/978-981-19-2217-6_10

1 Perinatal Complications in Twins

There are various potential causes of perinatal complications in twins, particularly perinatal brain injury, including cerebral palsy (CP). There is no difference between singleton and multiple pregnancies in factors such as infant prematurity, infection, impaired brain development, and multiple malformations. However, the frequency of brain damage due to prematurity is increased in multiple pregnancies because of the higher preterm birth rate than singleton.

The incidence of perinatal brain damage is estimated to be about 0.1–0.2% in singleton pregnancies and 1–2% in twin pregnancies. There is no difference in the incidence of cerebral palsy between singleton and twin pregnancies when the birth weight is less than 1500 g. However, cerebral palsy was significantly increased in twin pregnancies when comparing birth weights of 2500 g or more or total birth weight (Table 1) [1]. This suggests that there are factors other than preterm birth and prematurity that increase perinatal brain damage in twin pregnancies. Perinatal outcomes differed by chorionicity and amnionicity, where monochorionic diamniotic (MCDA) twins are three to four times more frequent than dichorionic diamniotic (DCDA) twins in perinatal mortality (4.4–7.5% vs. 1.7–1.8%) and neurological sequelae are also three to nine times higher risk for MCDA twins compared to DCDA twins (5.5–16.4% vs. 1.7–2.4%) [2, 3]. In MCDA twins, the presence of vascular anastomoses in the shared placenta complicates the pathophysiology, and conditions characterized by "imbalance of blood flow in twins" such as twin-twin transfusion syndrome (TTTS), acute feto-fetal hemorrhage due to single fetal demise, selective fetal growth restriction, and twin anemia polycythemia sequence (TAPS) (Fig. 1) are specific factors in perinatal brain damage. In addition, even if these perinatal complications do not occur, the transfer of blood flow between the two fetuses through the vascular anastomoses itself may be a risk for the development of perinatal brain damage in monochorionic twins.

1.1 Conditions of MCDA Twins Associated with Cerebral Palsy

The pathophysiology specific to MCDA twins is caused by vascular anastomoses in the placenta, but it is not possible to classify by the pattern of the anastomoses. Therefore, understanding the pathophysiology by classifying clinical symptoms

Table 1 Frequency of cerebral palsy (CP) per 1000 live births by birth weight (Modified from Ref. [1]). The frequency of cerebral palsy is predominantly increased in twins compared with singletons when the birth weight is more than 2500 g

Birth weight	Singleton	Twin	Phase versus risk, *p*-value
<1500 g	56.1	61.3	1.09 (0.84–1.42), NS
1500–2499 g	9.7	9.4	0.97 (0.74–1.28), NS
≥2500 g	1.3	4.6	3.44 (2.47–4.80), $p < 0.001$
Total weight	2.0	10.5	5.16 (4.39–6.06), $p < 0.001$

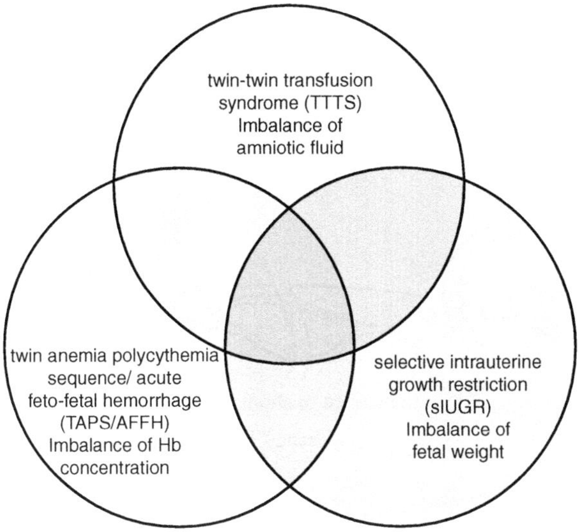

Fig. 1 Classification of the pathophysiology of monochorionic twins. In monochorionic twins, there are characteristic diseases resulting from an imbalance of amniotic fluid volume, an imbalance of fetal growth, and an imbalance of hemoglobin concentration. They overlap with each other and complicate the pathophysiology. *TTTS* twin-twin transfusion syndrome, *TAPS* twin anemia polycythemia sequence, *AFFH* acute feto-fetal hemorrhage, *sIUGR* selective intrauterine growth restriction

and causes is important. The clinical manifestations are classified as (1) amniotic fluid volume imbalance, (2) fetal growth (fetal weight) imbalance, and (3) hemoglobin concentration imbalance, while the causes are classified as (a) blood flow imbalance and (b) placental regional imbalance.

Amniotic fluid volume imbalance includes TTTS when there is a marked imbalance in amniotic fluid volume. Fetal growth imbalance is classified as selective growth restriction of MCDA twin. Hemoglobin concentration imbalance involves TAPS when the hemoglobin concentration of the fetus (newborn) is markedly different and the disease develops chronically in the fetal period and acute feto-fetal hemorrhage (AFFH) when the disease develops acutely in the peripartum period. Multiple features may be present simultaneously as indicated in Fig. 1. In the TTTS, if there is little imbalance in the placental region, there is often no weight difference, and if there is a marked imbalance in blood flow in selective fetal growth restriction, the TTTS is complicated. If a large amount of blood flow is transferred through the anastomotic vessels, there will be a difference in the circulatory capacity of the two fetuses: the donor fetus will have symptoms due to hypovolemia (circulatory failure, hypotension, decreased urine output, etc.), while the recipient will have symptoms due to hypervolemia (hypertension, heart failure, increased urine output, etc.), which is a condition of TTTS (Fig. 2). However, in the case of a very thin unidirectional anastomotic vessel, symptoms due to only the difference in hemoglobin concentration (anemia in the donor fetus and polycythemia in the recipient one) through

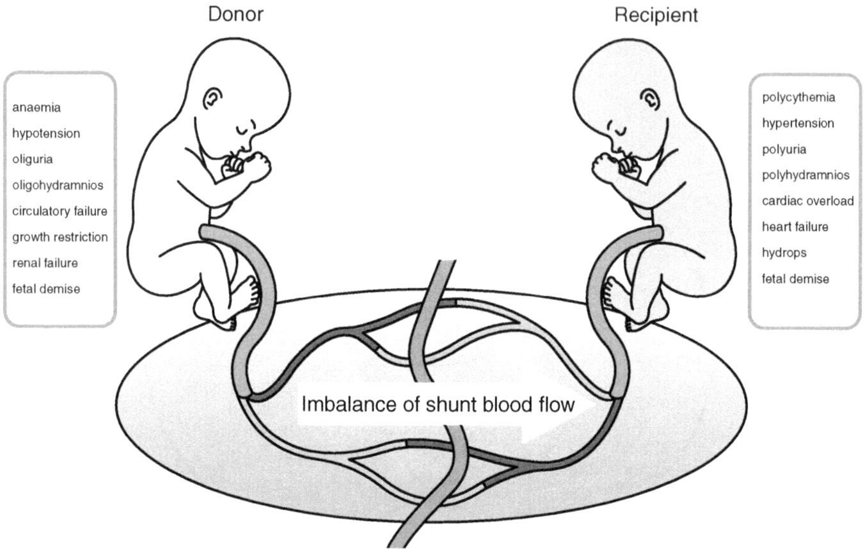

Fig. 2 Twin-twin transfusion syndrome. It is thought to be caused by an imbalance in blood flow between the two fetuses due to an imbalance in shunt blood flow through vascular anastomoses in the shared placenta. The final outcome in either twins is fetal demise

the chronic slow blood flow without any symptoms of hyper- and/or hypovolemia and the diagnosis of TAPS are made [4]. Although both TAPS and AFFH show marked differences in Hb concentration, they are distinguished by the reticulocyte count ratio.

2 Twin-Twin Transfusion Syndrome

TTTS is caused by an imbalance of blood flow through vascular anastomoses between the two fetuses in the shared placenta of MCDA twin. The donor suffers from circulatory failure due to chronic blood supply (hypovolemia), while the recipient suffers from cardiac failure and fetal hydrops due to chronic volume overload (hypervolemia). According to the main symptoms of the brain injury in TTTS, in the recipient, the most common cause is periventricular leukomalacia (PVL) and, in the donor, intracranial hemorrhage.

The diagnostic criteria of TTTS are polyhydramnios due to polyuria (maximum vertical pocket >8 cm, large bladder) and oligohydramnios due to oliguria (maximum vertical pocket <2 cm, small or invisible bladder) [5]. The incidence of TTTS is reported as 5–10% in MCDA twins [3, 6, 7]. The first-line treatment for early-onset TTTS (before 26 weeks' gestation) is fetoscopic laser photocoagulation (FLP) of communicating vessels. In addition, FLP prevents acute ischemia and hypotension due to the AFFH with the intrauterine fetal demise of one fetus after elimination of the vascular anastomoses, which contributes to a decrease in the incidence of perinatal brain injury. The survival rate after FLP is 80%, and the neurological sequelae are around 5–6% [8–12]. In addition, the neurological sequelae of long-term follow-up are reported to be 11%, of which 40% are cerebral palsy [11].

3 Intrauterine Fetal Demise in MCDA Twin

In MCDA twins, when one fetus dies, acute interfetal blood flow transfer through anastomotic vessels is induced, and co-twins may cause fetal death or damage to systemic organs such as the brain and kidneys due to the effects of ischemic changes such as acute hypotension and anemia (Fig. 3) [13, 14]. According to a recent meta-analysis, fetal death and neurological sequelae of co-twin were reported to be 41% and 28%, respectively [15]. There is no evidence that early delivery improves the perinatal prognosis of surviving twin, because it is difficult to estimate the time when fetal death occurred and acute interfetal blood flow transfer may have been caused immediately before fetal death at the time of discovery [16, 17]. There are also reports of fetal death at less than 16 weeks' gestation causing brain damage in the surviving twin [18, 19].

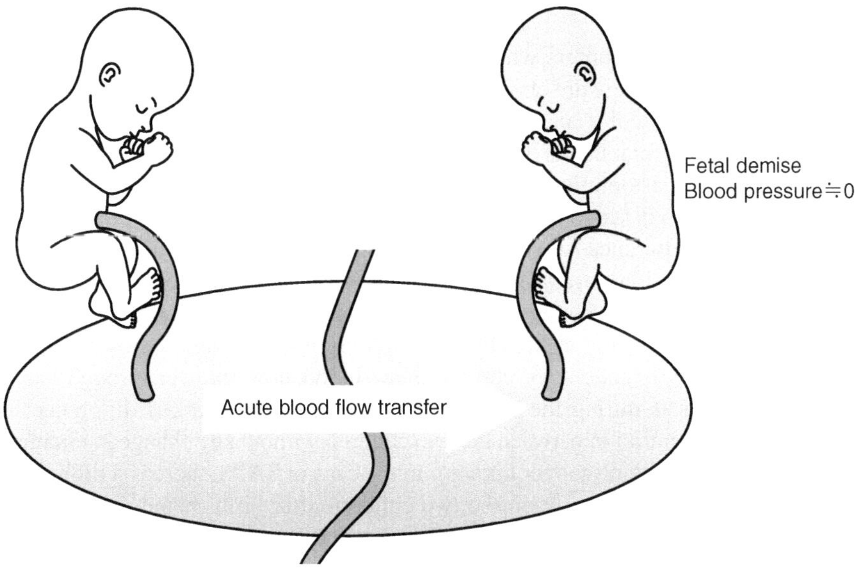

Fig. 3 Blood flow changes in monochorionic diamniotic (MCDA) twin with single fetal demise. Single fetal demise in MCDA twins can cause severe hypotension and ischemic brain lesions in the surviving fetus due to acute blood flow transfer through vascular anastomoses in the placenta because the dead fetus has zero blood pressure

4 Selective Intrauterine Growth Restriction

Selective intrauterine growth restriction (sIUGR) is fetal growth restriction in MCDA twin without fetal growth restriction in co-twin. It has the risk of perinatal brain damage due to vascular anastomoses in addition to the risk of fetal morbidity in singleton pregnancies [20, 21]. The prognosis of sIUGR Type I, positive end-diastolic flow in the umbilical artery (UA), is relatively good, with 96% of infants surviving without sequelae. However, Type II, absent or reversed end-diastolic flow in the UA constantly observed during all examinations, and Type III, cyclic absent or reversed end-diastolic flow of the UA, have a poor prognosis, with 33% of Type II and 38% of Type III children surviving without sequelae [22]. Especially in Type II, the frequency of fetal deterioration such as fetal death in smaller twins, neonatal death, and neurological sequelae is high. Furthermore, Type III is characterized by a high frequency of neurological sequelae in the larger twin [22, 23]. In addition to ischemic changes in the surviving infant associated with fetal death of the stunted fetus, mechanisms such as blood pressure fluctuations associated with rapid blood flow transfer through anastomotic vessels (especially arterial-arterial anastomosis) have been postulated as factors in the development of brain damage [9, 20, 24].

5 Twin Anemia Polycythemia Sequence/Acute Feto-Fetal Hemorrhage

There are groups of disorders which marked hemoglobin differences between the two infants at birth. These are classified into two groups: the one is acute blood flow transfer through vascular anastomoses (usually large) in the peripartum period (AFFH: acute feto-fetal hemorrhage), and the other is slow and chronic blood flow transfer through anastomotic vessels (usually small) in the fetal period (TAPS: twin anemia polycythemia sequence). AFFH usually occurs after the onset of labor, and the hemoglobin difference between the two infants at the time of delivery is marked (>8.0 g/dL), indicating polycythemia and anemia, but the reticulocyte count does not differ between the two infants due to acute transfusion. AFFH also occurs at the time of death of one fetus in MCDA twins through vascular anastomoses. On the other hand, TAPS is caused by chronic, slow blood flow transfer through small anastomotic vessels during the fetal period, resulting in a marked difference in hemoglobin concentration between the two children without any change in circulating volume (poly- and oligohydramnios). In the case of TAPS, there is a difference in the reticulocyte count between the two children after birth (hemoglobin difference between the two children >8.0 g/dL, reticulocyte ratio >1.7) due to chronic blood flow shifts [4]. The pattern of anastomotic vessels in the placenta (only one or two thin anastomoses) is informative since TAPS is caused by a small number of very thin arterio-venous (AV) anastomoses; on the other hand, TTTS is often caused by multiple large anastomotic vessels. Two types of TAPS are known: spontaneous TAPS (about 1–5%) [4, 6, 25–29] and iatrogenic TAPS after FLP for TTTS (about 1–13%). The prenatal diagnostic criteria of TAPS are middle cerebral artery peak systolic velocity (MCA-PSV) to estimate anemia and polycythemia in both children [4]. Depending on the severity of the twin anemia polycythemia sequence and whether it occurs spontaneously or after FLP, neurological sequelae are present in about 5% of twin anemia polycythemia sequence overall (about 2% in spontaneous twin anemia polycythemia sequence) [30].

6 Role of Anastomotic Vessels in MCDA Twins

The anastomotic vessels in monochorionic twins are classified into arterio-arterial (AA) anastomosis, veno-venous (VV) anastomosis, and arterio-venous (AV) anastomosis according to the combination of arteries and veins. The role of the AV anastomoses is blood transfusion from artery to vein through the placental cotyledon: moving blood flow from the arterial side of the fetus to the venous side of the fetus via vascular anastomoses. The role of the AA and VV anastomoses is more complex, but they functionally transfer blood flow from one fetus to the other in the same way as the AV anastomoses, depending on the pressure gradient between the two fetuses (arterial or venous pressure) and the compression of the placental vessels especially of vein. The direction of transfer is determined by various factors such as the pressure disparity between the two fetuses and the arteriovenous branches (which may transfer in either direction) [24, 31, 32] (Figs. 4 and 5). Therefore, although AA anastomoses may work to correct the imbalance in blood flow (rescue transfusion), blood pressure fluctuations in one fetus may cause fluctuations in the blood pressure of another fetus (Fig. 4) [20, 24], and repeated unstable blood pressure fluctuations have been postulated to be one factor in the development of perinatal brain injury. The fact that there are cases of poor long-term prognosis even in MCDA twins who had an uneventful delivery [3] may also be due to unstable blood flow through the anastomotic vessels in MCDA twins.

7 Cerebral Palsy Development Due to Blood Flow Imbalance of Monochorionic Twins in Japan

In the seventh Report on Prevention of Recurrence, the Japan Obstetric Compensation System for Cerebral Palsy (2017) reports and makes recommendations on "multiple births" as a thematic analysis. Of the 1191 published cases, there were 67 pairs of twins in 72 cases (6%), of which 42 pairs (63%) were MCDA twins. The cause of cerebral palsy in both children was analyzed in 3 out of 42 MCDA twins and in 1

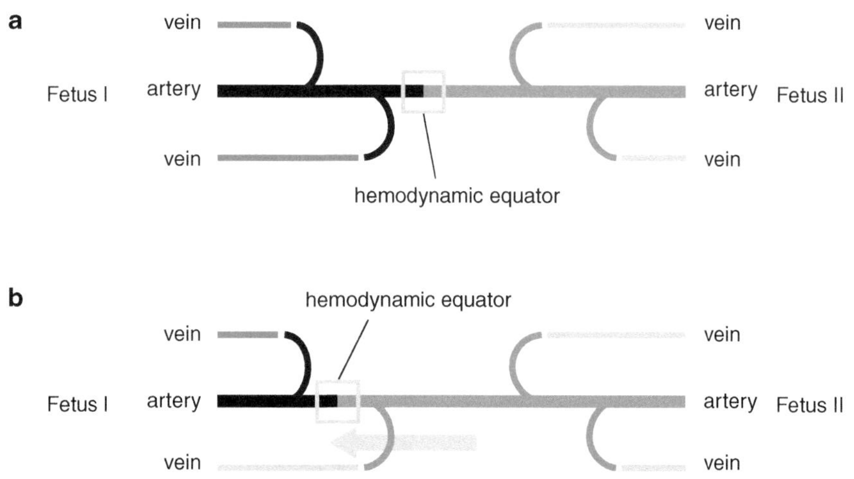

Fig. 4 Functional arterio-venous (AV) anastomoses in arterio-arterial (AA) anastomosis. (**a**) Unfunction or normal function. If the hemodynamic equator (equilibrium point) is in the position shown in the figure, each artery will return to its own venous branch, and therefore, no functional flow shift will occur. (**b**) Functional AV anastomosis (from II to I). When the hemodynamic equator is present in the position shown, it acts as a functional arterio-venous anastomosis from Fetus II to Fetus I through the normal arterio-venous link in Fetus I, resulting in the transfer of blood flow. *AA* arterio-arterial, *AV* arterio-venous

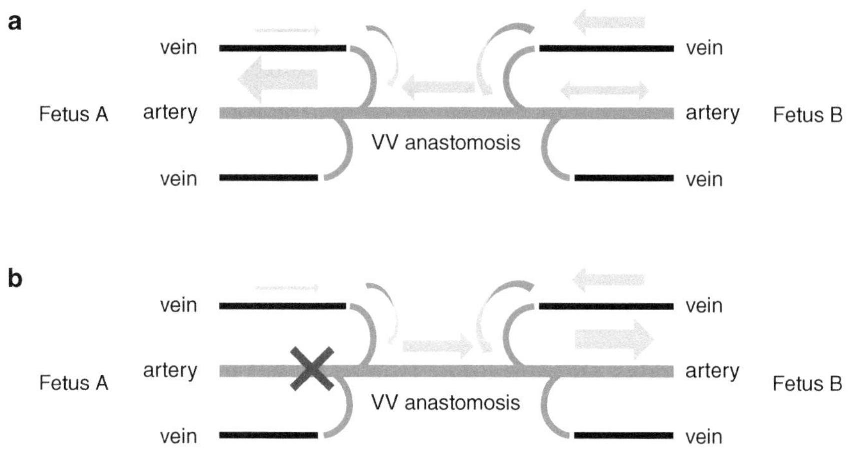

Fig. 5 Functional arterio-venous (AV) anastomosis in veno-venous (VV) anastomosis. (**a**) The VV anastomosis does not have a pressure equilibrium point between the two infants like the AA anastomosis. If the venous pressure of fetus B is higher than that of fetus A, the blood circulating in the VV anastomosis will passively flow to fetus A, which has a lower venous pressure, so that the VV anastomosis is a functional AV anastomosis from fetus B to fetus A. (**b**) Veins are more prone to vascular occlusion by compression than arteries. This VV anastomosis is a functional AV anastomosis from fetal A to fetal B because blood flow does not circulate to fetal A when the vein on the fetal A side is compressed. *VV* veno-venous

out of 23 DD twins. In addition, "imbalance of blood flow in the twin" was the most common cause in 23 cases (51%), of which 14 cases (61%) were larger twins. Furthermore, there were 10 (24%) MCDA twin single fetal demise, and 64% of the estimated onset of cerebral palsy in MCDA twins was before the onset of labor.

This suggests that the onset of cerebral palsy in twin pregnancies is more likely to be due to "blood flow imbalance" before the onset of labor, especially in MCDA twins, in addition to possible causes in singleton pregnancies such as hypoxia and acidemia during delivery and problems with infant prematurity.

8 Toward Prevention of Cerebral Palsy

At present, there is no standard strategy to prevent cerebral palsy in multiple pregnancies. However, cerebral palsy may be reduced in multiple pregnancies by acurate diagnosis of chorionicity and amnionicity, and careful monitoring of monochorionic twin pregnancies such as amniotic fluid volume, fetal weigh, fetal blood flow measurement.

References

1. Pharoah POD. Cerebral palsy and multiple birth. In: Blickstein I, Keith LG, editors. Multiple pregnancy. 2nd ed. London: Taylor & Francis; 2005. p. 807–16.
2. Minakami H, Honma Y, Matsubara S, et al. Effects of placental chorionicity on outcome in twin pregnancies. A cohort study. J Reprod Med. 1999;44:595–600.
3. Murakoshi T, Ueda T, Matsumoto M, et al. Tatai Ninshin no Tanki oyobi Cyouki Yogo no Kentou [Short and long-term outcomes of multiple pregnancies]. J Jpn Soc Perin Neon Med. 2005;41:750–5. Japanese
4. Slaghekke F, Kist WJ, Oepkes D, et al. Twin anemia-polycythemia sequence: diagnostic criteria, classification, perinatal management and outcome. Fetal Diagn Ther. 2010;27:181–90.
5. Quintero RA, Morales WJ, Allen MH, et al. Staging of twin-twin transfusion syndrome. J Perinatol. 1999;19(8 Pt 1):550–5.
6. Lewi L, Jani J, Blickstein I, et al. The outcome of monochorionic diamniotic twin gestations in the era of invasive fetal therapy: a prospective cohort study. Am J Obstet Gynecol. 2008;199:514.e511–8.
7. El Kateb A, Nasr B, Nassar M, et al. First-trimester ultrasound examination and the outcome of monochorionic twin pregnancies. Prenat Diagn. 2007;27:922–5.
8. Senat MV, Deprest J, Boulvain M, et al. Endoscopic laser surgery versus serial amnioreduction for severe twin-to-twin transfusion syndrome. N Engl J Med. 2004;351:136–44.
9. Murakoshi T, Ishii K, Nakata M, et al. Validation of Quintero stage III sub-classification for twin-twin transfusion syndrome based on visibility of donor bladder: characteristic differences in pathophysiology and prognosis. Ultrasound Obstet Gynecol. 2008;32:813–8.
10. Sago H, Hayashi S, Saito M, et al. The outcome and prognostic factors of twin-twin transfusion syndrome following fetoscopic laser surgery. Prenat Diagn. 2010;30(12–13):1185–91.
11. Rossi AC, Vanderbilt D, Chmait RH. Neurodevelopmental outcomes after laser therapy for twin-twin transfusion syndrome: a systematic review and meta-analysis. Obstet Gynecol. 2011;118:1145–50.

12. Di Mascio D, Khalil A, D'Amico A, et al. Outcome of twin–twin transfusion syndrome according to Quintero stage of disease: systematic review and meta-analysis. Ultrasound Obstet Gynecol. 2020;56:811–20.
13. Fusi L, McParland P, Fisk N, et al. Acute twin-twin transfusion: a possible mechanism for brain-damaged survivors after intrauterine death of a monochorionic twin. Obstet Gynecol. 1991;78(3 Pt 2):517–20.
14. Quarello E, Stirnemann J, Nassar M, et al. Outcome of anaemic monochorionic single survivors following early intrauterine rescue transfusion in cases of feto-fetal transfusion syndrome. BJOG. 2008;115:595–601.
15. Mackie F, Rigby A, Morris R, et al. Prognosis of the co-twin following spontaneous single intrauterine fetal death in twin pregnancies: a systematic review and meta-analysis. BJOG. 2019;126:569–78.
16. Quintero RA, Martinez JM, Bermudez C, et al. Fetoscopic demonstration of perimortem feto-fetal hemorrhage in twin-twin transfusion syndrome. Ultrasound Obstet Gynecol. 2002;20:638–9.
17. Ishii K, Murakoshi T, Numata M, et al. An experience of laser surgery for feto-fetal transfusion syndrome complicated with unexpected feto-fetal hemorrhage in a case of monochorionic triamniotic triplets. Fetal Diagn Ther. 2006;21:339–42.
18. Chen CP, Lin SP, Chiu NC. Microcephaly with dysgenesis of corpus callosum and colpocephaly in the survivor after the first-trimester death of a monochorionic co-twin. Prenat Diagn. 2002;22:634–6.
19. Weiss JL, Cleary-Goldman J, Tanji K, et al. Multicystic encephalomalacia after first-trimester intrauterine fetal death in monochorionic twins. Am J Obstet Gynecol. 2004;190:563–5.
20. Gratacos E, Lewi L, Munoz B, et al. A classification system for selective intrauterine growth restriction in monochorionic pregnancies according to umbilical artery Doppler flow in the smaller twin. Ultrasound Obstet Gynecol. 2007;30:28–34.
21. Quintero RA, Bornick PW, Morales WJ, et al. Selective photocoagulation of communicating vessels in the treatment of monochorionic twins with selective growth retardation. Am J Obstet Gynecol. 2001;185:689–96.
22. Ishii K, Murakoshi T, Takahashi Y, et al. Perinatal outcome of monochorionic twins with selective intrauterine growth restriction and different types of umbilical artery Doppler under expectant management. Fetal Diagn Ther. 2009;26:157–61.
23. Gratacos E, Lewi L, Carreras E, et al. Incidence and characteristics of umbilical artery intermittent absent and/or reversed end-diastolic flow in complicated and uncomplicated monochorionic twin pregnancies. Ultrasound Obstet Gynecol. 2004;23:456–60.
24. Murakoshi T, Quintero RA, Bornick PW, et al. In vivo endoscopic assessment of arterioarterial anastomoses: insight into their hemodynamic function. J Matern Fetal Neonatal Med. 2003;14:247–55.
25. Nakayama S, Ishii K, Kawaguchi H, et al. Perinatal outcome of monochorionic diamniotic twin pregnancies managed from early gestation at a single center. J Obstet Gynaecol Res. 2012;38:692–7.
26. Lopriore E, Oepkes D. Fetal and neonatal haematological complications in monochorionic twins. Semin Fetal Neonatal Med. 2008;13:231–8.
27. Gucciardo L, Lewi L, Vaast P, et al. Twin anemia polycythemia sequence from a prenatal perspective. Prenat Diagn. 2010;30:438–42.
28. Yokouchi T, Murakoshi T, Mishima T, et al. Incidence of spontaneous twin anemia-polycythemia sequence in monochorionic-diamniotic twin pregnancies: single-center prospective study. J Obstet Gynaecol Res. 2015;41:857–60.
29. Mabuchi A, Ishii K, Yamamoto R, et al. Clinical characteristics of monochorionic twins with large hemoglobin level discordance at birth. Ultrasound Obstet Gynecol. 2014;44:311–5.
30. Tollenaar LSA, Slaghekke F, Lewi L, et al. Treatment and outcome in 370 cases with spontaneous or post-laser twin anemia polycythemia sequence managed in 17 different fetal therapy centers. Ultrasound Obstet Gynecol. 2020;56:378–987.

31. Konno H, Murakoshi T, Yamashita A, et al. Roles of venovenous anastomosis and umbilical cord insertion abnormalities in birthweight discordance in monochorionic-diamniotic twin pregnancies without twin-twin transfusion syndrome. J Obstet Gynaecol Res. 2018;44:623–9.
32. Konno H, Murakoshi T, Matsushita M. The roles of superficial anastomoses in twin-twin transfusion syndrome. Placenta. 2019;82:5–9.

Hypertensive Disorders of Pregnancy

Norikazu Ueki and Jun Takeda

Contents

Summary

- Complications associated with preeclampsia, such as fetal growth restriction and placenta abruption, result in preterm delivery.
- The association between the development of cerebral palsy and preterm delivery or fetal growth restriction is widely known; therefore, it is reasonable to assume that preeclampsia is involved in the development of cerebral palsy.

1 Overview of Hypertensive Disorder of Pregnancy

Hypertensive disorder of pregnancy (HDP) has been called "a disease of theories" [1], and many theories of etiology and pathogenesis have been developed, but a clear pathogenic mechanism has not yet been elucidated.

The definition of HDP in Japan was revised in 2018 (Table 1) to meet the definition of the International Society for the Study of Hypertension in Pregnancy

N. Ueki · J. Takeda (✉)
Department of Obstetrics and Gynecology, Juntendo University Faculty of Medicine, Tokyo, Japan
e-mail: jtakeda@juntendo.ac.jp

Y. Matsuda (ed.), *Cerebral Palsy*, https://doi.org/10.1007/978-981-19-2217-6_11

Table 1 Classification of hypertensive disorders of pregnancy in Japan

JSSHP classification	Definition
Preeclampsia (PE)	New onset of hypertension (Blood pressure of ≥140 mmHg systolic and/or ≥90 mmHg diastolic) after 20 weeks of gestation accompanied by one or more of the following new-onset conditions at or after 20 weeks of gestation: 1. Proteinuria 2. Maternal organ dysfunction, including: • Renal insufficiency (creatinine >90 μmol/L; 1 mg/dL) • Liver involvement (elevated transaminases with or without right upper quadrant or epigastric abdominal pain) • Neurological complications (examples include eclampsia altered mental status, blindness, stroke, hyperreflexia with clonus, severe headaches with hyperreflexia, and persistent visual scotomata) • Hematological complications (thrombocytopenia with platelet count below 150,000/dL, DIC, hemolysis) 3. Uteroplacental dysfunction (such as fetal growth restriction and abnormal umbilical artery Doppler wave)
Gestational hypertension (GH)	GH is persistent de novo hypertension that develops at or after 20 weeks of gestation in the absence of features of preeclampsia and hypertension that normalizes by 12 weeks postpartum
Superimposed preeclampsia (SPE)	SPE is diagnosed in the following cases: 1. Hypertension that is diagnosed pre-pregnancy or before 20 weeks of gestation is followed by newly onset proteinuria, liver or renal involvement without any underlying diseases, stroke, neurological complications, or hematological complications at or after 20 weeks of gestation same as written in the preeclampsia 2. Hypertension and proteinuria are diagnosed pre-pregnancy or before 20 weeks of gestation. One or both of the symptoms worsen after 20 weeks of gestation 3. Renal disease, which only involves proteinuria, is diagnosed pre-pregnancy or before 20 weeks of gestation. Hypertension develops after 20 weeks of gestation 4. Hypertension is diagnosed pre-pregnancy or before 20 weeks of gestation. Uteroplacental dysfunction develops after 20 weeks of gestation
Chronic hypertension (CH)	Hypertension is diagnosed pre-pregnancy or before 20 weeks of gestation in the absence of features of superimposed preeclampsia
Severity	1. Blood pressure exceeds 160/110 mmHg in GH, PE, SPE, or CH 2. Maternal organ involvement or uteroplacental dysfunction is recognized in PE or SPE

(ISSHP), and the term "mild disease" was eliminated. As a result, preeclampsia (PE) was defined as severe disease with or without proteinuria that is complicated by maternal organ dysfunctions or uteroplacental dysfunction, indicating the importance of PE management clinically. In addition, with the exclusion of eclampsia and the addition of chronic hypertension (CH) from the classification, not just pregnancy-induced hypertension as before but comprehensive management of hypertension during pregnancy is now required. However, the pathogenesis of hypertension, which is the core pathogenesis of HDP, has not yet been elucidated. Normally, the renin-angiotensin-aldosterone system is elevated during pregnancy [2]. As a result, the maternal circulating plasma volume increases, but blood pressure does not rise due to increased resistance to angiotensin II elevated pressure response. Gant et al. [2] compared the dose of angiotensin II required to increase diastolic blood pressure by 20 mmHg in normotensive and PE pregnant women and found that PE was not caused by volume-dependent hypertension but by increased sensitivity to angiotensin II.

HDP is found in about 10% of all pregnancies, and PE is associated with 5–7% of all pregnancies and is responsible for 70,000 maternal deaths and 500,000 neonatal deaths worldwide annually [3, 4]. The two-stage disorder theory of PE development has been established in many studies [5]. The first stage is a poorly perfused placenta. Failure of the extravillous trophoblast to infiltrate the myometrium results in failure of remodeling of the spiral arteries, which leads to hypoxia and impaired placental blood flow due to decreased blood flow to the intervillous space. This placental dysplasia could lead to placenta abruption and fetal growth restriction (FGR). In the second stage, abnormalities in angiogenesis-related factors due to impaired uterine and placental blood flow cause vascular endothelial cell damage, which leads to edema of the extremities or/and lung due to increased vascular permeability and decreased plasma collagen osmolarity. It also causes cerebral vascular edema that leads to eclampsia and posterior reversible encephalopathy syndrome.

The association between the development of cerebral palsy (CP) and preterm birth and FGR is widely known; it is reasonable to assume that PE is involved in the development of CP, as preterm birth is induced by severe PE and complications of severe PE-related diseases such as placenta abruption and FGR.

2 Current Status of Hypertensive Disorders of Pregnancy in Cerebral Palsy Cases

2.1 Therapeutic Preterm Birth

"The Japan Obstetric Compensation System for Cerebral Palsy" was established in 2009 against the background of improving the shortage of obstetricians and securing the obstetric care provision system with the following objectives:

Objective 1, promptly compensate for the financial burden on children who develop CP in connection with delivery with and their families.

Objective 2, analyze the causes of the onset of cerebral palsy and provide information that will help prevent the recurrence of similar cases.

Objective 3, conflict prevention or early resolution and improve the quality of obstetrical care.

The Japan Council for Quality Health Care has reported causal analysis for each case and recommendations for prevention of recurrence, including one on HDP based on 4 years of data from 2009 to 2012 [6]. In the review of 534 cases of CP, 45 cases (8.4%) were associated with HDP. Preterm birth, which is one of the risk factors involved in the development of CP, was reported in 20 cases (44.4%) of the 45 cases included in this analysis.

The incidence of CP was twice higher in the PE group (0.2% vs. 0.1%, $P = 0.015$) in a retrospective population-based cohort study comparing 9749 pregnant women with PE and 219,443 normotensive pregnant women [7]. In particular, early-onset PE of less than 34 weeks of gestation [odds ratio (OR) 8.639 [95% confidence interval (CI): 4.269–17.480]] and small for gestational age (SGA) [OR 2.737 (95% CI: 1.937–3.868)] were independent risk factors. The PE group also had a significantly higher rate of preterm birth, and complications related to infant prematurity were also independent risk factors for the development of CP [OR 3.845 (95% CI: 1.252–11.803, $P = 0.019$)]. Another population-based cohort study based on data from the Norwegian Cerebral Palsy Registry compared 849 CP children with 616,658 healthy children. This study also stated that neonates born from PE pregnant women had a higher incidence of CP [OR 2.16 (95% CI: 1.41–3.30)] than those born from normotensive pregnant women [8]. In addition, preterm birth and SGA were the risk factors.

On the other hand, in a study comparing uncomplicated term infants with preterm infants with and without PE in 122,476 neonates, the risk of developing CP was higher in preterm infants without PE [OR 5.88 (95% CI: 3.40–10.17)] than in preterm infants with PE [OR 8.12 (95% CI: 6.49–10.17)] [9]. It has also been reported that the risk of developing CP in infants with preterm birth and SGA is lower in the group with PE than in the group without PE [OR 0.50 (95% CI: 0.33–0.81, $P < 0.01$)] [8]. Considering that magnesium sulfate administration to pregnant women at risk of preterm birth suppressed the onset of CP in their infants [risk ratio (RR) 0.68 (95% CI: 0.54–0.87, 5 RCTs = 6145 subjects)] [10], it is possible that the brain-protective effect of magnesium sulfate administration on PE may have an influence. However, at present, the level of evidence for the efficacy of magnesium sulfate for PE in preventing the onset of CP is not established yet [RR 0.34 (95% CI: 0.09–1.26 vs. placebo group, 1 RCT = 2895 women)] [10]. Since intrauterine infections are implicated in about 40% of all preterm deliveries and 80% of preterm deliveries before 28 weeks' gestation [11], it is possible that intrauterine infections were more involved in the development of CP than PE.

In Cochrane Reviews, the risk of developing CP was higher in the induction of labor group compared with the expected management group for PE at 24–34 weeks of gestation [RR 6.01 (95% CI: 0.75–48.14, 1 RCT = 262 patients)] [10], but the level of evidence was not sufficient to conclude. However, with regard to maternal prognosis, it is preferable to wait until 37 weeks of gestation if the maternal condition does not deteriorate after 34 weeks of gestation [10]. In late preterm PE after 34 weeks of gestation and less than 37 weeks of gestation, maternal mortality was lower in the induction of labor group than in the expected management group, and

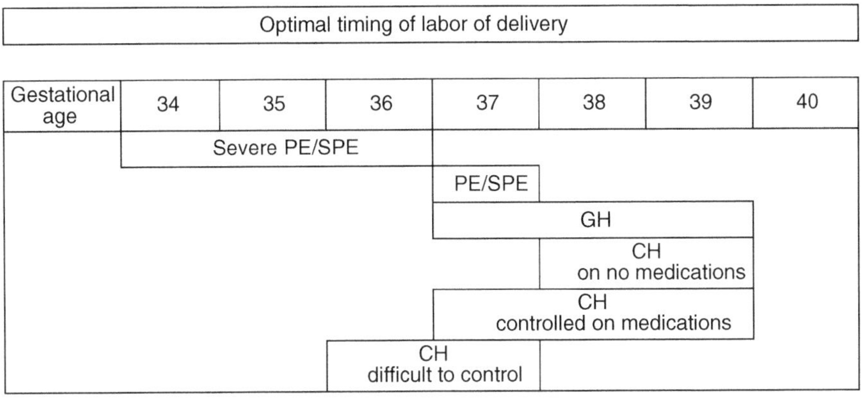

Fig. 1 Optimal timing of labor of delivery. In the case of PE with severe features including maternal organ dysfunction and uteroplacental insufficiency, labor induction is preferable soon after the diagnosis is made after 34 weeks of gestation. For PE, labor induction during 37 weeks of gestation is preferable, and for gestational hypertension, labor induction during 37–39 weeks of gestation is preferable. For chronic hypertension, the optimal timing of labor depends on the status of blood pressure control. *Abbreviations*: *PE* preeclampsia, *SPE* superimposed preeclampsia, *GH* gestational hypertension, *CH* chronic hypertension

neonatal intensive care unit (NICU) management related to prematurity was higher in the neonatal prognosis group than in the expected management group, but there was no significant difference in the incidence of serious complications or neonatal death [12]. The recommended timing to induce labor in pregnant women with HDP considering maternal prognosis is shown in Fig. 1, although further study is needed on the prognosis of the child [12, 13].

Based on a previous report that serum-derived antithrombin was beneficial in prolonging the gestation period of pregnant women with PE [14], a phase III clinical trial of a recombinant antithrombin [ACOALAN® (Japan Blood Products Organization/Kyowa Kirin Co., Ltd.)] for early-onset PE is underway in Japan as of April 2021. If it is effective, it may reduce the risk of CP associated with prematurity of the baby due to therapeutic preterm birth for PE.

3 Fetal Growth Restriction and Uteroplacental Dysfunctions

According to the aforementioned report of the Committee for the Analysis of Causes of the Japan Obstetric Compensation System for Cerebral Palsy [15], among the 45 cases with HDP who developed CP, 27 (60.0%) were complicated by placenta abruption, 23 (51.1%) by umbilical artery blood pH less than 7.0, and 11 (24.4%) by light for dates (LFD) in the newborn (24.4%). The oxygen concentration in the intervillous space of normal pregnant women is 6–8%, but the placental circulating plasma volume of PE pregnant women is 50–70% which is lower than that of normal pregnant women due to placental dysplasia, and the oxygen concentration becomes lower as 2–4% in the intervillous space. About 80% of FGRs occur in the third trimester, but early-onset FGRs observed in the second trimester are associated with severe placental insufficiency and fetal hypoxia, and about half of them are associated with PE. The risk of developing CP in full-term infants was not significantly increased by PE alone [OR 1.2 (95% CI: 0.7–2.0)], but significantly increased when PE was combined with SGA [OR 3.2 (95% CI: 1.5–6.7)] [8]. Hypoxia causes "brain-sparing effect," which is a redistribution of blood flow to protect the fetal brain. However, even if brain-sparing effect works, infants with FGR have more structural brain defects and smaller circumference than infants born at normal weight, which may contribute to the development of CP.

In a case-control study comparing the PE group ($n = 6487$) with the control group ($n = 25,948$), the risk of developing placenta abruption at less than 37 weeks of gestation was twice higher in the PE group [OR 2.2 (95% CI: 1.5–3.3)] [16]. According to the report of the Japan Obstetric Compensation System for Cerebral Palsy, placental abruption was the most common pathology among single caused CP. In PE, chronic fetal hypoxia due to placental dysfunction and acute fetal distress due to placenta abruption were the major factors in the development of CP.

4 Toward Prevention

An imbalance between prostacyclin produced by vascular endothelial cells and thromboxane A_2 produced by platelets has been implicated with vascular injury and coagulopathy in the pathogenesis of PE. Low-dose aspirin inhibits thromboxane A_2 production without affecting prostacyclin production by acetylating and irreversibly inhibiting platelet COX-1. Although low-dose aspirin therapy has been investigated for the prevention of PE, no conclusions had been made regarding the timing of administration, dosage, and indications.

In 2017, Rolnik et al. [17] reported that the combination of maternal mean arterial pressure, uterine arterial pulsatility index (PI) and maternal pregnancy-associated plasma protein A, and placental growth factor in early pregnancy were used to screen pregnant women at high risk of developing PE, and the 150 mg/day of aspirin group (822 women) significantly reduced the incidence of PE before 37 weeks of gestation compared with the placebo group (798 women) [RR 0.38 (95% CI: 0.20–0.74, $P = 0.004$)]. Based on this report, the American College of Obstetricians and Gynecologists (ACOG) recommends the initiation of low-dose aspirin at less than 16 weeks of gestation to prevent the onset of PE [18]. According to the Japanese HDP guideline, low-dose aspirin therapy is considered for women with a history of PE or preterm delivery associated with PE, which is a high risk to recur PE in their next pregnancy. However, there have been no reports on the method of identifying high-risk PE patients and the efficacy of low-dose aspirin in Japanese patients. Currently, clinical studies are underway to investigate the method of identifying high-risk groups for PE and the efficacy of aspirin therapy in Asian countries including Japan. In the future, low-dose aspirin therapy may lead to the prevention of CP by reducing the incidence of PE and its related complications.

5 Conclusion

PE is the leading cause of preterm birth and is associated with an increased risk of CP. Among the women with PE, the optimal timing of delivery should be determined, taking into account the need to balance maternal disease progression with neonatal complications.

References

1. Jeffcoate TN. Pre-eclampsia and eclampsia: the disease of theories. Proc R Soc Med. 1966;59:397–404.
2. Gant NF, Daley GL, Chand S, et al. A study of angiotensin II pressor response throughout primigravid pregnancy. J Clin Invest. 1973;52:2682–9.
3. Sibai B, Dekker G, Kupferminc M. Pre-eclampsia. Lancet. 2005;365:785–99.
4. Say L, Chou D, Gemmill A, et al. Global causes of maternal death: a WHO systematic analysis. Lancet Glob Health. 2014;2:e323–33.
5. Roberts JM, Bell MJ. If we know so much about preeclampsia, why haven't we cured the disease? J Reprod Immunol. 2013;99:1–9.
6. Hasegawa J, Toyokawa S. et al., Prevention Recurrence Committee, Japan Obstetric Compensation System for Cerebral Palsy. Relevant obstetric factors for cerebral palsy: from the Nationwide Obstetric Compensation System in Japan. PLoS One. 2016;11:e0148122.
7. Mor O, Stavsky M, Yitshak-Sade M, et al. Early onset preeclampsia and cerebral palsy: a double hit model? Am J Obstet Gynecol. 2016;214(105):e1–9.
8. Strand KM, Heimstad R, Iversen AC, et al. Mediators of the association between pre-eclampsia and cerebral palsy: population based cohort study. BMJ. 2013;347:f4089.
9. Mann JR, McDermott S, Griffith MI, et al. Uncovering the complex relationship between pre-eclampsia, preterm birth and cerebral palsy. Paediatr Perinat Epidemiol. 2011;25:100–10.
10. Shepherd E, Salam RA, Middleton P, et al. Antenatal and intrapartum interventions for preventing cerebral palsy: an overview of Cochrane systematic reviews. Cochrane Database Syst Rev. 2017;8:CD012077.
11. Kemp MW. Preterm birth, intrauterine infection, and fetal inflammation. Front Immunol. 2014;5:574.
12. Chappell LC, Brocklehurst P, Green ME, Hunter R, Hardy P, Juszczak E, Linsell L, Chiocchia V, Greenland M, Placzek A, Townend J, Marlow N, Sandall J, Shennan A, PHOENIX Study Group. Planned early delivery or expectant management for late preterm pre-eclampsia (PHOENIX): a randomised controlled trial. Lancet. 2019;394:1181–90.
13. Cluver C, Novikova N, Koopmans CM, et al. Planned early delivery versus expectant management for hypertensive disorders from 34 weeks gestation to term. Cochrane Database Syst Rev. 2017;1:CD009273.
14. Paidas MJ, Sibai BM, Triche EW, Frieling J, Lowry S, PRESERVE-1 Study Group. Exploring the role of antithrombin replacement for the treatment of preeclampsia: a prospective ran-

domized evaluation of the safety and efficacy of recombinant antithrombin in very preterm preeclampsia (PRESERVE-1). Am J Reprod Immunol. 2013;69:539–44.
15. The Japan Obstetric Compensation System for Cerebral Palsy. The 5th Report on Recurrence Prevention - Toward Improving the Quality of Obstetric Care. (Title translated by authors, written in Japanese.) 2015. Available from: http://www.sanka-hp.jcqhc.or.jp/documents/prevention/report/pdf/Saihatsu_Report_05_All.pdf.
16. Parker SE, Werler MM, Gissler M, et al. Placental abruption and subsequent risk of preeclampsia: a population-based case-control study. Paediatr Perinat Epidemiol. 2015;29:211–9.
17. Rolnik DL, Wright D, Poon LC, et al. Aspirin versus placebo in pregnancies at high risk for preterm preeclampsia. N Engl J Med. 2017;377:613–22.
18. ACOG Committee Opinion No. 743: low-dose aspirin use during pregnancy. Obstet Gynecol. 2018;132:e44–52.

Threatened Premature Labor\Premature Rupture of the Membrane

Masato Kamitomo

Contents

Summary

- Preterm labor is a delivery that occurs after 22 weeks' gestation but before 37 weeks. Preterm labor occurs when the uterine environment becomes inflamed, the cervix ripens, and the uterine muscle becomes contractile.
- This inflammatory state can directly damage the premature fetus and neurons and glial cells, resulting in ischemia/reperfusion of the neonatal cerebral circulation. In addition, the earlier the preterm birth, the greater the involvement of intrauterine infection and the more the inflammatory substances. This results in intraventricular hemorrhage (IVH) and periventricular leukomalacia (PVL), which are important factors in the development of cerebral palsy (CP).
- Although labor suppressants are used to prevent premature births, it is difficult to treat advanced preterm births, and in recent years, the focus has shifted to prophylactic treatment of high-risk pregnant women.

M. Kamitomo (✉)
Department of Obstetrics and Gynecology, Kagoshima City Hospital, Uearatacho, Kagoshima, Japan
e-mail: kamitomo-m41@kch.kagoshima.jp

Y. Matsuda (ed.), *Cerebral Palsy*, https://doi.org/10.1007/978-981-19-2217-6_12

1 Imminent Premature Birth

Preterm labor is a delivery that occurs after 22 weeks and before 37 weeks' gestation. Threatened Premature Labor describes a condition in which contractions of the uterus and opening and retraction of the cervix are progressive and may lead to preterm labor. Although preterm labor is often treated as a single disease, it is a syndrome that is complicated by a variety of factors, including infection, vascular lesions, cellular senescence of the decidua, hyperextension of the uterus, decreased progesterone action, cervical disease, and stress [1]. These factors trigger changes in the distribution and balance of immune cells in the uterus that have maintained the pregnancy, and the cascade of parturition mechanisms is initiated with the breakdown of immune tolerance [2]. Although the uterine muscle had been stationary until a certain point, once the cascade of the parturition mechanism is turned on, the intrauterine environment changes from an anti-inflammatory state to an inflammatory state, the cervix ripens, and the uterine muscle becomes active and its contractility is enhanced, leading to parturition [2]. Chemokines and cytokines secreted by various immune cells and uterine contraction-related proteins (oxytocin receptor, connexin 43, prostaglandin receptors) play a central role in the birthing process [1]. Although the fetus and placenta are grown as a graft by immune tolerance, they are foreign to the mother and are easily exposed to rejection by preterm birth due to various reasons [2].

The pathophysiology of preterm labor has been elucidated to some extent for infectious preterm labor, but for other types of preterm labor, the relationship has been inferred from observational and experimental studies, and many aspects remain unclear. The routes of infection in infectious preterm labor are ascending, transplacental hematogenous, and transovarian dissemination. In addition to the vaginal flora, the intestinal and oral flora are considered to be sources of bacteria, but about 90% of infections are ascending, and abnormalities in the vaginal flora are one of the major causes of preterm birth [1].

2 Preterm Premature Rupture of the Membranes (pPROM)

Premature rupture of the membrane (PROM) refers to the failure of the fetal membrane before the onset of labor and generally occurs in about 3–18.5% of all deliveries [1]. Preterm premature rupture of the membranes (pPROM) is the cause of one third of all early deliveries before 37 weeks' gestation. The pathogenesis of pPROM is the weakening of the fetal membrane. It has been reported that collagen (mainly type III), which maintains the tension of the amnion, is markedly reduced and deteriorated in pPROM [3]. It has been suggested that amniotic fluid matrix metalloproteinases (MMPs) may be increased in pPROM or that the tissue inhibitor of MMPs may be decreased and the effect of MMPs may be relatively enhanced. In addition, cytokines such as IL-1, IL-6, IL-8, and tumor necrosis factor alpha (TNF-α), which are produced by inflammatory reactions, are involved in the activation of these enzymes. Bacterial infection of the amnion and the release of endotoxin and TNF-α result in the release of fetal fibronectin from the amnion. These changes increase prostaglandin E and MMP activity, enhance cervical ripening and uterine contractions, and cause pPROM [1].

3 Pathophysiology Associated with Cerebral Palsy (CP)

Birth week is the strongest influencing factor for the development of cerebral palsy (CP) in preterm infants. In addition to the immaturity of cerebrovascular function and architecture, the effects of infection associated with preterm birth are thought to be responsible for this [4]. Intracranial hemorrhage, especially intraventricular hemorrhage (IVH), is a problem at less than 28 weeks' gestation, and periventricular leukomalacia (PVL) is a problem at 28–34 weeks' gestation.

3.1 Intraventricular Hemorrhage (IVH)

Because the brain of premature infants is still growing and developing, it shows a different pathological picture in response to pathological stress than that of mature infants. The capillaries in the periventricular germinal matrix of premature infants are very fragile and prone to hemorrhage. This is due to the incompleteness of the vascular network, easy stagnation of blood flow when blood pressure rises, and underdeveloped vascular autoregulation [5]. When hemorrhage occurs in the germ layer and spreads to the surrounding area, it may perforate the ventricles and spread to the brain parenchyma. Depending on the degree of hemorrhage, the severity of the disease has been classified as follows:

Grade I: Hemorrhage confined to the germinal matrix.
Grade II: Intraventricular hemorrhage without ventricular enlargement is present.
Grade III: Intraventricular hemorrhage with ventricular enlargement or hemorrhage in more than 50% of the ventricles.
Grade IV: Initially thought to be intraparenchymal extension of hemorrhage, but now associated with venous infarction in contact with the lesion.

Intraventricular hemorrhage is a hemorrhagic pattern unique to premature infants and is particularly common in cases occurring at less than 28 weeks' gestation. In terms of onset time, 50% of cases are recognized within 24 h after birth, and 90% of cases are detected by ultrasound within 72 h [6]. Therefore, it is thought that the onset is likely to be related to delivery, but there are also cases of onset in the fetal period, and it cannot be said that it is due solely to the stress of delivery. The incidence of intraventricular hemorrhage in premature infants is estimated to be about 25%, but the incidence of grade III–IV hemorrhage, which tends to have a poor neurological prognosis, is about 5%, and the incidence of cerebral palsy is about five times higher than in the group without intraventricular hemorrhage. The smaller the birth week and birth weight, and the stronger the inflammatory changes such as fetal infection, the more severe the grade III–IV is likely to be [7, 8].

3.2 White Matter Disorder, Periventricular Leukomalacia

Periventricular leukomalacia is a condition caused by cerebral ischemia and is a common white matter disorder in preterm infants, especially in infants born before 32 weeks' gestation. The vascular network in the deep white matter of preterm infants before 32 weeks' gestation is not fully developed, and the autoregulation function is inadequate. If cerebral circulatory pressure decreases for any reason during this period, deep white matter is easily ischemic. It is also known that increased cytokine levels, such as chorioamnionitis and neonatal sepsis, directly cause white matter damage and periventricular leukomalacia [1, 9]. The earlier the onset of preterm labor and pPROM, the more likely it is to be associated with a high degree of intrauterine inflammation (histological chorioamnionitis). As mentioned above, preterm labor and pPROM induce inflammation of the intrauterine environment, resulting in increased levels of chemokines (IL-8) and cytokines (IL-1 and IL-6). Inflammatory substances secreted by immune cells due to infection act on capillaries and cause impaired blood circulation. These substances also enhance uterine contractions and directly affect oligodendrocytes and myelination, resulting in abnormal axonal myelination. Increased cytokines due to hemorrhage, ischemia, reperfusion, tissue hypoxia, and infection increase glutamate and free radicals, which stimulate NMDA receptors and promote intracellular calcium influx, leading to widespread neuronal cell death and disruption of neural network architecture [1, 9].

Figure 1 shows the pathogenesis of preterm birth and cerebral palsy. There is a strong association between preterm birth and intraventricular hemorrhage and periventricular leukomalacia due to the common pathway of inflammatory changes. Ischemia, infection, and immaturity act alone or in combination to form brain lesions, but the degree of cerebral white matter vascular control and the degree of maturation of the subependymal germ layer vary with the number of weeks of fetal life, so that intraventricular hemorrhage tends to occur at less than 28 weeks of fetal life and periventricular leukomalacia at 28–32 weeks of fetal life [9].

4 Current Status of Underlying Diseases in Cerebral Palsy

According to the "Statistics of Maternal and Child Health in Japan 2019" [10], out of a total of 918,400 live births in 2018, 51,732 were born at less than 37 weeks' gestation, with a preterm birth rate of 5.6%. While the total number of births has

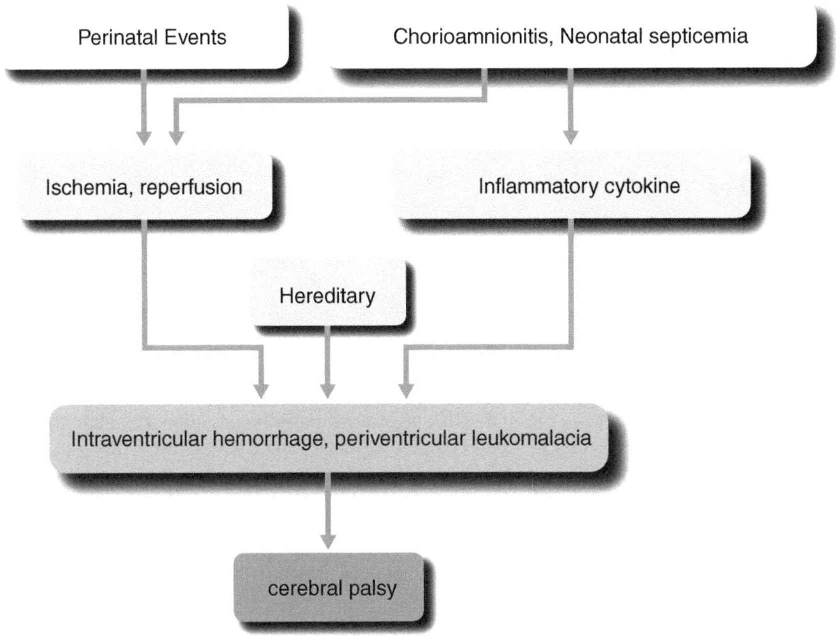

Fig. 1 Association between cerebral palsy (CP) and preterm birth. In the development of intraventricular hemorrhage and periventricular leukomalacia, inflammation (cytokines) damages neurons indirectly and directly through changes in blood flow

been decreasing, the preterm birth rate has been gradually increasing since 1980, but has remained unchanged in recent years. With the development of perinatal care, the survival rate of premature infants has increased, and the neurological prognosis is improving. However, although the life expectancy has improved in cases of preterm birth in the first half of the 20th week of pregnancy, the neurological prognosis is not always favorable, and as a result, the frequency of cerebral palsy has not changed significantly [11].

5 Toward Prevention

The treatment of preterm labor has shifted from the administration of uterine contraction inhibitors such as ritodrine and magnesium sulfate to prophylactic treatment of high-risk cases of preterm labor. This is because it is difficult to treat preterm labor that has already progressed to a certain degree and it is difficult to improve the perinatal prognosis [12]. In recent years, factors such as a history of miscarriage, family history, cervical length, and vaginal flora have been evaluated, and pregnant women who require progesterone administration, cervical suture, and treatment of vaginitis in the first trimester of pregnancy have been managed from an anti-inflammatory perspective, contributing to a decrease in the incidence of preterm birth [12].

References

1. Romero R, Dey SK, Fisher SJ. Preterm labor: one syndrome, many causes. Science. 2014;345:760–5.
2. Areia A, Vale-Pereira S, Alves V, et al. Membrane progesterone receptors in human regulatory T cells: a reality in pregnancy. BJOG. 2015;122:1544–50.
3. Kanayama N, Teral T, Kawashima Y, et al. Collagen types in normal and prematurely ruptured amniotic membranes. Am J Obstet Gynecol. 1985;153:899–903.
4. Smith DD, Sagaram D, Miller R, et al. Risk of cerebral palsy by gestational age among pregnancies at-risk for preterm birth. J Matern Fetal Neonatal Med. 2020;33:2059–63.
5. Verhagen EA, Hummel LA, Bos AF, et al. Near-infrared spectroscopy to detect absence of cerebrovascular autoregulation in preterm infants. Clin Neurophysiol. 2014;125:47–52.
6. Paneth N, Pinto-Martin J, Gardiner J, et al. Incidence and timing of germinal matrix/intraventricular hemorrhage in low birth weight infants. Am J Epidemiol. 1993;137:1167–76.
7. Furukawa S, Sameshima H, Ikenoue T. Circulatory disturbances during the first 24 postnatal hours in extremely premature infants 25 weeks or less of gestation with histological fetal inflammation. J Obstet Gynaecol Res. 2008;34:27–33.
8. Stavsky M, Mor O, Mastrolia SA, et al. Cerebral palsy-trends in epidemiology and recent development in prenatal mechanisms of disease, treatment, and prevention. Front Pediatr. 2017;5:21.
9. Yoon BH, Kim CJ, Romero R, et al. Experimentally induced intrauterine infection causes fetal brain white matter lesions in rabbits. Am J Obstet Gynecol. 1997;177:797–802.
10. Ei T. Boshihoken no omonaru toukei 2019 [Statistics of maternal and child health in Japan 2019]. Tokyo: Maternal and Child Health Agency; 2020. p. 49, 44–5. Japanese.
11. O'Callaghan ME, MacLennan AH, Gibson CS, et al. Epidemiologic associations with cerebral palsy. Obstet Gynecol. 2011;118:576–82.
12. Newnham JP, White SW, Meharry S, et al. Reducing preterm birth by a statewide multifaceted program: an implementation study. Am J Obstet Gynecol. 2017;216:434–42.

Fetal Growth Restriction/Small for Dates

Yumi Kono

Contents

Summary

- Fetal growth restriction (FGR)/small for dates (SFD) is a general term for children whose growth in utero were suppressed due to multiple factors, including children who are constitutionally small.
- The prevalence of cerebral palsy (CP) is higher in children with a smaller birth weight *Z*-score, i.e., a more severe degree of FGR/SFD, born at after 32 weeks of gestation.
- The pathological conditions that may cause CP, such as birth defect, abnormal blood flow in multiple births, placental and umbilical cord anomalies or dysfunction, and intrauterine inflammation and/or infection, are closely related to FGR of the infants.

1 Overview of Fetal Growth Failure/SFD

When a fetus is smaller than normal, he/she is diagnosed as FGR. FGR is a general term for cases in which the growth of the fetus in the uterus is suppressed for some reason. The "Glossary of Obstetrics and Gynecology, 4th

---

Y. Kono (✉)
Department of Pediatrics, Jichi Medical University, Shimotsuke, Tochigi, Japan
e-mail: ykono@jichi.ac.jp

Y. Matsuda (ed.), *Cerebral Palsy*, https://doi.org/10.1007/978-981-19-2217-6_13

Edition" by the Japan Society of Obstetrics and Gynecology [1] states that FGR should be determined using the reference values for each gestational week of Japanese fetal weight, which included only healthy fetus born at full term. The terms often used by neonatologists, such as light for dates (LFD), SFD, and small for gestational age (SGA), are different from FGR because they are based on the values of body size at birth for each gestational week. In other words, FGR is determined using an intrauterine fetal growth curve for each gestational week [2], and SFD is determined using neonatal anthropometric charts at birth by gestational week [3].

The estimated fetal weight less than −1.5 SD for gestational age is defined FGR to be noted as a high-risk pregnancy in Japan. In contrast, SFD or also called SGA is judged as less than 10th percentile of the neonatal anthropometric standards for gestational age, which is one of the eligibility criteria of growth hormone (GH) treatment for SGA short stature. Because −1.5 SD is equivalent to 6.7 percentile, the criteria for FGR and SFD/SGA are different. There could be cases whose determination of FGR and SFD are not consistent in the same child. Because neonatologists and pediatricians treat children after birth, they usually have information about FGR with the expected weight of the fetus and then determine whether the child is SFD or appropriate for date (AFD) using the birth size standard by gestational age after birth [3].

2 Risk Factors for FGR

The risk factors for FGR are broadly categorized into fetal factors, maternal factors, and placental and umbilical cord factors. Table 1 shows the etiology of FGR listed in the guidelines of the American College of Obstetricians and Gynecologists (ACOG) [4]. However, about 70% of FGRs are related to constitutional predisposition, and clear etiology cannot be identified in many cases.

FGR is associated with a high risk of intrauterine fetal death and stillbirth. SFD infants have high rates of neonatal mortality and morbidity, such as hypoglycemia, hyperbilirubinemia, hypothermia, intraventricular hemorrhage (IVH), necrotizing enterocolitis, neonatal seizures, sepsis, and respiratory distress syndrome [5]. It is important to note that the neurodevelopmental outcome of infants depends on the risk factors of FGR/SFD as well as gestational age. FGR/SFD infants are a mixed population of infants exposed to adverse intrauterine conditions and small but normal infants. As a result of perinatal selection, the surviving cases may appear to have good neurodevelopmental outcomes. On the other hand, the outcomes may be unfavorable when chromosomal abnormalities, multiple births, or congenital infections are included as causes of FGR. In addition, the outcomes are affected by the intensive perinatal care and interventions to mothers and fetus with FGR. Finally, the gestational age could be critical to the adverse outcomes. Regardless of FGR,

Table 1 Etiology of fetal growth restriction [4]

• Maternal medical conditions
– Pregestational diabetes mellitus
– Renal insufficiency
– Autoimmune disease (e.g., systemic lupus erythematosus)
– Cyanotic cardiac disease
– Pregnancy-related hypertensive diseases of pregnancy (e.g., chronic hypertension, gestational hypertension, or preeclampsia)
– Antiphospholipid antibody syndrome
• Substance use and abuse (e.g., tobacco, alcohol, cocaine, or narcotics)
• Multiple gestation
• Teratogen exposure (e.g., cyclophosphamide, valproic acid, or antithrombotic drugs)
• Infectious diseases (e.g., malaria, cytomegalovirus, rubella, toxoplasmosis, or syphilis)
• Genetic and structural disorders (e.g., trisomy 13, trisomy 18, congenital heart disease, or gastroschisis)
• Placental disorders and umbilical cord abnormalities

preterm births are associated with a high incidence of morbidities associated to CP, such as IVH, periventricular leukomalacia (PVL), and necrotizing enterocolitis.

3 Pathophysiology Associated with CP

The risk of CP increased in FGR/SFD infants compared with non-FGR/AFD infants when they were born at full term, late preterm after 34 weeks, or moderate preterm after 32 weeks by the report from a large multicenter study (Surveillance of Cerebral Palsy in Europe) [6]. In this study, birth weight *Z*-scores were calculated based on the conventional standard or fetal standard, and correlation between *Z*-scores and prevalence of CP was evaluated according to the duration of pregnancy. In the group after 32 weeks of gestation, the smaller the *Z*-score, the higher the prevalence of CP, which was more evident when using the fetal standard (Fig. 1). When SGA children weighing less than the 10th percentile (corresponding to a *Z*-score of less than −1.28) were compared with appropriate for gestational age (AGA) children in the 25th–75th percentile (corresponding to a *Z*-score of −0.67 to 0.67), rates of CP increased in SGA children after 32 weeks of gestation. The SGA children born at 32–42 weeks are four- to sixfold more likely to have CP than the AGA children born at the same gestational weeks. The association between SGA and CP in infants born at less than 32 weeks was not clear, possibly because the risk of brain damage associated with prematurity, such as IVH or PVL, outweighs the risk of that associated with FGR/SFD at birth.

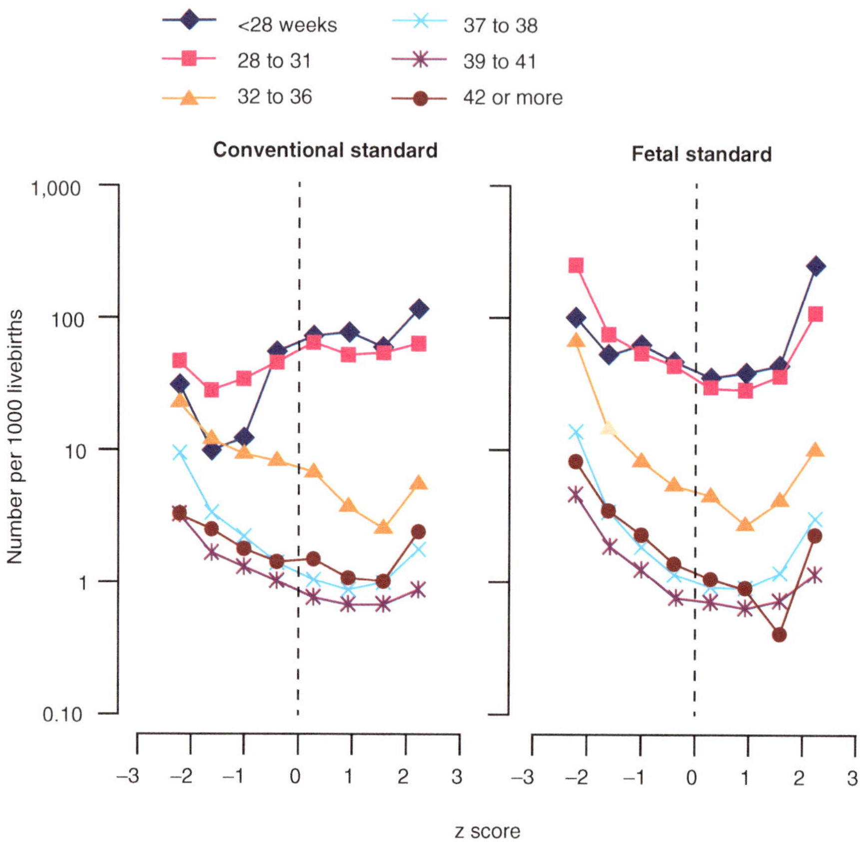

Fig. 1 Prevalence of cerebral palsy by Z score of weight for gestation: effect of different growth standards [6]

In cases of FGR with placental insufficiency or FGR associated with hypertensive disorders of pregnancy (HDP), the pathophysiology associated with CP remains unclear. The uterine artery ligation in rodent causes placental insufficiency and FGR. This model has been aimed at replicating findings seen in human FGR [7]. Brain sparing (a mild decrease in brain weight compared to body weight), ventricular enlargement, white matter damage, and decreased basal ganglia and hippocampal volume found in this FGR model were similar to those found in human FGR. Adult animals with growth restriction at birth demonstrated deficits in gait, memory, object recognition, and spatial processing. Histologically, neuronal necrosis and astrogliosis were observed in the hippocampus, parahippocampal cortex, cingulate gyrus, cerebral white matter, and cerebellum. In addition, white matter injury involved oligodendrocyte precursor maturation arrest. This animal model can provide pathophysiological evidence for studies of CP and other pathological outcomes of placental insufficiency in human FGR/SFD infants.

On the other hand, several studies suggest that preeclampsia may be associated with a decreased risk of CP in preterm and low birth weight infants [8]. Increased endogenous corticosteroid secretion would promote maturation of the infant's cerebral nervous system and reduce the risk of IVH, which is a compelling cause of CP in preterm infants, although there was no significant difference in the rate of IVH in preterm extremely low birth weight infants between with and without preeclampsia. In a recent population-based study of infants born after 35 weeks of age, severe FGR (<−2SD) infants born to normotensive mothers showed a significantly increased risk of CP compared with AGA infants born to normotensive mothers [odds ratio (OR) 4.81 [95% confidence interval (CI): 2.7–8.5]], whereas severe FGR infants of HDP mothers were not associated with a significant increased risk of CP compared to AGA infants of normotensive mothers [OR 2.56 (95% CI: 0.78–8.4)] [9].

Many studies have reported the usefulness of ultrasound pulsed Doppler as an examination of fetal well-being in FGR. The presence or absence of disruption or regurgitation of umbilical artery blood flow and pulsatility index (PI) values are used for evaluation. Interruption or regurgitation of umbilical artery blood flow is an indicator of chronic hypoxemia, increased placental vascular resistance, and progression to fetal dysfunction (non-reassuring fetal status) and stillbirth. In a French prospective cohort study (EPIPAGE-2) of singleton infants associated with suspected FGR or a maternal HDP from 22 to 31 weeks of gestation, an association between the neurological outcomes at 2 years of age and umbilical cord blood flow using ultrasound pulsed Doppler was evaluated [10]. By the last ultrasound examination before delivery, umbilical artery Doppler waveform was classified into absent or reversed end-diastolic flow (ARED, $n = 179$) group and normal or reduced end-diastolic flow (NORED, $n = 305$) group. The morbidity rate of CP with GMFCS level 2 or higher was significantly high in the ARED group: 2.7% in the ARED group versus 0.2% in the NORED group. After adjustment for gestational age, ARED was associated significantly with severe or moderate neuromotor and/or sensory disability (adjusted OR, 11.3; 95% CI, 1.4–93.2). These results suggested the usefulness of evaluating umbilical artery blood flow in relation to an elevated risk of neurosensory disability in children born very preterm due to FGR or maternal HDP.

4 FGR/SFD in CP in Recent Reports

Like the wide variety of risk factors for FGR/SFD, the etiology of CP diagnosed based on symptoms and syndromes is diverse, and multiple factors are often involved. Among 2457 cases for which a causal analysis report was sent to the Japan Obstetric Compensation System for Cerebral Palsy, the results of an analysis of cases born between 2009 and 2014 and 0–1 years old at the time of diagnosis were reported in detail [11, 12]. Up to birth in 2014, the reported cases were either with a birth weight ≥2000 g and a gestational age of ≥33 weeks or those with a gestational age of ≥28 weeks with the specified requirements. In the 999 analyzed cases, the proportion of LFD defined as birth weight less than the 10th percentile of the birth size standard by gestational age was 134 cases (13.4%) [11]. Within the conditions listed as the primary cause of CP in the causal analysis report, no case listed FGR as a cause of single condition, and only 8 (0.8%) cases listed FGR as a cause of multiple conditions. In an overview of the 2457 cases, the proportion of LFD was 376 (15.3%) [12]. The proportion of LFD in moderate-to-severe CP covered by the Japan Obstetric Compensation System for Cerebral Palsy was higher than that of LFD in the general population. However, the rate of FGR as the main cause of CP was low, which may reflect FGR was accompanied with other main causes listed in the repots, such as placental or umbilical cord anomalies, blood flow imbalance in multiple births, and infections or inflammations.

Nelson et al. [13] proposed four perinatal factors for CP in singleton infants born at full term or near term: asphyxia, inflammation, restricted growth, and birth defect (malformations, deformities, or injuries present at birth regardless of cause) (Fig. 2). Birth defect was the most frequent factor in the CP group compared with the control group without CP matched for length of gestation (≤1 week), date of birth (≤12 months), and number of fetuses. When combined with birth defect with FGR

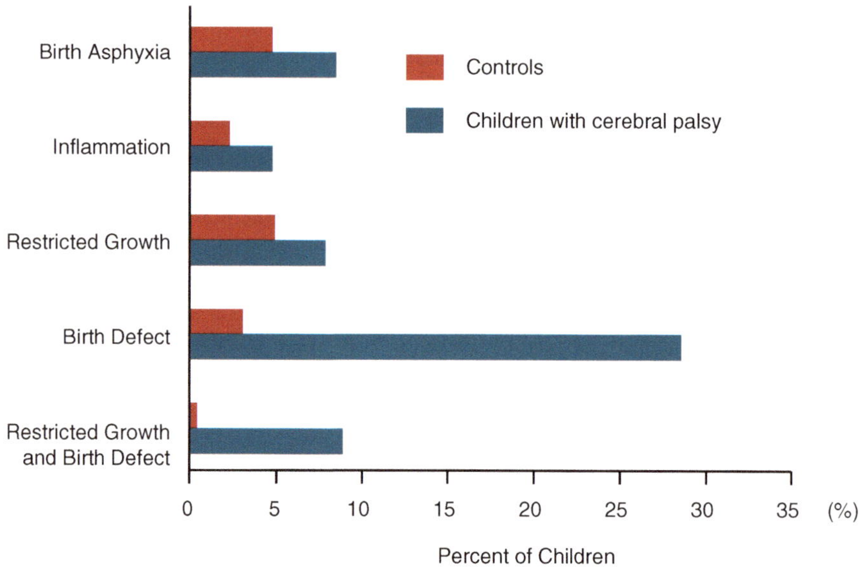

Fig. 2 Distribution of four major risk factors in singleton children with cerebral palsy born at a gestational age of at least 35 weeks, 1980–1995 [13]. Data are from a study of 496 children with cerebral palsy and 508 controls. The four risk factors were a potentially asphyxiating intrapartum event, evidence of inflammation, fetal growth restriction (defined as a birth weight that was more than 2 SD below the optimal weight for gestation, sex, maternal height, and parity, or a neonatal diagnosis of fetal growth restriction), and a major birth defect. Data shown are for one or more of these risk factors in at least 2% of children with cerebral palsy or controls. Major birth defects were the most frequently occurring risk factor in children with cerebral palsy, and when combined with fetal growth restriction, they were associated with the highest relative risk

of less than −2 SD, it was associated with the highest relative risk for CP. They suggested birth defect, that is, a risk factor for FGR as well, was the most strongly associated with CP in infants born after 35 weeks of gestation.

5 Toward the Prevention of CP

Epidemiological data on FGR/SFD suggested that the risk of CP increases with more severe restricted growth in children born at full term or late preterm. Although preventive measures may differ depending on the cause of growth restriction, assessment of fetal well-being by ultrasound pulse Doppler could be useful in predicting brain damage from placental insufficiency. In the case of FGR with birth defect, it is difficult to find effective strategies to prevent FGR. At least, we should carefully manage prenatal and perinatal conditions related to CP in mothers, fetus, and newborns. In addition, we should inform patients to eliminate causal risk factors for FGR, such as smoking, alcohol, and high caffeine intake.

References

1. Japan Society of Obstetrics and Gynecology. Sanfujinka yougoshuu/yougo kaisetsushuu [Glossary of obstetrics and gynecology]. 4th ed. Tokyo: Japan Society of Obstetrics and Gynecology; 2018. p. 225–6. Japanese.
2. Perinatal Committee of the Japan Society of Obstetrics and Gynecology. Iinnkai Teiann: Cyouompa Taijikeisoku no Hyoujyunnka to Nihonjinn no Kijyunchi [Committee proposal: standardization of ultrasound fetal measurements and reference values for Japanese]. Acta Obstet Gynaecol Jpn. 2005;57:92–117. Japanese.
3. Itabashi K, Fujimura M, Kusuda S, et al. Nihon shounika gakkai shinseiji taikaku hyoujyunchi no Dounyuu ni Tsuite [Committee on Neonates of the Japan Pediatric Society. Report of the Neonatal Committee of the Japan Pediatric Society: introduction of a new standard for anthropometric measurements at birth according to the duration of pregnancy]. J Jpn Pediatr Soc. 2010;114:1271–93. Japanese.
4. ACOG. ACOG practice bulletin no. 204: fetal growth restriction. Obstet Gynecol. 2019;133:e97–109.
5. Yanney M, Marlow N. Paediatric consequences of fetal growth restriction. Semin Fetal Neonatal Med. 2004;9:411–8.
6. Jarvis S, Glinianaia SV, Torrioli M, et al. Cerebral palsy and intrauterine growth in single births: a European Collaborative Study. Lancet. 2003;362:1106–11.
7. Basilious A, Yager J, Fehlings MG. Neurological outcomes of animal models of uterine artery ligation and relevance to human intrauterine growth restriction: a systematic review. Dev Med Child Neurol. 2015;57:420–30.
8. Xiong X, Saunders LD, Wang FL, et al. Preeclampsia and cerebral palsy in low-birth-weight and preterm infants: implications for the current "ischemic model" of preeclampsia. Hypertens Pregnancy. 2001;20:1–13.
9. Blair EM, Nelson KB. Fetal growth restriction and risk of cerebral palsy in singletons born after at least 35 weeks' gestation. Am J Obstet Gynecol. 2015;212(520):e1–7.
10. Delorme P, Kayem G, Lorthe E, et al. Neurodevelopment at age 2 and umbilical artery Doppler in cases of preterm birth after prenatal hypertensive neurodevelopment at age 2 and umbilical artery Doppler in cases of preterm birth after prenatal hypertensive disorder or suspected fetal

growth restriction: the EPIPAGE 2 prospective population-based cohort study. Ultrasound Obstet Gynecol. 2020;56:557–65. https://doi.org/10.1002/uog.22025.
11. Japan Council for Quality Health Care. 10th Report on prevention of recurrence, the Japan Obstetric Compensation System for Cerebral Palsy. Tokyo: Japan Council for Quality Health Care; 2020. p. 77–9. Japanese.
12. Japan Council for Quality Health Care. 10th Report on prevention of recurrence, the Japan Obstetric Compensation System for Cerebral Palsy. Tokyo: Japan Council for Quality Health Care; 2020. p. 93. Japanese.
13. Nelson KB, Blair E. Prenatal factors in singletons with cerebral palsy born at or near term. N Engl J Med. 2015;373:946–53.

Cases Probably Considered as Intrauterine Onset

Kotaro Fukushima

Contents

Summary

- A study using the Japan Obstetric Compensation System for Cerebral Palsy has revealed that at least some cases of cerebral palsy (CP) without acidemia are due to central nervous system damage caused by transient hypoxia and ischemia in utero and that some cases show a certain phenotype along the time course from onset.
- Although it is difficult to predict the onset of the disease, accurately diagnose it in utero, and avoid it by prophylactic intervention, it is essential to confirm the presence of acidemia at the time of delivery by umbilical artery blood gas analysis in order to estimate the onset of central nervous system dysfunction.
- In cases with decreased fetal movement, abnormal baseline thin variation of fetal cardiotocography (CTG), and amniotic fluid overload, it was necessary to follow the neurological prognosis carefully even if there was no evidence of paresis or acidemia at delivery.

In the fetal cardiotocography (CTG), which is currently the most widely used method for evaluating fetal well-being, it is assumed that the central nervous system of the fetus is normally developed and the physiological heart rate control

K. Fukushima (✉)
Fukushima Clinic, Fukuoka, Japan
e-mail: k-fukushima@fukushima-clinic.jp

Y. Matsuda (ed.), *Cerebral Palsy*, https://doi.org/10.1007/978-981-19-2217-6_14

mechanism is functioning in order to recognize the pattern of the fetal heart rate pattern. Conversely, if this control mechanism is disrupted or developmental disorders occur, the fetus is not considered for CTG examination, and the condition of the fetus cannot be evaluated correctly [1]. A typical case is when the fetal heart rate pattern is altered by transplacental transfer of some drugs administered to the mother and the CTG pattern deviates from the original fetal well-being.

In recent years, it has become known that CTG patterns may not fully reflect the well-being of the fetus even in the presence of diseases or maternal environments that affect the functional development of the fetus itself, such as in conditions such as cardiac disease, congenital diseases of the central nervous system, fetal growth failure, and intrauterine infection, where the relationship between CTG findings and intrauterine oxygenation and neurological prognosis is different from normal [2, 3]. It is now known that CTG patterns may not adequately reflect the well-being of the fetus [2, 3]. In utero-onset cerebral palsy caused by irreversible damage to the central nervous system due to transient hypoxia and ischemia in utero is another condition in which the CTG pattern does not assess the well-being of the fetus. In this section, we review the characteristics and frequency of CTG findings and clinical images in such cases.

1 Overview and Pathophysiology of In Utero-Onset CP

Hypoxic-ischemic encephalopathy (HIE) is one of the major causes of perinatal brain injury, including cerebral palsy (CP). Although HIE was classically thought to occur mostly around delivery, it is now known that in many cases HIE occurs in utero before onset of delivery. In Japan, the analysis of a large number of CP cases has been made possible by reports on the analysis of the causes of CP in the Japan Obstetric Compensation System for Cerebral Palsy, and new findings have been obtained [4, 5].

In the causal analysis report of the Japan Obstetric Compensation System for Cerebral Palsy, using the method of excluding cases in which a condition that could cause general hypoxia and acidemia existed and cases in which the cause of the onset of the disease was in the neonatal period, the authors extracted cases presumed to be HIE caused by transient circulatory disturbances in utero and examined their clinical images [5]. Among 596 cases of cerebral palsy with singleton delivery after 33 weeks of gestation analyzed by the Japan Obstetric Compensation System for Cerebral Palsy by the end of June 2015, there were 137 cases with a gas analysis value of pH ≥ 7.2. Among them, 53 cases were presumed to have CP due to HIE caused by transient circulatory disturbance in utero, and abnormalities of cardiotocography (CTG) (transient tachycardia and decreased variability) were observed in 74%, fetal movement decreased in 15 cases, and amniotic fluid volume increased in 5 cases (Fig. 1). When the patients were divided into two groups according to the presence or absence of abnormalities in the baseline variability of CTG, those with

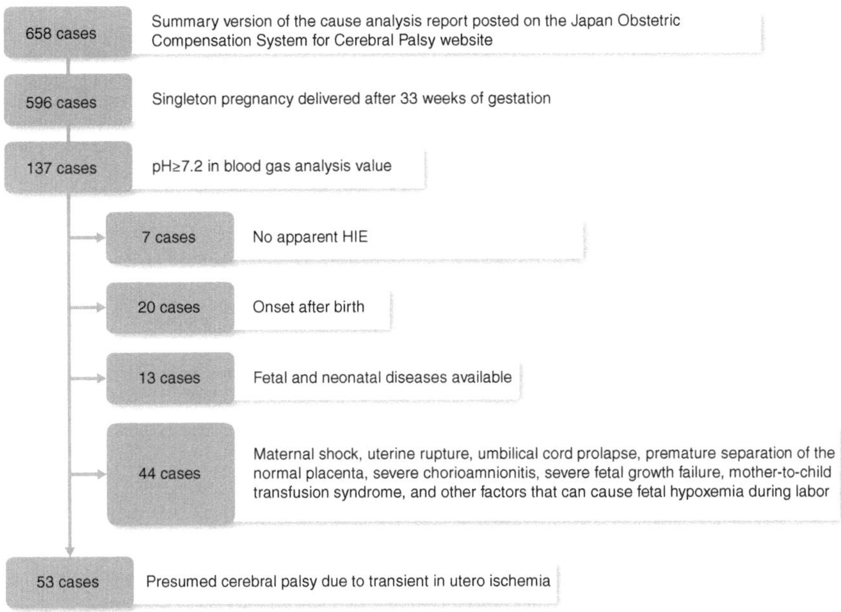

Fig. 1 Flowchart of case selection for presumed hypoxic-ischemic encephalopathy (HIE) due to transient circulatory disturbance in utero (modified from Ref. [5]). Among 596 cases of cerebral palsy in singleton deliveries after 33 weeks of gestation analyzed by cases with gas analysis pH $\geq$ 7.2, with findings of HIE on imaging, onset not in the neonatal period. We selected cases of HIE presumed to be caused by transient circulatory disturbance in utero

abnormalities in fine variation had earlier weeks of labor, lower Apgar score values, more cases with decreased fetal movement, and fewer cases with excessive amniotic fluid than those without abnormalities in variability [5].

When these cases were compared with cases in which the time from the presumed hypoxic event to delivery of the baby was around or within 1 week, around 2 weeks, or longer, it was found that cases in which delivery occurred around or before 1 week from the event suggesting the onset of the hypoxic event, such as decreased fetal movement, showed more cases of CTG abnormalities and decreased variability. On the other hand, there was an increase in amniotic fluid volume in cases where the time between the event and delivery was around 2 weeks or longer. This suggests that a transient intrauterine ischemic event that causes irreversible changes in the central nervous system may result in decreased fetal movement and abnormal CTG during the first few days to a week, and if the baby is referred to obstetricians during this period, it may be diagnosed as non-reassuring fetal status (NRFS) or delivered. Despite that, after a certain period of time, the baby gradually recovers, and CTG abnormalities disappear, while some patients may have findings reflecting amniotic fluid overload and spastic paralysis due to dysphagia (Fig. 2).

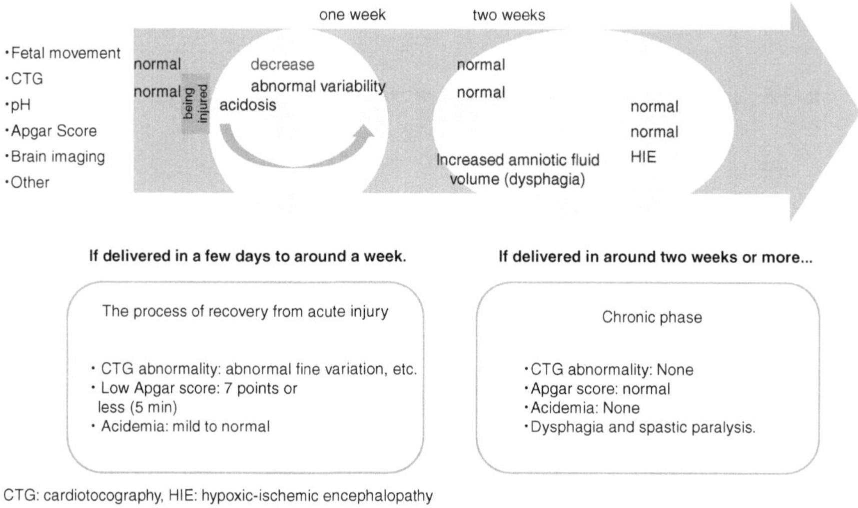

Fig. 2 Time course from injury and phenotypic differences in fetuses and newborns (hypothesis). We modeled and hypothesized the phenotypes of cases that are recognized and delivered relatively early after injury and those that are delivered relatively long after injury

2 Current Status of Prenatal Onset CP

In a review of reported cases in the Japan Obstetric Compensation System for Cerebral Palsy, HIE due to transient circulatory disturbance in utero was presumed to be the cause of CP in 9% of singleton deliveries of CP after 33 weeks of gestation. Therefore, it is inferred that central nervous system disorders caused by transient circulatory disturbances in utero, including movement disorders other than CP, developmental disorders, and those with unknown causes, are more frequent. In a questionnaire survey conducted among the facilities participating in the maternal-fetal intensive care unit (MFICU) (29 facilities responded), the same study was conducted in 12 facilities (total of 25,777 singleton deliveries after 33 weeks of gestation during 3 years) where a secondary survey was available. It was estimated that at least two cases of CP were due to transient intrauterine ischemia (frequency of about 1 in 13,000 deliveries) [6].

The incidence of CP in full-term births is about 2.5/1000 [1], and if about 10% of these babies are affected by CP, the incidence is about 1 in 4000 deliveries. The accuracy of our study is limited by the fact that it is a retrospective study based on information from a database. However, since they avoided overestimating the incidence, it is estimated that there is at least one or more cases of transient in utero CP due to HIE in several thousand to about 10,000 deliveries. Considering that, depending on the area of injury, circulatory disturbances may be expressed as motor or developmental disorders other than CP, it is possible that a higher percentage of developmental disorders, including those that are undiagnosed or of unknown cause, are caused by transient circulatory disturbances in utero.

In developmental disorders, it is known that a characteristic disposition such as difficulty in raising children is already observed in the newborn and infant periods [7]. In fact, the Japan Environment and Children's Study, a large-scale epidemiological study in Japan, reported the possibility that the presence of an umbilical artery blood pH of 7.2 and an Apgar score of 7 or more on the 5-min scale, despite the diagnosis of fetal dysfunction, was associated with the disposition of neonatal irritability [8].

In other words, transient circulatory disturbance in utero, which cannot be captured in general clinical practice, may be a factor that has a significant impact on "development." On the other hand, this phenomenon is not necessarily negative, but can be considered as one of the mechanisms that give rise to diversity in humans, such as the creation of "individuality."

3 Toward Prevention

It is clinically difficult to choose not to intervene in cases of abnormal CTG during delivery, and therefore, in order to avoid cesarean sections that do not improve the prognosis, such as prenatal-onset CP, it is important to accurately diagnose such conditions before birth, to detect such conditions before they occur, and to identify and prevent high-risk cases.

Differentiation of prenatally onset CP is not easy because many cases show a decrease or disappearance of baseline variability, as if hypoxia or ischemia occurred at that time. However, there is a reason for the change in CTG findings. In other words, there are cases in which transient tachycardia is no longer seen in a child with a reactive pattern in the previous non-stress test (NST), even though there is no cause for deterioration in fetal well-being, and cases in which transient bradycardia appears that did not exist before without other factors. In such cases, we can infer the presence or absence of hypoxia or acidemia in a relatively short time by Doppler flowmetry or biophysical profile. For this reason, it is essential to perform cord blood gas analysis at the time of delivery.

In addition, not only cases with the NRFS phenotype but also those with a long time since the injury may have a worse-than-expected condition of the baby after delivery, despite the absence of fetal heart rate abnormalities. Therefore, it is important to be reminded of this condition. In addition, depending on the area of injury, developmental disorders other than CP may be the cause.

The goal of current perinatal care is not only the safe birth of the mother and child but also the subsequent child care and healthy growth and development of the child.

Fortunately, even in the absence of abnormalities in the peripartum period, careful follow-up for developmental and neurological prognosis and future parental support should be considered in the future, even in cases of decreased fetal movement, unexplained CTG abnormalities, and amniotic fluid overload, even in the absence of paresis or acidemia at delivery [7, 8]. Although the limitations of CTG in improving the prognosis of CP have long been pointed out, this association with postnatal growth and development may be a new role for CTG.

This chapter is based on Refs. [5, 6] with some additions and corrections.

References

1. Nelson KB, Ellenberg JH. Antecedents of cerebral palsy: multivariate analysis of risk. N Engl J Med. 1986;315:81–6.
2. Blair EM, Nelson KB. Fetal growth restriction and risk of cerebral palsy in singletons born after at least 35 weeks' gestation. Am J Obstet Gynecol. 2015;212(520):e1–7.
3. Scher AI, Petterson B, Blair E, et al. The risk of mortality or cerebral palsy in twins: a collaborative population-based study. Pediatr Res. 2002;52:671–81.
4. Matsuda Y, Umezaki H, Ogawa M, et al. Umbilical arterial pH in patients with cerebral palsy. Early Hum Dev. 2014;90:131–5.
5. Fukushima K, Morokuma S, Kitadai Y, et al. Analysis of antenatal-onset cerebral palsy secondary to transient ischemia in utero using a national. J Obstet Gynaecol Res. 2016;42:1297–303.
6. Fukushima K. Tainaideno Ikkaseikyoketsu niyoru chusushinkeishougai nikannsuru Kentou—Sankairyouhosyouseido Geninbunsekishourei narabini MFICU Renrakukyougikai Sankashisetsusyourei deno Kento kara [A study on central nervous system disorders caused by transient ischemia in utero: an analysis of cases in the Japan Obstetric Compensation System for Cerebral Palsy and cases in facilities participating in the MFICU liaison council]. Obstet Pract. 2017;66:113–20. Japanese.
7. Garon N, Zwaigenbaum L, Bryson S, et al. Temperament and its association with autism symptoms in a high-risk population. J Abnorm Child Psychol. 2016;44:757–69.
8. Morokuma S, Michikawa T, Kato K, et al. Non-reassuring foetal status and neonatal irritability in the Japan Environment and Children's Study: a cohort study. Sci Rep. 2018;8:15853.

Reduced Fetal Movement

Hironori Takahashi

Contents

H. Takahashi (✉)
Department of Obstetrics and Gynecology, Jichi Medical University,
Shimotsuke, Tochigi, Japan
e-mail: hironori@jichi.ac.jp

Y. Matsuda (ed.), *Cerebral Palsy*, https://doi.org/10.1007/978-981-19-2217-6_15

Summary

- Some infants who develop cerebral palsy (CP) are born with the mother aware of reduced fetal movement.
- In 2009, Japan started the Obstetric Compensation System for Cerebral Palsy, and a considerable number of cases related to reduced fetal movement have been reported among those applying for the system.
- Observation of fetal movement is the only way to provide free, continuous assessment without the need for medical equipment.
- On the other hand, only the pregnant woman herself can make a judgment, and it lacks objectivity.
- There are many known risk factors for cerebral palsy, including low body weight, prematurity, infection, and multiple births. In cases of reduced fetal movement and postnatal cerebral palsy, the infant may be severely hypoxic or even acidotic at delivery. Premature detachment of the normal placenta and maternal-infant transfusion syndrome are representative diseases. In these diseases, reduced fetal movement is often the trigger for detection of the disease.
- In addition, some fetal abnormalities may include fetal movement abnormalities, which require attention. However, the extent to which fetal movement observation reduces cerebral palsy has not yet been clarified.

1 Actual Fetal Movement

Fetal movement is usually perceived at 16–20 weeks of gestation [1]. Multiparous pregnant women experience fetal movement 2–3 weeks earlier than first-time mothers. Although there is no clear evidence [2], the fetus is said to be most active at 28–34 weeks of gestation, after which fetal movements decrease [3]. In a healthy fetus, 4–100 fetal movements per hour are observed [4]. When the fetal condition deteriorates, the fetus attempts to store energy, and oxygen consumption decreases. It is speculated that redistribution of blood flow occurs in utero, and as fetal oxygen consumption decreases, fetal movements decrease. Reduced fetal movement may be caused temporarily by sleep, but also by low amniotic fluid, maternal overweightness, and sedation.

2 Difficulties in Observing Fetal Movement

The measurement of fetal movement differs from other tests in that it can only be perceived by the mother. Medical practitioners advise pregnant women to pay attention to fetal movement and tell them if it decreases or disappears. However, if this is strictly enforced for pregnant women, they may feel overwhelmed. This may be justified if fetal movement monitoring leads to an improvement in the perinatal outcome, but there is no clear evidence for this. The reasons for the lack of evidence are as follows: (1) the time between the decrease in fetal movement and fetal death is short; (2) there are various evaluation methods for fetal movement observation, but they are not standardized and the criteria for fetal movement decrease are not consistent; and (3) pregnant women are not aware of all fetal movements.

3 Fetal Movement Evaluation Method

Various methods of fetal movement assessment have been proposed to make the assessment consistent. The most famous method is Cardiff's count to 10 method [5]. In this method, the time required to feel ten movements of the fetus at a fixed time each day is recorded. In this method, the patient is placed in a relaxed lateral recumbent position with the bladder empty and the hand on the abdomen to count the fetal movements. On the other hand, the Sadovsky method [6] requires the fetal movement count to be performed after each meal. In addition, a modified version of the method, which does not restrict the time of fetal movement counting or the position of counting, is widely used [7]. The average time required for fetal movement counting is 10 min [2], but the time required increases with the number of weeks of pregnancy: the 90th percentile time is 25 min at 22–36 weeks of gestation, whereas it is 35 min at 37–40 weeks of gestation [7]. A significant increase in the number of pregnant women taking more than 30 min has been reported after 39 weeks of gestation or at birth weights of 3000 g or more [8]. If the fetal movement count takes longer, the patient should be told to contact medical staff.

4 Evidence on Fetal Movement Counting

Studies on fetal movement counting have been spasmodic since the 1980s. Only high-quality randomized controlled trials (RCTs) were selected, and there are two systematic reviews or meta-analyses of whether fetal movement counting improves perinatal outcomes.

4.1 Cochrane Systematic Review [1]

4.1.1 Method

Cochrane searched for studies related to fetal movement, and only those RCTs that were judged to have a good design were included. Most of the studies were two-arm comparisons, one with and one without fetal movement counting, but the control group was different, as described below.

4.1.2 Results

Five RCTs (totaling 71,458 participants) were reviewed [5, 9–12]. One study with a cluster RCT was the largest, with 68,654 participants entered in that study alone. The setting of the control group differed, with two of the five articles comparing standard obstetric care, two comparing methods of fetal movement counting, and the remaining one comparing perinatal outcomes by fetal movement counting and placental hormone production (hPL) levels.

Fetal Movement Count Group vs. Usual Obstetric Care Group

There was no difference in the stillbirth rate [risk ratio (RR): 0.93 [95% confidence interval (95% CI): −0.61 to 1.07]] or cesarean section rate [RR: 0.93 (95% CI: 0.60–1.44)] between the two groups. Maternal anxiety was significantly increased in the normal fetal movement count group [standardized mean difference (SMD): −0.22 (95% CI: −0.35 to 0.10)]. There was no significant difference in attachment formation to the fetus [SMD: −0.02 (95% CI: −0.15 to 0.11)]. Hospitalization for fetal movement reduction was significantly more frequent in the fetal movement count group [RR: 2.72 (95% CI: 1.34–5.52)], and another study found a trend toward more prenatal hospitalization in the fetal movement count group [SMD: 0.38 (95% CI: −0.17 to 0.93)] [10]. There was no significant difference between the two groups for children with a birth weight below the 10th percentile [RR: 0.98 (95% CI: 0.66–1.44)]. The most important outcome, "perinatal death or morbidity," was not reported.

Once-Daily Fetal Movement Count Group vs. After-Meal Fetal Movement Count Group

A total of 1400 patients were entered into the study. There was no significant difference in the cesarean section rate [RR: 2.33 (95% CI: 0.61–8.99)]. No "perinatal death or morbidity" was reported.

In summary, this Cochrane review concludes that there is insufficient evidence to show that fetal movement counting significantly improves perinatal outcomes.

Fetal Count Group vs. Human Placental Lactogen Measurement Group

This study involved 1191 patients. There was no difference in the cesarean section rate [RR 1.18 (95% CI: 0.83–1.69)]. The number of hospital visits was significantly lower in the fetal movement count group than in the lactogen measurement group [RR: 0.26 (95% CI: 0.20–0.35)], but the frequency of an Apgar score of less than 7 points per quintile was significantly higher [RR: 1.72 (95% CI: 1.01–2.93)]. This study also did not report on "perinatal death or morbidity."

4.2 A Systematic Review by Bellussi et al. [13]

4.2.1 Method

We reviewed RCTs on fetal movement counts and perinatal outcomes. Five RCTs among 1290 articles related to fetal movement published up to May 2019 were selected for meta-analysis [9, 11, 14–16]. All of the articles advised telling the patients to contact the hospital if they felt anxious about fetal movement. We studied the perinatal outcomes of 261,691 fetuses subjected to fetal movement counting and 196,094 fetuses managed according to standard obstetric management. Fetal anomalies were excluded, but two papers that included twin pregnancies were included in the study.

4.2.2 Results (Table 1)

There were no significant differences in perinatal death, neonatal death, stillbirth rate, neonatal intensive care unit (NICU) admission rate, preterm birth rate, or small for gestational age (SGA). There was a significant increase in preterm birth [RR: 1.07 (95% CI: 1.05–1.10)], induced labor [RR: 1.15 (95% CI: 1.09–1.22)], and cesarean section [RR: 1.11 (95% CI: 1.10–1.12)] in the fetal movement count group. However, these differences may not be clinically meaningful.

5 Findings on Reduced Fetal Movement Identified Through the Japan Obstetric Compensation System for Cerebral Palsy [17]

Among 658 cases of cerebral palsy (CP) registered in the Japan Obstetric Compensation System for Cerebral Palsy by June 2015, 53 cases involving singleton pregnancies, deliveries after 33 weeks of gestation, and umbilical artery blood pH $\geq$7.2 at birth were included. In this study, 53 patients with congenital morphological abnormalities, fetal growth failure, or infection were included. In 14 of 37 cases (38%), fetal movement was reported to have disappeared, indicating that the clinical picture may differ depending on the time between the episode and delivery.

Table 1 Summary of the meta-analysis of Bellussi et al. Each parameter is listed as "number of cases in fetal movement count group (%) vs. number of cases in control group (%)"

Author	Perinatal death	SGA (<10%)	Premature birth	Induction of childbirth	Cesarean section
Neldam [14]	14/1583 (0.88) vs. 21/1569 (1.34)	120/1583 (7.6) vs. 110/1569 (7)	48/1562 (3.1) vs. 41/1549 (2.7)	Not mentioned	206/1583 (13) vs. 175/1569 (11.2)
Grant [9]	Not mentioned	Not mentioned	Not mentioned	Not mentioned	Not mentioned
Saastad [11]	0/544 vs. 1/532	46/543 (8.5) vs. 46/530 (8.7)	20/544 (3.7) vs. 24/532 (4.5)	77/544 (14.2) vs. 76/532 (14.3)	36/544 (6.6) vs. 38/532 (7.1)
Delaram [15]	Not mentioned	Not mentioned	0/100 vs. 0/108	Not mentioned	53/100 (53) vs. 58/108 (53.7)
Norman [16]	1238/227,816 (0.54) vs. 923/157,654 (0.58)	10,853/227,860 (4.7) vs. 8444/157,692 (5.4)	17,376/227,860 (7.6) vs. 11,228/157,692 (7.1)	83,499/227,860 (36.6) vs. 49,952/157,692 (31.7)	64,572/227,860 (28.3) vs. 40,231/157,692 (25.5)
Total	1252/229,943 (0.54) vs. 944/159,755 (0.59)	11,019/229,986 (4.8) vs. 8600/159,791 (5.4)	17,444/230,066 (7.6) vs. 11,293/159,881 (7.1)	83,576/228,404 (36.6)/50,028/158,224 (31.6)	64,867/230,087 (28.2)/40,502/159,901 (25.3)
RR (95% CI)	0.92 (0.85–1.00)	0.92 (0.83–1.02)	1.07 (1.05–1.10)	1.15 (1.09–1.22)	1.11 (1.10–1.12)

SGA small for gestational age

6 Recent Research Findings Related to Fetal Movement

In addition to the above, other studies related to fetal movement have been reported, and we will introduce some of the most interesting ones.

6.1 Association Between Reduced Fetal Movement and Long-Term Prognosis of the Child [18]

6.1.1 Objective

(1) To investigate whether reduced fetal movement is associated with perinatal outcome and (2) whether reduced fetal movement is associated with long-term neurological morbidity in the child.

6.1.2 Method

A single-center case-control study in Israel.

Study Group (Reduced Fetal Movement Group)

A total of 439 women who complained of reduced fetal movement from the late second trimester to end of pregnancy.

Comparison Group

A total of 241,903 women who did not complain of reduced fetal movement.

6.1.3 Results

1. Perinatal prognosis

   The reduced fetal movement group had significantly more first-time mothers (38.7% vs. 23.6%, respectively, $P < 0.001$), more in vitro fertilization (IVF) (4.8% vs. 1.1%, respectively, $P < 0.001$), more amniotic fluid deficiency (14.6% vs. 2.3%, respectively, $P < 0.001$), and more fetal growth restriction (FGR) (4.8% vs. 1.8%, respectively, $P < 0.001$) than the comparison group. Induction of labor was more common in the reduced fetal movement group (74.0% vs. 26.0%, respectively, $P < 0.001$), cesarean section was more common (34.9% vs. 13.5%, respectively, $P < 0.001$), and there were fewer patients with a 5-min Apgar score of less than 7 (0.2% vs. 2.3%, respectively, $P = 0.042$). There were no cases of perinatal death in the reduced fetal movement group.

2. Neurological morbidity in children

   The reduced fetal movement group had more movement disorders (3.2% vs. 1.8%, respectively, $P = 0.036$) and a higher hospitalization rate (4.8% vs. 3.1%, respectively, $P = 0.044$). No significant difference was found in cerebral palsy. Cox proportional hazards model analysis of neurological factors associated with child hospitalization showed that they were associated with reduced fetal movement [hazard ratio (HR): 1.54 (95% CI: 1.0–2.37), $P = 0.048$], gestational week [HR: 0.93 (95% CI: 0.92–0.94), $P < 0.001$], and under-amniotic fluid [HR: 1.2 (95% CI: 1.04–1.38), $P = 0.012$].

6.2 Association Between Fetal Movement Changes and Stillbirth [19]

6.2.1 Objective

To identify fetal movement changes associated with stillbirth.

6.2.2 Method

A questionnaire on fetal movement was administered to patients managed between April 2014 and March 2016 in 41 perinatal centers in the UK. Conducted in the form of a case-control study, mothers experiencing stillbirths were interviewed about fetal movement in the 2 weeks before fetal death, and controls were interviewed about fetal movement in the last 2 weeks.

Study Group (Stillbirth Group)

A total of 291 stillbirths after 28 weeks of gestation.

Comparison Group

A total of 733 successfully continuing their pregnancies.

6.2.3 Results

Multivariate analysis showed that the frequency of fetal movement was significantly decreased in the stillbirth group [adjusted OR (aOR): 4.51 (95% CI: 2.38–8.55)]. Conversely, no changes in fetal movement [aOR: 0.18 (95% CI: 0.13–0.26)] or hiccup awareness [aOR: 0.31 (95% CI: 0.17–0.56)] were risk-reducing factors for stillbirth.

6.3 *Reduced Fetal Movement Cases and Placental Findings [20]*

6.3.1 Objective

To clarify whether reduced fetal movement at full term is associated with placental abnormalities and neonatal prognosis.

6.3.2 Method

A case-control study of managed deliveries between January 2008 and May 2019 at a single center in Israel.

Study Group (Reduced Fetal Movement Group)

Among pregnant women with full-term deliveries who were aware of reduced fetal movement within 2 weeks before delivery, 203 had placental pathology results.

Comparison Group

A total of 203 patients adjusted for maternal age, weeks of delivery, and proportion of vaginal births versus cesarean sections with the study group.

6.3.3 Results

In the reduced fetal movement group, the time from awareness of decreased movement to delivery was 8.2 ± 4.4 days (mean ± SD). Induction of labor (19.2% vs. 10.8%, respectively, $P = 0.02$), cesarean section (23.6% vs. 13.7%, respectively, $P = 0.01$), placenta weight <10th percentile (22.6% vs. 3.9%, respectively, $P < 0.001$), and neonatal morbidity (15.7% vs. 6.8%, respectively, $P = 0.007$) were all significantly higher in the reduced fetal movement group than the comparison group. As for placental pathological findings, composite maternal vascular malperfusion (MVM)[1] (46.3% vs. 33.4%, respectively, $P = 0.01$) and inflammatory findings (43.3% vs. 29.5%, respectively, $P = 0.005$) were both observed significantly more frequently in the reduced fetal movement group. Multivariate analysis showed that factors associated with infant morbidity were reduced fetal movement [aOR: 1.7 (95% CI: 1.1–4.8)] and placental MVM [aOR: 1.2 (95% CI: 1.0–2.9)].

---

[1] Dysfunction of maternal vascular perfusion is one of the five major findings added as new guidelines for the diagnosis of placental pathology (Amsterdam Placental Workshop Group Consensus Statement, 2016). Specific pathological findings include chorionic hypoplasia, chorionic hyperplasia, and desmoplastic membrane vasculopathy.

6.4 Effect of Reduced Fetal Movement on Induction of Labor [21]

6.4.1 Objective

To clarify the current status of induction of labor among pregnant women who are aware of reduced fetal movement.

6.4.2 Method

A prospective study conducted in Stockholm in 2014. A questionnaire was administered to pregnant women with reduced fetal movement.

Study Group (Reduced Fetal Movement Group)

Two thousand six hundred and eighty-three women with singleton pregnancies after 28 weeks of gestation without fetal abnormalities who were aware of reduced fetal movement.

Comparison Group

A total of 26,041 patients who were managed at the same time and not aware of reduced fetal movement.

6.4.3 Results

(1) The frequency of labor induction increased in the reduced fetal movement group [RR: 1.4 (95% CI: 1.3–1.5)]. (2) The frequency of labor induction increased as the severity of reduced fetal movement increased: 1.3-fold increase in the number of times perceived decreased fecundity, compared with 3.2-fold increase in the number of times perceived decreased fecundity in pregnant women who perceived decreased fecundity five or more times. (3) The rate of fetal problems was significantly higher in the reduced fetal movement group [RR: 3.9 (95% CI: 3.00–5.21)], and the rate of induced labor due to fetal indications, including low amniotic fluid and fetal growth restriction (FGR), was significantly higher in the reduced fetal movement group [RR: 1.6 (95% CI: 1.4–1.8)].

6.5 *Characteristics of Fetal Movement in Obese Pregnant Women [22]*

6.5.1 Objective

To determine the characteristics of fetal movement in obese pregnant women.

6.5.2 Method

We performed a secondary analysis of RCTs conducted for other purposes related to obesity in New Zealand between April 2015 and June 2017 and a case-control study examining risk factors for stillbirth between February 2012 and December 2015.

Study Group (Obese Group)

A total of 233 obese (BMI >30) pregnant women. Pregnancies with diabetic complications were excluded.

Comparison Group

A total of 149 non-obese (BMI <25) pregnant women.

6.5.3 Results

In the obese group, there was a significant difference in (1) more active fetal movements before meals and (2) fewer fetal movements within 1 h of meal consumption (47.4% in the obese group vs. 32.0% in the non-obese group, $P < 0.001$).

There is no clear evidence that fetal movement counting improves perinatal outcomes. However, we would like to emphasize that fetal movement counting itself is not meaningless. In other words, pregnant women naturally observe fetal movements without active fetal movement counting, so it is difficult to show the effect of fetal movement counting. On the other hand, it is still unclear how many pregnant women are aware of fetal hypotonia among children with a poor perinatal prognosis and cerebral palsy, the kind of diseases that cause fetal hypotonia, and their proportion. In addition, we do not know the characteristics of cases with a good prognosis among those with reduced fetal movement. It is necessary to clarify these issues in a well-designed study.

References

1. Mangesi L, Hofmeyr GJ, Smith V, et al. Fetal movement counting for assessment of fetal well-being. Cochrane Database Syst Rev. 2015;10:CD004909. https://doi.org/10.1002/14651858.CD004909.pub3.
2. Winje BA, Saastad E, Gunnes N, et al. Analysis of 'count-to-ten' fetal movement charts: a prospective cohort study. BJOG. 2011;118:1229–38.
3. Pearson JF, Weaver JB. Fetal activity and fetal wellbeing: an evaluation. Br Med J. 1976;1(6021):1305–7.
4. Cronje HS, Grobler CJF, Visser AA. Obstetrics in southern Africa. Pretoria: van Schaik Publishers; 1996.
5. Gómez LM, De la Vega G, Padilla L, et al. Compliance with a fetal movement chart by high-risk obstetric patients in a Peruvian hospital. Am J Perinatol. 2007;24:89–93.
6. Sadovsky E, Ohel G, Havazeleth H, et al. The definition and the significance of decreased fetal movements. Acta Obstet Gynecol Scand. 1983;62:409–13.
7. Kuwata T, Matsubara S, Ohkusa T, et al. Establishing a reference value for the frequency of fetal movements using a modified 'count to 10' method. J Obstet Gynaecol Res. 2008;34:318–23.
8. Koshida S, Ono T, Tsuji S, et al. Fetal movement frequency and the effect of associated perinatal factors: a multicenter study. Women Birth. 2019;32:127–30.
9. Grant A, Elbourne D, Valentin L, et al. Routine formal fetal movement counting and risk of antepartum late death in normally formed singletons. Lancet. 1989;2:345–9.
10. Mikhail MS, Freda MC, Merkatz RB, et al. The effect of fetal movement counting on maternal attachment to the fetus. Am J Obstet Gynecol. 1991;165(4 Pt 1):988–91.
11. Saastad E, Winje BA, Stray Pedersen B, et al. Fetal movement counting improved identification of fetal growth restriction and perinatal outcomes—a multi-centre, randomized, controlled trial. PLoS One. 2011;6:e28482.
12. Thomsen SG, Legarth J, Weber T, et al. Monitoring of normal pregnancies by daily fetal movement registration or hormone assessment. A random allocation study. J Obstet Gynaecol. 1990;10:189–93.
13. Bellussi F, Po' G, Livi A, et al. Fetal movement counting and perinatal mortality: a systematic review and meta-analysis. Obstet Gynecol. 2020;135:453–62.
14. Neldam S. Fetal movements as an indicator of fetal well-being. Dan Med Bull. 1983;30:274–8.
15. Delaram M, Jafarzadeh L. The effects of fetal movement counting on pregnancy outcomes. J Clin Diagn Res. 2016;10:SC22–4.
16. Norman JE, Heazell AEP, Rodriguez A, et al. Awareness of fetal movements and care package to reduce fetal mortality (AFFIRM): a stepped wedge, cluster-randomised trial. Lancet. 2018;392:1629–38.
17. Fukushima K, Morokuma S, Kitadai Y, et al. Analysis of antenatal-onset cerebral palsy secondary to transient ischemia in utero using a national. J Obstet Gynaecol Res. 2016;42:1297–303.
18. Zamstein O, Wainstock T, Sheiner E. Decreased fetal movements: perinatal and long-term neurological outcomes. Eur J Obstet Gynecol Reprod Biol. 2019;241:1–5.
19. Heazell AEP, Budd J, Li M, et al. Alterations in maternally perceived fetal movement and their association with late stillbirth: findings from the Midland and North of England stillbirth case-control study. BMJ Open. 2018;8:e020031.
20. Levy M, Kovo M, Izaik Y, et al. Reduced fetal movements at term in singleton low risk pregnancies-is there an association with placental histopathological findings? Acta Obstet Gynecol Scand. 2020;99:884–90.
21. Akselsson A, Lindgren H, Georgsson S, et al. Increased labor induction and women presenting with decreased or altered fetal movements—a population-based survey. PLoS One. 2019;14:e0216216.
22. Bradford B, Cronin R, McKinlay C, et al. Maternally perceived fetal movement patterns: the influence of body mass index. Early Hum Dev. 2019;140:104922.

Placental Abruption

Shunji Suzuki

Contents

Summary

- Placental abruption (PA) is a condition in which the placenta separates from the normal implanted site of uterine body before the delivery of the fetus. It has been identified as the most common cause of cerebral palsy (CP) among those registered in the Japan Obstetric Compensation System for Cerebral Palsy (JOCS-CP).
- They are classified into two groups: revealed hemorrhage/abruption type with external hemorrhage and concealed hemorrhage/abruption type with-

S. Suzuki (✉)
Department of Obstetrics and Gynecology, Nippon Medical School,
Bunkyo-ku, Tokyo, Japan
e-mail: shun@nms.ac.jp

Y. Matsuda (ed.), *Cerebral Palsy*, https://doi.org/10.1007/978-981-19-2217-6_16

out external hemorrhage. The latter has a poorer prognosis for the mother and infant.
- Because there has been no evidence-based prevention method for AP, it is required to inform pregnant women about AP and to establish a fetal emergency transport system.
- When acute-onset AP where fetal survival has been confirmed is diagnosed based on clinical symptoms, the baby should be delivered as soon as possible.

1 Definition and Pathogenesis of Placental Abruption (PA)

1.1 *Definition*

Placental abruption (PA, premature separation of the normally implanted placenta) is a condition in which the placenta detaches from the normal implanted site of uterine body before the delivery of the fetus. Placental separation will begin when ischemic necrosis occurs in the basal decidua and maternal blood vessels in the decidua fail, and the hematoma formed along the decidua (retroplacental hematoma) further separates the adjacent placenta, eventually separating the entire placenta from the uterine wall. If the separation area becomes large, non-reassuring fetal status (NRFS) or fetal demise will occur [1].

On the maternal side, tissue thromboplastin enters the bloodstream and promotes blood coagulation (microthrombosis) in blood vessels throughout the body, resulting in disseminated intravascular coagulation (DIC) due to significant consumptive coagulopathy and increased fibrinolysis.

1.2 *Clinical Progress*

The time course of AP varies depending on whether the failed vessel is an artery or a vein and its size. The placental findings of AP are characterized by hemorrhage in the basal decidua, which is accompanied by hemorrhagic degeneration and necrosis of the decidua plate, and by the fact that the hematoma adheres to the decidua plate and becomes difficult to remove manually as time passes after the formation of the posterior placental hematoma. The maternal surface of the placenta where the hematoma is present sometimes shows “indentation,” as if the chorionic tissue has caved in. Histopathologically, an infiltration of blood cells from the hematoma will be observed to be into the decidua. As a cause of vascular disruption, it has been reported that morphological abnormalities in the uterine spiral arteries occur during the invasion of trophoblast cells into the desquamation membrane in cases of premature desquamation [2] and that granulocyte elastase, a proteolytic enzyme activated by inflammation in intrauterine infection (= chorioamnionitis, CAM). In the case of CAM, it has been reported that granulocyte elastase, a proteolytic enzyme activated by inflammation, may cause a decrease in the adhesiveness of the decidua to the uterine wall or the vascularity of the decidua may be disrupted by the weakening of the chorionic and/or decidual membranes where the inflammation has been spread. In addition, an arterial hemorrhage caused by the former tends to occur suddenly and progress rapidly, whereas in the latter case, a venous hemorrhage associated with CAM tends to be triggered by symptoms of preterm labor or premature rupture of the membranes (PROM) and tends to progress relatively slowly.

Furthermore, when slow venous hemorrhage occurs in mid-pregnancy, chronic PA sometimes progress to a poor prognosis complicated by chronic abruption-oligohydramnios sequence (CAOS), in which the amniotic fluid level is low due to the decrease in fetal renal circulation; however, in this section, we will focus only on the acute-onset AP.

2 Symptoms of Placental Abruption (PA) Associated with Cerebral Palsy (CP)

2.1 Relation to Cerebral Palsy (CP)

In cases of PA, residual neurological sequelae have been reported to be noted in 15–20% of surviving infants [1]. PA is the most common disease for cerebral palsy (CP) among those registered in the Japan Obstetric Compensation System for Cerebral Palsy (JOCS-CP) [3]. About 20% of the main causes of CP are PA (about 35% in preterm infants). On the other hand, according to the overview of PA in the Japan Society of Obstetrics and Gynecology Perinatal Registry (2001–2010), the average onset time of PA was 34.2 weeks of gestation, and about 36% of the cases occurred at less than 34 weeks of gestation [4]. In a previous study by Pariente et al. [5] on the long-term prognosis of children with PA, PA did not lead to an increase in hospitalization due to neurological symptoms in infants; however, PA was associated with an increased incidence of cerebral palsy and developmental disabilities (hazard ratio: 6.71 and 3.36, respectively).

About 10% of the cases of CP registered in the JOCS-CP have been reported to have no problem with the findings of umbilical artery blood gases; however, in all cases of CP caused mainly by PA, the umbilical artery pH was low suggesting the presence of fetal hypoxia (ischemia) [6]. The fetus receives oxygen and nutrients from the mother through the placenta, and if the placenta is separated before fetal delivery, the oxygen supply to the fetus will be insufficient resulting in fetal hypoxia. The prognosis of the infant is correlated with the size of area of PA. If the area is large, neonatal death or CP may be resulted even if the fetus is rapidly delivered. Once in Japan, a modified version of Page's classification, which includes the degree of PA, had been frequently used for a wide range of symptoms of PA. This classification can be used only for a retrospective review of the cases because of the low evidence on the degree of PA. For example, there is the possibility of loss of fetal beat even in the mild Page's classification. Therefore, the classification will not be useful in clinical practice to achieve desirable neonatal outcomes.

2.2 Brain MRI Findings of the Neonates Associated with Cerebral Palsy (CP)

Brain MRI findings in infants with CP due to PA include hypoxic-ischemic encephalopathy (HIE) in full-term infants and periventricular leukomalacia (PVL) in preterm infants. The former is subdivided according to the severity and duration of hypoxia/ischemia as follows: (1) total asphyxia, in which both the brainstem and mesencephalon are affected, which is caused by a short but severe episode of acidemia/ischemia due to PA associated with arterial hemorrhage and (2) profound asphyxia, in which the basal ganglia and thalamus are affected. The prognosis of full-term infants correlates with the severity and duration of fetal bradycardia. On the other hand, in preterm infants, the gestational weeks and the presence of intrauterine infection (inflammation) are major confounding factors for CP. This is also related to the fact that preterm deliveries with PA have been often managed as preterm labor associated with chorioamnionitis and have a high prevalence of PA with revealed hemorrhage in which the placenta is separated from the marginal side associated with PROM [3, 4]. In preterm infants, hypercytokinemia has been observed to be associated with the development of PVL, even if PA does not develop, and also has caused multiple organ failure such as chronic lung disease and/or necrotizing enterocolitis as fetal inflammatory response syndrome (FIRS).

2.3 Clinical Manifestations Associated with Cerebral Palsy (CP)

The first subjective symptoms of PA in pregnant women are genital bleeding, abdominal pain, abdominal distension, and decreased or absent fetal movements suggesting severe fetal asphyxia. PA is characterized by two types of hemorrhage depending on the site of separation: (1) revealed hemorrhage/abruption (Fig. 1a), in which the separation proceeds from the marginal side of the placenta and external bleeding is observed, and (2) concealed hemorrhage/abruption (Fig. 1b), in which blood accumulates between the placenta and the uterine wall and no external bleeding is observed [7]. The latter type, which accounts for 20–40% of all PA, has adverse neonatal outcomes and is associated with a high incidence of intrauterine fetal demise. Conversely, genital bleeding is the first clinical symptom in the

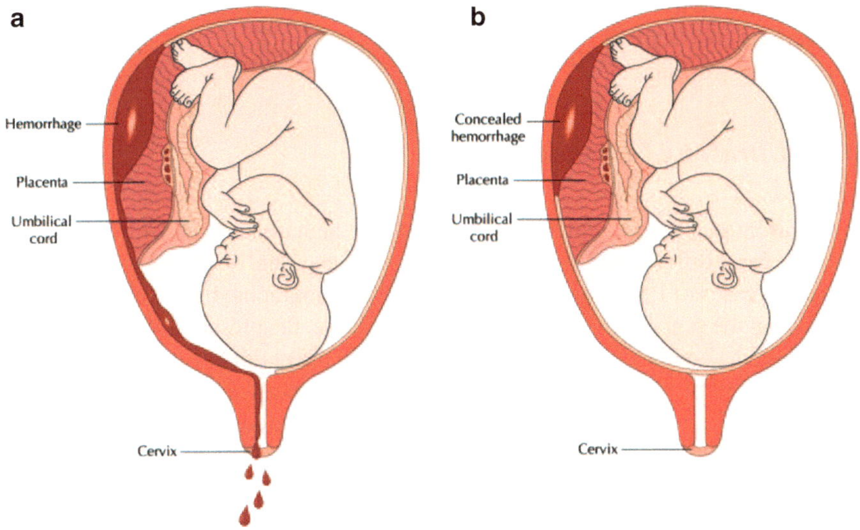

Fig. 1 Types of hemorrhage in placental abruption. (Reproduced with permission from [7]). (**a**) External bleeding in placental abruption (revealed hemorrhage/abruption). (**b**) No external bleeding in placental abruption (concealed hemorrhage/abruption)

majority of PA cases; however, intrauterine fetal death or severe neonatal asphyxia is not common in cases of massive hemorrhage. In cases of revealed hemorrhage/abruption, in which bleeding is discharged outside the uterus, it can be expected that external bleeding may prevent the separation toward the center of the placenta; however, in cases of concealed hemorrhage/abruption, separation toward the center of the placenta may proceed and result in the formation of a posterior placental hematoma increasing intrauterine pressure. In addition, the absence of external bleeding tends to delay the diagnosis of PA, which worsens the neonatal outcomes. Bloody amniotic fluid is often absent at the time of cesarean section in the absence of PROM [8]. The risk of developing DIC is also increased because tissue thromboplastin is more likely to enter the maternal circulation in cases of concealed hemorrhage/abruption.

3 Diagnosis of Placental Abruption (PA)

3.1 Clinical Findings

The diagnosis of PA begins with the suspicion of PA based on the various clinical findings such as genital bleeding (often non-coagulative), abdominal pain (plate-like hardness, often sustained contractions with no distinct intervals), abnormal fetal heart rate patterns in cardiotocogram (CTG), cyclic uterine contractions, uterine tachysystole, similar contractions with preterm labor, and irregular wave-like uterine contractions.

3.2 Ultrasound Examination

In ultrasonography, placental thickening and/or hematoma between the placenta and uterine wall (= retroplacental hematoma) may be observed in typical or advanced cases of PA. The specificity of the ultrasonographic findings in PA is high (96%), but the sensitivity is low (24%) [9]. Therefore, the presence of a retroplacental hematoma on ultrasonography can lead to a definitive diagnosis of PA; however, the possibility of PA cannot be ruled out even if no abnormal findings are observed in ultrasound examination. If the placenta is located at the anterior wall of the uterus, abdominal pain can be noticed immediately after the onset of the PA, and it may be relatively easy to identify the findings of PA by the palpation with the palm (plate-like hardness) and/or ultrasonography.

3.3 Fetal Heart Rate Monitoring

According to a retrospective study of low-risk pregnant women in Miyazaki Prefecture, Japan [10], when fetal heart rate abnormalities (repeated late decelerations or bradycardia) were already present at the time of admission, PA was common (46% of them), and 73% of the PA cases resulted in CP or stillbirth. Therefore, if a fetal heart rate abnormality is observed in women with symptoms of impending preterm labor, the management should be performed with the assumption of PA. In addition, since abnormal fetal heart rate patterns may become apparent or develop after the admission, it is necessary to re-observe the fetal heart rate patterns and confirm that there is no fetal heart rate abnormality if subjective symptoms change during the management of preterm labor.

3.4 Case Report of Placental Abruption (PA)

Figure 2 shows the findings of CTG in a case of preterm labor complicated by PA with revealed venous hemorrhage. At 39 weeks and 0 days of gestation, she visited her primary care midwifery home because of PROM. She complained frequent uterine contractions, and bloody amniotic fluid was observed. She was transferred to a regional perinatal center due to suspicion of PA. At the time of arrival to the perinatal center, she had an external hemorrhage of 160 g. However, ultrasonography did not reveal the presence of retroplacental hematoma or placental thickness. She was

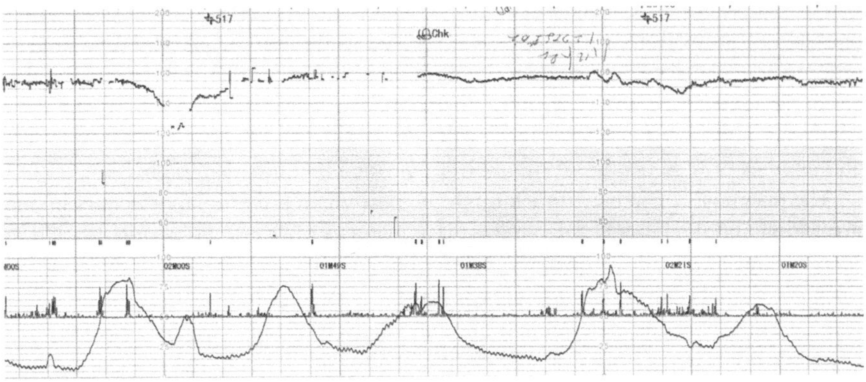

Fig. 2 Fetal heart rate in the cardiotocogram in a case of placental abruption due to venous hemorrhage

monitored with CTG. An emergent cesarean section was performed because of decreased baseline variability and repeated late decelerations in the CTG. During surgery, a large amount of hemorrhage with clots in the uterus and a retroplacental hematoma were observed. The neonatal Apgar scores were 8 and 9 at 1 and 5 min, respectively, and the umbilical artery pH was 7.170. According to the case, it is important not to overestimate the findings of ultrasonography and to suspect PA based on clinical symptoms.

On the other hand, in cases of PA with arterial hemorrhage, the fetal heart rate usually shows bradycardia at the time of admission, and a decision to perform an emergent cesarean section often has to be performed before installing CTG.

Ideally, PA should be suspected based on clinical findings before fetal heart rate abnormalities are detected. It is also important not to deny the possibility of PA in any situation where fetal heart rate abnormalities are detected. In cases of transporting pregnant women on suspicion of PA, it is important to share information and not to waste time in confirming the diagnosis of PA in the receiving facilities.

4 Treatment and Prevention of Placental Abruption (PA)

4.1 What to Do at Diagnosis

When PA occurs, the fetus should be delivered as soon as possible in cases where the fetus is alive. In particular, if the fetus has a potential for intact survival and a forced vaginal delivery is not possible, an emergent cesarean section should be performed. The golden time for intact survival has been suggested within 1 h of the onset of PA, and the risk of maternal critical obstetric hemorrhage and DIC increases after 2–3 h of PA onset. Therefore, although it is necessary to pay attention to the risk of maternal DIC during and after cesarean section, it is advisable to omit preoperative examinations as much as possible and to shorten the preoperative time in order to expect a good neonatal outcome. In addition, in cases of severe fetal bradycardia or fetal death, the CTG may misrecord the maternal heart rate as the fetal heart rate. If it is difficult to differentiate between the two heart rates, the presence and number of fetal heart rate should be confirmed by ultrasonography.

The prognosis of fetus with PA might be best when preterm labor occurs in one institution and the fetus is delivered rapidly, but about 70% of PA resulted in CP in Japan occurred outside of obstetric institutions [3]. Because about half of all deliveries are managed in private clinics in Japan, it is important to inform pregnant women about AP and to establish an emergency transport system especially for women who develop PA at home. Specifically, for the former, all pregnant women should be informed by around 30 weeks of gestation so that they should contact obstetric institutes as soon as possible if they have unusual symptoms such as abdominal pain or bleeding. In the latter case, the following points should be mentioned: (1) clarification of the decision criteria for transport according to the function and role, (2) smooth provision and understanding of information between the transporting and receiving facilities, and (3) advance preparation of delivery based on the premise of forced delivery at the receiving institute [3].

It is advisable for each institute and region to make arrangements and simulate the response to PA in advance, including the call of staff, emergent cesarean section, and preparation for maternal transport. In addition, because it is often impossible to record medical records during the response, the record should be kept over time, and a detailed record should be noted after treatment is completed.

4.2 *Risk Factors and Prevention*

There is no evidence-based prevention for PA. Risk factors for the development of PA include a history of PA and younger and older pregnancies [10]. A review in Europe and the United States [11] reported that there is a large regional difference in the involvement of smoking and that the use of magnesium sulfate decreases the risk of PA, whereas the risk of PA is increased in hypertensive disorders. On the other hand, it has been reported that the risk of recurrence of PA in the next pregnancy tends to be lower in patients with hypertensive pregnancy. In contrast to these findings, 9.7% of pregnant women registered in the JOCS-CP who developed PA have been reported to smoke during pregnancy, and 18.8% have been reported to have hypertensive disorders.

In addition, epidemiological studies have shown that inadequate folic acid intake was associated with an increased incidence of PA; Ruiter et al. in the Netherlands [12] found that the overall incidence of PA was about 0.2% and the incidence of PA increased to 5.8% if there was a history of PA (0.06% if there was no history; odds ratio 93). The incidence of recurrent PA in the second pregnancy was 2.3% and 3.3% for women who had PA at 22–31 and 32–36 weeks of first gestation, respectively; however, it was 11% for women who had PA at 37 weeks or later of the first gestation. About half of the recurrent PA occurred before 37 weeks of next gestation. Therefore, planned delivery at 37 weeks of gestation may be an option for women with a history of PA after 37 weeks of previous gestation.

References

1. Cunningham FG, Leveno KJ, Bloom SL, et al. Williams obstetrics. 25th ed. New York: McGraw Hill Education; 2018. p. 767–73.
2. Dommisse J, Tiltman AJ. Placental bed biopsies in placental abruption. Br J Obstet Gynaecol. 1992;99:651–4.
3. Japan Council for Quality Health Care. Placental abruption. 6th report on prevention of recurrence, the Japan Obstetric Compensation System for Cerebral Palsy. Japanese. Available from: http://www.sanka-hp.jcqhc.or.jp/documents/prevention/index.html. Accessed 13 May 2020.
4. Nakai A. Jyouitaiban soukihakuri—shusankidamashii no misedokoro [Placental abruption—the focus of the perinatal soul]. J Jpn Soc Perinat Neonat Med. 2016;52:1346–8. Japanese.
5. Pariente G, Wainstock T, Walfisch A, et al. Placental abruption and long-term neurological hospitalisations in the offspring. Paediatr Perinat Epidemiol. 2019;33:215–22.
6. Matsuda Y, Umezaki H, Ogawa M, et al. Umbilical arterial pH in patients with cerebral palsy. Early Hum Dev. 2014;90:131–5.
7. Oyelese Y, Ananth CV. Placental abruption. Obstet Gynecol. 2006;108:1005–16.
8. Suzuki S. Clinical significance of preterm singleton pregnancies complicated by placental abruption following preterm premature rupture of membranes compared with those without p-PROM. ISRN Obstet Gynecol. 2012;2012:856971.
9. Glantz C, Purnell L. Clinical utility of sonography in the diagnosis and treatment of placental abruption. J Ultrasound Med. 2002;21:837–40.
10. Doi K, Furukawa S, Samejima H. Taiji shinpakusuu monitoring [Fetal heart rate monitoring]. Obstet Gynecol. 2014;63:1959–63. Japanese.
11. Ananth CV, Keyes KM, Hamilton A, et al. An international contrast of rates of placental abruption: an age-period-cohort analysis. PLoS One. 2015;10:e0125246.
12. Ruiter L, Ravelli AC, de Graaf IM, et al. Incidence and recurrence rate of placental abruption: a longitudinal linked national cohort study in the Netherlands. Am J Obstet Gynecol. 2015;213(573):e1–8.

Intrauterine Infection/Chorioamnionitis

Yoshio Matsuda

Contents

Summary

- Definitions and diagnostic criteria for intrauterine infection/chorioamnionitis (CAM) have not been standardized.
- Regarding the association between CAM and cerebral palsy, there is a difference between the backward approach (involvement of CAM as an underlying disease from the viewpoint of cerebral palsy) and the forward approach (onset of cerebral palsy from the viewpoint of the presence of CAM). This may be related to the fact that the diagnostic criteria are not always consistent.
- Cytokines are important factors that link the two. In sensitized or preconditioned fetuses, inflammation may lead to brain damage even when the hypoxic stress is minimal.

Y. Matsuda (✉)
Tokyo Healthcare University, Hogashi-Gotanda, Shinagawa, Tokyo, Japan

Y. Matsuda (ed.), *Cerebral Palsy*, https://doi.org/10.1007/978-981-19-2217-6_17

1 Diagnosis and Problems of Intrauterine Infection/Chorioamnionitis

Normally, the uterus is a sterile environment, and the fetus is protected from the outside world by the uterus, placenta, and fetal membrane. Intrauterine infection is a condition in which pathogens (such as bacteria and viruses) invade the uterus, placenta, amniotic fluid, and fetus. Bacterial infections of the uterus are mainly ascending infections caused by indigenous vaginal bacteria and are classified into the following four stages:

Stage I: Bacterial vaginosis or cervicitis, in which the vaginal flora is altered and invades the cervix.

Stage II: Placental, fetal membranous, or decidual infection (so-called chorioamnionitis: CAM), in which the bacteria reach the uterus and inhabit the decidua.

Stage III: Choriovasculitis or intra-amniotic infection, in which bacteria have invaded the fetal blood vessels or amniotic fluid.

Stage IV: Fetal infection in which bacteria invade the fetus by swallowing or other means [1].

On the other hand, from a pathological point of view, the term histological chorioamnionitis (hCAM) is used as an indicator of intrauterine infection, which is a condition in which inflammatory cells infiltrate either the fetal membrane, chorionic plate, subchorionic space, chorionic vessels, umbilical cord, or Walton's jelly [2].

1.1 Inflammatory Reaction

Inflammatory reactions associated with bacterial invasion can be divided into two groups: maternal and fetal. The leukocytes in the amniotic fluid, umbilical cord, and chorionic surface vessels are of fetal origin, whereas those in the placenta are of maternal origin. Not surprisingly, the presence of inflammation on the fetal side is associated with more complications in the fetus/neonate.

These inflammations can be classified as acute or chronic (subacute). Chronic inflammations can cause more severe neonatal complications because of the longer duration of fetal inflammation.

1.1.1 Findings Indicative of Chronic (Subacute) Inflammation

Necrotizing funisitis and necrotizing chorioamnionitis are known as clinical entities of chronic (subacute) inflammation. Necrotizing funisitis refers to the presence of bands or calcification around the umbilical vessels caused by degeneration of inflammatory cells, while necrotizing chorioamnionitis refers to the presence of necrotic tissue under the amnion.

Stillbirth, fetal growth restriction, neonatal infection, and necrotizing enterocolitis are more common in cases with necrotizing funisitis than in cases with acute funisitis [3].

In 2003, the Society for Pediatric Pathology, Perinatal Section, Amniotic Fluid Infection Nosology Committee tried the classification of placental and umbilical cord inflammation according to the maternal and fetal side, the degree of progression, and the duration. They proposed the stage and grade classification as shown in Table 1 [4]. In other words, inflammation in the placenta (decidua, chorionic plate) is classified as inflammation of maternal origin, while vasculitis of the chorionic surface and funisitis are classified as inflammation of fetal origin.

Table 1 Placenta reaction patterns related to amniotic fluid infection: nomenclature and definitions (reproduced with permission from [4])

Diagnostic categories	Suggested diagnostic terminology	Definitions
Maternal inflammatory response		
Stage		
1—Early	Acute subchorionitis or chorionitis	PMN in subchorionic fibrin and/or membrane trophoblast
2—Intermediate	Acute chorioamnionitis	Diffuse-patchy PMN in fibrous chorion and/or amnion
3—Advanced	Necrotizing chorioamnionitis	PMN karyorrhexis, amniocyte necrosis, and/or amnion basement membrane thickening/hypereosinophilia
Grade		
1—Mild–moderate	No special terminology required	Not severe as defined below
2—Severe	Severe acute chorioamnionitis *or* with subchorionic microabscesses	Confluent PMN (≥10 × 20 cells in extent) between chorion and decidua; ≥3 isolated foci or continuous band
Other	Chronic (or subacute) chorioamnionitis	Subamnionic mononuclear cell infiltrate with occasional PMN (meconium and hemosiderin-laden macrophages excluded)
Fetal inflammatory response		
Stage		
1—Early	With chorionic vasculitis *or* umbilical phlebitis	Intramural PMN-chorionic vessels and/or umbilical vein
2—Intermediate	With umbilical vasculitis (one or two arteries ± vein) *or* umbilical panvasculitis (all vessels)	Intramural PMN-umbilical artery or arteries (±umbilical vein)
3—Advanced	With (subacute) necrotizing funisitis *or* with concentric umbilical perivasculitis	PMN ± associated debris in concentric bands-rings-halos around one or more umbilical vessels

(continued)

Table 1 (continued)

Diagnostic categories	Suggested diagnostic terminology	Definitions
Grade		
1—Mild–moderate	No special terminology required	Not severe as defined below
2—Severe	With a severe fetal inflammatory response *or* with intense chorionic (umbilical) vasculitis	Near confluent intramural PMN-chorionic and/or umbilical vessels with attenuation/degeneration of VSMC
Other	With associated fetal vessel thrombi	Recent thrombosis associated with intramural PMN
Other specific features	Peripheral funisitis	Focal aggregates of PMN at the umbilical cord surface
	Acute villitis	PMN in villous stroma (or between trophoblast and stroma)
	Acute intervillositis with intervillous abscesses	Patchy-diffuse PMN in intervillous space
	Decidual plasma cells	Unequivocal plasma cells in decidua basalis or capsularis

PMN polymorphonuclear leukocyte, *VSMC* vascular smooth muscle cell

As mentioned above, the infection moves from the outside to the inside of the placenta, and the closer the infection is to the fetus, the more severe the disease becomes, and the longer the infection is present, the more chronic (subacute) the inflammation becomes.

1.2 Clinical Chorioamnionitis (cCAM)

The term clinical chorioamnionitis (cCAM) is used interchangeably with intrauterine infection when the infection manifests itself as maternal symptoms.

As a diagnostic criterion, "maternal fever of 38°C or higher with maternal or infant tachycardia, uterine tenderness, foul odor of amniotic fluid or vaginal discharge, or increased maternal leukocytes" by Lenki et al. [5] has been widely used, but it is not without its problems.

1.3 Introduction of Triple I

In fact, there is still confusion concerning the distinction between cCAM and hCAM and its use in relation to intrauterine infection. A workshop was held in 2015 on the diagnosis and management strategies for CAM. As the terminology used for CAM so far is not uniform, Triple I (intrauterine inflammation or infection or both) was newly proposed as a more general and descriptive term [6].

In addition to fever, one or more of the following four items:

1. Fetal tachycardia (>160 bpm for 10 min or longer)
2. Maternal WBC >15,000 in the absence of corticosteroids
3. Purulent fluid from the cervical os (cloudy or yellowish thick discharge confirmed visually on speculum exam to be coming from the cervical canal)
4. Biochemical or microbiologic amniotic fluid results consistent with microbial invasion of the amniotic cavity

And pregnant women with fever can be divided into three types as follows.

A. Isolated maternal fever (documented fever)
B. Suspected Triple I: 1–3 above
C. Confirmed Triple I: If all of the following are satisfied in addition to 1–3 above

    Amniocentesis confirms infection (gram stain).
    Low levels of sugar in amniotic fluid or positive amniotic fluid bacterial culture.
    Histopathological examination of the placenta shows findings of infection.

- Fever was defined as follows: Measured orally, 39 °C or more (102.2 °F), or 38 °C or more (100.4 °F) and less than 39 °C, retested 30 min later if the same is true.

Confirmed Triple I is diagnosed after delivery, and appropriate antimicrobial agents (ampicillin + gentamicin is described here) are started in suspected Triple I. However, it is necessary to distinguish between suspected and confirmed Triple I for the management of neonates. Reports on the association with cerebral palsy based on such classifications are awaited.

2 Association with Cerebral Palsy

2.1 Current Situation in Japan

In 2009, the Japan Obstetric Compensation System for Cerebral Palsy (JOCS-CP) was launched in 2009 to provide financial compensation for children with CP, as well as to investigate the causes and make recommendations for preventing recurrence, and 2457 cases were reported in a report by the Committee for Prevention of Recurrence after analyzing the causes [7].

As maternal complications, chorioamnionitis accounted for 14.5% (357 cases). However, the term "chorioamnionitis" in this case is annotated as "chorioamnionitis (hCAM)" diagnosed by placental histopathological examination. Moreover, the number of cases in which this infection was considered to be the sole or combined cause was 60 or 2.4% of all cases (the infection is only described as being other than GBS or herpes infection, such as chorioamnionitis or intrauterine infection).

2.2 A Systematic Review

2.2.1 Relationship Between cCAM/hCAM and CP

Meta-analyses and systematic reviews of the association between cCAM/hCAM and CP have been published in 2017, and these associations have been examined from two perspectives [8]: (1) a comparison of the incidence of CP in the presence or absence of CAM (forward perspective study, forward approach) and (2) a comparison of the incidence of CAM in the presence or absence of CP (backward perspective study, backward approach).

In the former study, 17 references were reviewed (with CAM: 125,256 vs. without CAM: 5,994,722) and were found that CP in preterm with hCAM increased (risk ratio [RR] = 1.34, $P < 0.01$), but did not differ between those with and without cCAM. On the other hand, in the latter study, 22 references were reviewed (with CP: 2513 vs. without CP: 8135) and found that cCAM (RR = 1.43, $P < 0.01$) increased in the CP group compared with the group without CP, but there was no increase in hCAM in preterm CP. Increased hCAM was found (RR = 4.26, $P < 0.05$), as well as cCAM in term/near-term CP (RR = 3.06, $P < 0.01$).

This means that there was no difference in the incidence of CP between patients with and without CAM, but there was a difference in the frequency of CAM between patients with and without CP. The overdiagnosis of CAM has been pointed out as a reason for this. As mentioned above, the diagnostic criteria of Lenki et al. that are currently widely used for the diagnosis of cCAM do not correlate with severe infection/inflammation of the fetus.

As a future perspective, the authors emphasize the need for a unified study of the diagnosis of CAM using the aforementioned concept of Triple I (intrauterine inflammation or infection or both).

2.2.2 Association of CP with Maternal Infections Other Than CAM

On the other hand, there are not many reports on the relationship between maternal infection other than CAM and CP.

Bear and Wu [9] compared the incidence of CP in CAM and non-CAM extra-amniotic infections (other genitourinary and respiratory) that occurred in the 12 months before delivery from a California birth cohort (1991–2001) of 6 million cases. Multivariate analysis adjusting for infant sex, maternal age, race, education, socioeconomic status, and obesity showed that the frequencies of CAM, genitourinary, and respiratory infections were 2.0%, 3.1%, and 0.6%, respectively. An infection diagnosis was more common in mothers of the 8473 infants with cerebral palsy than in mothers of unaffected children (13.7% vs. 5.5%, $P < 0.001$). All three types of maternal infections (chorioamnionitis, OR 3.1, 95% CI 2.9–3.4; other genitourinary infection, OR 1.4, 95% CI 1.3–1.6; and respiratory infection, OR 1.9, 95% CI 1.5–2.2) were associated with cerebral palsy in multivariable analyses. Maternal extra-amniotic infections, whether diagnosed during prenatal or birth hospitalizations, conferred an increased risk of cerebral palsy.

The reason for this is that severe respiratory infections that require hospitalization induce a systemic inflammatory response, leading to fetal brain damage by the same mechanism as CAM. Furthermore, maternal hypoxia can also lead to fetal brain damage if it is prolonged. In addition, antimicrobial agents used for the treatment of infection can also lead to fetal brain damage, as shown in the ORACLE II study [10].

2.2.3 Report by Freud et al.

Freud et al. [11] examined neurological morbidity (outcome) up to 18 years of age in a population-based retrospective cohort analysis. Of the 238,622 neonates, 0.5% had maternal CAM, and 3.1% were hospitalized for neurological morbidity. There was no difference between patients with and without CAM (3.8% vs. 3.1%), but there was an association in CP (0.5% vs. 0.1%, OR 5.77, 95% CI 2.5–13.0). The association was also found after adjusting for preterm birth, birth weight, maternal complications such as diabetes and HDP, and mode of delivery (HR = 2.78, 95% CI 1.20–6.43). Based on these results, it is essential to deliver the baby as soon as possible after the diagnosis of CAM, and this will lead to prevention.

2.2.4 Report by Shevell et al.

Shevell et al. [12] analyzed 455 CPs with placental pathology from the Quebec birth cohort in Canada. Of these, 12% had findings of hCAM. These placentas were more frequently above the 90th percentile for placental weight than placentas without hCAM (53.7% vs. 30.7%) and more often delivered at less than 32 weeks (51.9% vs. 24.1%). Children with hCAM had more spastic paraplegia (37% vs. 19.2%), and MRI findings showed more periventricular white matter injury (PWMI) (52.9% vs. 35.8%), suggesting the need for a case-control study is necessary.

2.3 Pathophysiology

Although the causal relationship between CAM and CP has not been fully elucidated, it is generally inferred as follows.

1. Infection activates inflammation-related pathways and releases various inflammatory markers (cytokines, interleukins, etc.). Inflammatory cytokines directly damage oligodendroglial cells and neurons through the activation of microglial cells and neurotoxicity, resulting in neurobehavioral abnormalities [13].
2. There is a known interaction between subthreshold injury, such as inflammatory cytokines, and other severe injuries, such as subsequent hypoxia [14], and the interval between both injuries determines whether the brain damage is reduced (tolerance) or becomes worse (sensitization) [15].
3. In sensitized or preconditioned fetuses, inflammation may lead to brain damage even if the hypoxic stress is minimal [16].
4. Furthermore, in relation to preterm birth, the increase in cytokines leads to enhanced uterine contractions, resulting in preterm birth, and IVH (intraventricular hemorrhage) and PVL (periventricular leukomalacia), which are associated with CP in preterm infants, are more likely to occur. The involvement of cytokines has also been shown here [17] (Fig. 1). Similar to systemic inflammatory response syndrome (SIRS) in adults, fetal inflammatory response syndrome (FIRS) was proposed based on the idea that fetal hypercytokinemia causes multiple organ failure in infants is considered to be the most severe form of CP as well as neonatal/infant death.

3 Toward Prevention

The authors examined the umbilical arterial blood pH in cases of CAM based on a report prepared by the Committee for Analysis of Causes of the Japan Obstetric Compensation System for Cerebral Palsy (JOCS-CP). Comparing the pH values of 168 cases divided by major causes, the mean pH of 17 CAM cases was 7.02 (6.8–7.19), which was lower than that of 42 cases of placental abruption 6.72 (6.43–6.99) [18]. Furthermore, when the frequency of severe acidosis ($pH < 7.0$) was compared between patients with and without CAM, 26.3% (5/19) of the cases with CAM were less than 74.6% (50/67) in the group without CAM [19]. This result confirms the finding of basic research that even mild hypoxia can cause brain damage if CAM is coexistent with acidosis.

In actual clinical practice, it may be an option to consider early delivery even if the nonreassuring fetal status is not severe on CTG while administering antimicrobial agents when CAM is detected.

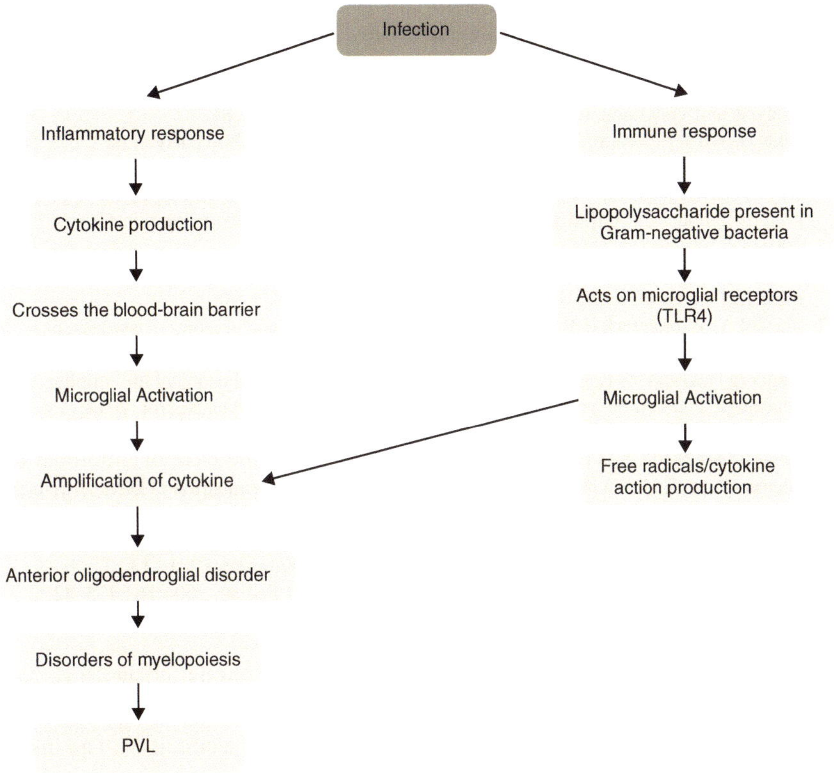

Fig. 1 Pathogenesis of cerebral palsy and neurocognitive deficits in the preterm infant. (Reproduced with permission from [17])

References

1. Romero R, Chaiworapongsa T, Espinosa J. Micronutrients and intrauterine infection, preterm birth and the fetal inflammatory response syndrome. J Nutr. 2003;133:1668S–73S.
2. Faye-Petersen OM, Heller DS, Joshi VV. Lesions of the membrane. In: Placental pathology. 2nd ed. Oxford: Taylor & Francis; 2006. p. P135–53.
3. Craver RD, Baldwin VJ. Necrotizing funisitis. Obstet Gynecol. 1992;79:64–70.
4. Redline RW, Faye-Petersen O, Heller D, et al., Society for Pediatric Pathology, Perinatal Section, Amniotic Fluid Infection Nosology Committee. Amniotic infection syndrome: nosology and reproducibility of placental reaction patterns. Pediatr Dev Pathol. 2003;6:435–48.
5. Lenki SG, Maciulla MB, Eglinton GS. Maternal and umbilical cord serum interleukin levels in preterm labor with clinical chorioamnionitis. Am J Obstet Gynecol. 1994;170:135–51.
6. Higgins RD, Saade G, Polin RA, et al. Chorioamnionitis workshops participants: evaluation and management of women and newborns with a maternal diagnosis of chorioamnionitis: summary of a workshop. Obstet Gynecol. 2016;117(3):426–36.

7. Japan Council for Quality Health Care. 10th Report on prevention of recurrence, the Japan Obstetric Compensation System for Cerebral Palsy. Tokyo: Japan Council for Quality Health Care; 2020. Japanese.
8. Shi Z, Ma L, Luo K, et al. Chorioamnionitis in the development of cerebral palsy: a meta-analysis and systematic review. Pediatrics. 2017;139(6):e20163781.
9. Bear JJ, Wu YW. Maternal infections during pregnancy and cerebral palsy in the child. Pediatr Neurol. 2016;57:74–9.
10. Keyon SL, Taylor DJ, Tarnow-Mordi W, et al. Broad-spectrum antibiotics for spontaneous preterm labour: the ORACLE II randomized trial. ORACLE Collaborative Group. Lancet. 2001;357:989–94.
11. Freud A, Wainstock T, Sheiner E, et al. Maternal chorioamnionitis & long term neurological morbidity in the offspring. Eur J Paediatr Neurol. 2019;23:484–90.
12. Shevell A, Wintermark P, Benini R, et al. Chorioamnionitis and cerebral palsy: lessons from a patient registry. Eur J Paediatr Neurol. 2014;18:301–7.
13. Hagberg H, Gressens P, Mallard C. Inflammation during fetal and neonatal life: implication for neurologic and neuropsychiatric disease in children and adults. Ann Neurol. 2012;71:444–57.
14. Fleiss B, Tann CJ, Degos V, et al. Inflammation-induced sensitization of the brain in term infants. Dev Med Child Neurol. 2015;57(3):17–28.
15. Hansen-Pupp I, Hallin A-L, Hellstroum-Westas L, et al. Inflammation at birth is associated with subnormal development in very preterm infants. Pediatr Res. 2008;64:183–8.
16. Hagberg H, Mallard C, Ferriero DM, et al. The role of inflammation in perinatal brain injury. Nat Rev Neurol. 2015;11:192–208. https://doi.org/10.1038/nrneurol.2015.13.
17. Blumenthal I. Periventricular leucomalacia: a review. Eur J Pediatr. 2004;163:435–42.
18. Matsuda Y, Umezaki H, Ogawa M, et al. Umbilical arterial pH in patients with cerebral palsy. Early Hum Dev. 2014;90:131–5.
19. Matsuda Y, Ogawa M, Nakai A, et al. Severe fetal acidemia in cases of clinical chorioamnionitis in which the infant later developed cerebral palsy. BMC Pregnancy Childbirth. 2015;15:124. https://doi.org/10.1186/s12884-015-0553-9. http://www.biomedcentral.com/1471-2393/15/124.

Fetomaternal Hemorrhage

Minoru Mitani and Yoshio Matsuda

Contents

Summary

- Fetomaternal hemorrhage is a serious condition that causes fetal circulatory failure and anemia due to the entry of fetal blood into the maternal circulation. Although it is infrequent, it can cause fetal death or neurological injury.
- Reduced or no fetal movement is the only symptom felt by the mother.
- Peak systolic velocity of the middle cerebral artery by ultrasound and maternal blood tests are useful for diagnosis. Although it is a rare disease, urgent diagnosis and treatment are necessary.

M. Mitani (✉)
Fukuda Hospital, Kumamoto, Japan
e-mail: ikyoku@fukuda-hp.or.jp

Y. Matsuda
Tokyo Healthcare University, Hogashi-Gotanda, Shinagawa, Tokyo, Japan

Y. Matsuda (ed.), *Cerebral Palsy*, https://doi.org/10.1007/978-981-19-2217-6_18

1 Overview

Fetomaternal hemorrhage (FMH) is a condition in which fetal blood enters the intervillous space of the maternal side due to damage or abnormality of the placental villi, resulting in anemia due to blood loss in the fetus. Depending on the volume of fetal blood into the maternal circulation, fetal and neonatal complications may vary. In severe cases, severe anemia and circulatory failure may occur, leading to sequelae and death. Since hydrops typically does not develop until the Hb deficit is >7 g/dL, severe fetal anemia is generally considered to be Hb <7 g/dL [1].

In all pregnancies, a very small amount of fetal blood may enter the maternal circulation, but this is not a problem in most cases. The circulating blood volume of the fetal placenta is 30 mL at about 20 weeks' gestation and 80–125 mL/kg of fetal weight near the expected date of delivery [2]. In normal pregnancies, the frequency and volume of entry into the maternal circulation increase with the gestational weeks, with a frequency of 53% and an average of 0.07 mL in the first trimester, 53% and 0.08 mL in the second trimester, 72% and 0.13 mL in the third trimester, and 76% and 0.19 mL at delivery [3]. Although there are no clear criteria for FMH, traditionally, it has been defined as hemorrhage of ≥30 mL fetal blood into the maternal circulation, as this is the volume of Rh-positive whole fetal blood that is covered by a standard 300 μg dose of RhIG to prevent alloimmunization, and this frequency has been reported to be about 0.3% [1]. Severe cases are considered to be more than 80–150 mL or more than 20 mL/kg [4]. The frequency of FMH of more than 80 mL was reported to be 0.9/1000 cases, and that of more than 150 mL was reported to be 0.2/1000 cases [2].

2 Causes and Risk Factors

The cause of the FMH is still unknown. In placental pathology, placental infarction, retroplacental hematoma, pallor, edema, increased number of nucleated erythrocytes on the fetal blood side, and intravascular thrombus on the fetal side are more frequently observed in cases of FMH compared with normal cases, and these findings are reported to be more frequent in severe cases [2, 4]. It is thought that the barrier mechanism in the placenta is disrupted or permeability is increased, causing fetal blood to flow into the intervillous space from the high-pressure fetal circulation. It is not clear what determines whether such a leak in the placental barrier will remain small, heal entirely, or result in massive acute blood loss. One theory is that the thrombosis represented a protective mechanism to limit the extent of the FMH and that the thrombotic lesions therefore represented prior episodes of FMH [2].

Factors reported to be associated with FMH include race, region, external cephalic version, abdominal trauma, abruption, umbilical vein anomalies, chorioamnionitis (CAM), monochorionic amniotic twins, preeclampsia, placental tumors, amniocentesis, and fetal laser therapy. Of these, abruption, abdominal trauma, and the presence of placental tumors are strongly related to FMH [2, 5]. In 1999, Ghidini and Korker [6] summarized the reports of external cephalic version showing FMH occurred in 16 (2.6%) of 664 cases of external rotation. The time lapse between the procedure and the onset of the FMH is unknown, but 1/4 of these patients had abnormal cardiotocography (CTG), and some had acidemia.

The association between choriocarcinoma of the placenta and FMH has also been noted. In 2018, She et al. [7] summarized a report of 24 cases of choriocarcinoma of the placenta with FMH. There were six cases of intrauterine fetal death (IUFD), and among the surviving cases, there were mild to severe cases, and, of note, 20% had metastasis to the fetus. Therefore, when the FMH is observed, pathological search of the placenta is necessary, and attention should be paid to the presence of choriocarcinoma.

In 2016, Stroustrup et al. [5] conducted a retrospective study of 23 cases of FMH and 92 cases in the control group. They found that there was no association between race, maternal age, pregnancy complications (such as diabetes, maternal hypercoagulopathy, hypertensive disorders of pregnancy, multiple pregnancy, placenta previa, CAM, etc.) and FMH and that in the FMH group, there are many cases in which the mothers work outside the home. As the number of cases is small, it is not a clear risk factor at present. In a study of 20 cases of FMH in the "Japan Council for Quality Health Care, 10th Report on Prevention of Recurrence, The Japan Obstetric Compensation System for Cerebral Palsy, March 2020," no specific maternal background was found [8]. The number of cases of FMH is small, and it is difficult to conduct a large-scale study, and the search for risk factors and causes is insufficient. About 80% of cases of FMH have no known cause [2], and further investigation is needed.

3 Symptoms

The symptoms of the FMH are listed in Table 1 [2]. Although there are no specific symptoms, many pregnant women complain of decreased or absent fetal movements. In the "Report on Prevention of Recurrence," 58% of the reasons for visiting the hospital were "decreased or absent fetal movements," 21% were onset of labor pain, 11% were rupture of membrane, 5% were abdominal pain and bleeding, and the other 21% were asymptomatic [8].

The diagnosis of FMH is not easy to make based on symptoms alone, but CTG may be the key to detection. It is well known that fetal anemia presents with a sinusoidal pattern, but as shown in Tables 1 and 2, there are few typical cases and a variety of CTG findings. Therefore, it is not easy to diagnose FMH by CTG alone, but it is necessary to keep FMH in mind as one of the differential diseases in cases of FMH with nonreassuring fetal status (NRFS).

Table 1 Summary of symptoms from a review of 120 cases of FMH [2]

	N (%)
Neonatal anemia	45 (35.0)
Decreased or absent fetal movement	32 (26.7)
Fetal death	15 (12.5)
Fetal hydrops	9 (7.5)
Nonreassuring fetal status (other than sinusoidal FHR pattern)	8 (6.7)
Fetal growth restriction	4 (3.3)
Sinusoidal FHR pattern	2 (1.7)
Fetal atrial fibrillation	1 (0.8)
Maternal transfusion reaction	1 (0.8)
Unknown	6 (5.0)

Table 2 Cardiotocogram findings on admission in 20 cases of FMH (modified from [8])

Cardiotocogram findings	*N* (%)
Minimal or undetectable of fetal heart rate baseline variability	14 (77.8)
Late deceleration	8 (44.4)
Absence of acceleration	7 (38.9)
Sinusoidal pattern	6 (33.3)
Prolonged deceleration	3 (16.7)
Variable deceleration	1 (5.6)
Bradycardia	1 (5.6)
Atypical deceleration	1 (5.6)
Unknown	1 (5.6)

Case Presentation (Provided from the Japan Council for Quality Health Care, 10th Report on Prevention of Recurrence, The Japan Obstetric Compensation System for Cerebral Palsy, March 2020) [8]
A multiparous woman visited the hospital because of the loss of fetal movement on the previous day. An abnormal CTG was shown (Fig. 1), and a cesarean section was performed on the same day.

Infant information: umbilical artery blood pH, 7.0; BE, −14 mmol/L; and Hb, 1.1 g/dL. The Apgar score at 1 and 5 min were 1 and 2.

Maternal postpartum blood tests: fetal Hb: 3.2%.

4 Diagnostic Tests

4.1 Hemoglobin F (HbF)

Hemoglobin F (HbF) quantification by the Kleihauer-Betke test and flow cytometry are commonly used for definitive diagnosis overseas. HbF quantification by flow

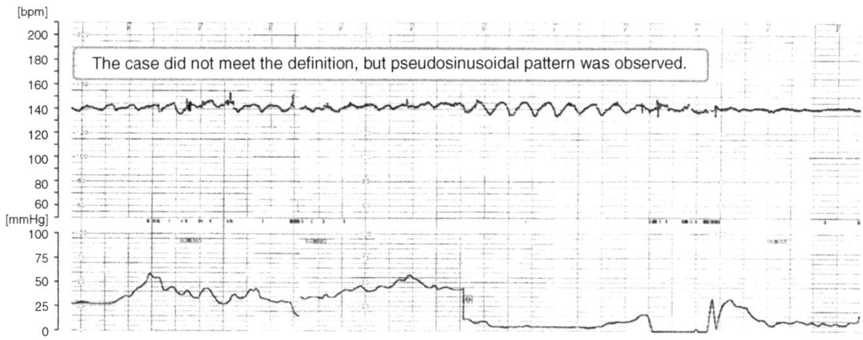

Fig. 1 Non-stress test on admission [8]

cytometry uses antibodies to fetal HbF to automatically and accurately measure the amount of fetal HbF and can distinguish between maternal and fetal HbF. In both methods, it is possible to calculate the entry volume of fetal blood by estimating the percentage of fetal blood and the maternal circulating blood volume.

In Japan, HbF is often measured by high-performance liquid chromatography (HPLC). The normal value is considered to be less than 1%, and it is elevated in diseases such as thalassemia, aplastic anemia, and leukemia. Maternal HbF is also measured by this method, and it has been reported that HbF by the HPLC method in normal pregnant women is 0.82 ± 0.25% in the first trimester, 0.66 ± 0.35% in the second trimester, 0.58 ± 0.38% in the third trimester, and 0.62 ± 0.31% 1 year after delivery [9]. In 1995, Tsuda et al. [10] measured maternal HbF values by the HPLC method in six patients with severe FMH (neonatal Hb: 2.3–7.1 g/dL). The authors reported that the maternal HbF values were 2.9–4.9%. In the "Report on Prevention of Recurrence," HbF was measured in all 20 cases, and HbF value was 1.1–10.0% (mean 5.4%) [8].

4.2 *Alpha-Fetoprotein*

Alpha-fetoprotein (AFP) is known to be elevated in FMH and is useful for diagnosis [11]. AFP was low in the early stages of pregnancy, but rose with gestational weeks of pregnancy, reached the highest level around 30–32 weeks' gestation, reached an average of 184–404 ng/mL, and then decreased again [12, 13]. The reference value of AFP in the FMH is not clear, and the "Report on Prevention of Recurrence" reported that AFP ranged from 236 to 9810 ng/mL (mean 4404.9 ng/mL) in 14 cases where it was measured [8].

Both of these methods are useful for diagnosis, but the problems are that it takes time to obtain the results and it is difficult to estimate the entry volume of fetal blood to maternal circulation at the bedside.

4.3 *Fetal Middle Cerebral Artery Peak Systolic Velocity (MCA-PSV)*

Fetal middle cerebral artery peak systolic velocity (MCA-PSV) is known to be useful in the diagnosis of fetal anemia and has been used to diagnose fetal anemia in pregnancies with blood type incompatibility. The sensitivity of MCA-PSV is 100% in the diagnosis of moderate or severe anemia, and the false-positive rate is reported to be 12% [14]. In 2017, Bellussi et al. [15] summarized 35 cases of FMH and MCA-PSV and reported that MCA-PSV was high in 34 of these cases, making it useful for diagnosis. Although it is difficult to estimate the amount of blood flow into the mother, it is useful as a rapid diagnostic method that can be performed at the bedside.

5 Management

When FMH is diagnosed, the treatment options are transfusion of blood to the fetus or delivery and neonatal care.

5.1 *Intrauterine Transfusion*

The only prenatal treatment for FMH may be improvement of anemia by intrauterine transfusion. In 2010, Wylie et al. [2] summarized 13 cases of intrauterine transfusion after diagnosis of FMH. They reported that one to five intrauterine transfusions were performed in each case, one case resulted in fetal death, two cases were delivered on the day of transfusion, two cases were delivered within 1 week after transfusion, and, in the remaining cases, the pregnancy could be prolonged for more than 1 week (range: 2–17 weeks). In 2019, Troia et al. [16] summarized 22 cases of intrauterine transfusion for FMH: 8 of 22 patients delivered within 72 h, of which 5 received multiple transfusions; 14 patients were able to prolong pregnancy beyond 72 h, of which 11 received multiple fetal transfusions (mean, 2.8 times; range, 1–8 times); and 2 patients had IUFD (mean, 2.8; range, 1–8). The mean time from the first transfusion to delivery in the remaining 12 patients was 53.6 days (range: 6–193 days). There were variable cases, from more than 10 weeks with a single transfusion to delivery within 72 h despite daily transfusions or IUFD, so the management of FMH is thought to be difficult.

In general, the following formulae provide fairly reliable estimates of the volume of blood needed for intrauterine transfusion.

$$\text{Intravascular transfusion} = \left(\text{target Hb} - \text{fetal Hb}\right) \times \text{fetal placental circulating blood volume} / \left(\text{donor Hb} - \text{target Hb}\right)$$

The fetal placental circulating blood volume is 125 mL/kg near the expected date, and the target Hb is about 17 g/dL [1, 3]. More than 20 mL/kg per transfusion is associated with fetal death, so several transfusions are necessary [1]. After transfusion, there is a risk of anemia again, and the fetus needs to be monitored, but transfusion of adult blood changes the viscosity of the blood and the blood flow rate. After intrauterine transfusion, it has been proposed to use a cut-off value of 1.69 MoM for severe anemia, with a false-positive rate of 6% [2].

5.1.1 Complications of Fetal Blood Transfusion Procedures

Complications of fetal transfusion procedures include NRFS, hemorrhage from the umbilical cord, hematoma, CAM, rupture of membrane, onset of labor, volume overload, and polycythemia, and fetal deaths have been reported to be 0.9–4.9% for all intrauterine transfusions [17]. The long-term prognosis of fetal blood transfusion cases has been reported to be favorable in maternal Rh(−) cases, but in FMH, the number of cases is small, and long-term prognosis is unknown [17, 18]. In the aforementioned report by Troia et al. [16] in 2019, two cases became IUFD, one with intraventricular hemorrhage and the other with hearing impairment. FMH has a small number of cases, so comparative studies are difficult. In addition, it is necessary to take into account that not all cases have been reported and the existence of unreported deaths and sequelae after fetal blood transfusion [2].

5.2 *Delivery or Fetal Transfusion?*

There are no definite criteria for the choice of delivery or intrauterine transfusion. Delivery is recommended after or near 37 weeks' gestation [11] and should also be considered if fetal hypoxia or acidemia is suspected on CTG. Intrauterine transfusion may be an option if the gestational age is early and there is enough time. Transportation to the tertiary center should also be considered, since the fetal blood transfusion requires specialized procedures and equipment.

It is also necessary to consult with the neonatologists and decide on the best course of action, taking into account the gestational age and the facilities of the hospital.

6 Cerebral Palsy and Related Conditions

In FMH, fetal blood loss leads to hypoxemia associated with circulatory failure and severe anemia, which can cause various complications such as cardiac failure, fetal hydrops, hypovolemic shock, IUFD, postnatal pulmonary hypertension, neurological sequelae, and neonatal death [2]. FMH accounts for 1.3–4.1% of all

IUFD cases [19–21], and the mortality rate in severe cases of FMH has been reported to be 26–42% [2, 21].

Complications and mortality are influenced by the entry volume, the speed of entry (chronic or acute), and the onset of gestational weeks [2]. In 2007, Rubod et al. reported that the mortality rate increased as the blood entry increased, and the mortality rate was 26% when the blood entry was 20 mL/kg or more, and 2/3 of the patients had IUFD when the blood entry was 80 mL/kg or more [21]. In animal experiments, it has been reported that if blood loss from the fetus is slow, it is compensated spontaneously, but if blood loss is rapid, hypoxia and acidemia occur, leading to death [2]. However, it is difficult to determine whether the FMH is chronic or acute from the clinical picture.

FMH is also a cause of cerebral palsy. In the 3 series reports combined, 2 of 98 surviving cases with long-term follow-up were reported to have cerebral palsy [2]. In the "Report on Prevention of Recurrence," 20 cases of cerebral palsy thought to be caused by FMH were recognized, which was reported to be 2.5% of all cases of cerebral palsy [8]. Although the exact frequency of cerebral palsy is unknown due to the small number of reported cases, it is considered to be an important cause of cerebral palsy. Intraventricular hemorrhage, periventricular leukomalacia, and cortical damage have been reported [16, 22].

7 Prevention of Cerebral Palsy

Regarding the FMH, the following recommendations have been made as fetal/perinatal management to prevent recurrence and improve the quality of obstetric care by the "Report on Prevention of Recurrence" as shown in Table 3 [8].

The cause of FMH is unknown in many cases, and its prevention and early detection are considered to be very difficult. We had better pay attention to causative events such as external rotation, maternal trauma, and placental tumors, which are currently reported as causes of FMH. Measurement of MCA-PSV and close

Table 3 Proposal of fetal management for prevention of recurrence and improvement of the quality of obstetric care according to the Report on Prevention of Recurrence (modified from [8])

(a) When a pregnant woman complains of decreased or absent fetal movement, the information is provided to the pregnant women in the outpatient clinic so as to contact the delivery institution.
(b) When a pregnant woman complains of decreased or absent fetal movement, confirm the fetal well-being by cardiotocogram and ultrasonography (biophysical profile score (BPS), amniotic fluid volume measurement, blood flow measurement, etc.).
(c) Become proficient in reading and responding to cardiotocogram by participating in in-hospital workshops and attending out-of-hospital workshops.
(d) If a sinusoidal pattern or loss of FHR variability is observed, the possibility of fetal anemia should be taken into consideration, and preparations should be made for maternal transport or rapid delivery, neonatal resuscitation, and neonatal management.

observation by CTG are necessary. However, it is unclear when these diseases cause FMH, and prevention and early detection are still difficult.

At present, the only possible management is not to overlook severe fetal anemia and treat it as soon as possible. It is necessary to keep in mind that FMH is a cause of decreased or absent fetal movements and that CTG findings of FMH may show various images other than the sinusoidal pattern. In Japan, there are few facilities that can diagnose FMH by maternal blood tests, so ultrasound measurement of MCA-PSV is useful for prompt diagnosis at the bedside. If fetal anemia is strongly suspected, delivery or fetal treatment should be considered, taking into account the condition of the fetus and the gestational weeks. If it is difficult to deal with, the patient should be transferred to a tertiary center. At present, no conclusion has been reached as to whether delivery or fetal therapy should be attempted, and the decision should be made at each facility.

References

1. Abbasi N, Johnson JA, Ryan G. Fetal anemia. Ultrasound Obstet Gynecol. 2017;50:145–53.
2. Wylie BJ, D'Alton ME. Fetomaternal hemorrhage. Obstet Gynecol. 2010;115:1039–51.
3. Cunningham FG, Leveno KJ, Bloom SL, et al. Fetal disorders. In: Williams obstetrics. 25th ed. New York: McGraw-Hill; 2019. p. 300–14.
4. Lewis NE, Marszalek L, Ernst LM. Placental pathologic features in fetomaternal hemorrhage detected by flow cytometry. Pediatr Dev Pathol. 2017;20:142–51.
5. Stroustrup A, Plafkin C, Tran TA, et al. Demographic and behavioral predictors of severe fetomaternal hemorrhage: a case-control study. Neonatology. 2016;109:248–54.
6. Ghidini A, Korker V. Fetal complication after external cephalic version at term: case report and literature review. J Maternal Fetal Med. 1999;8:190–2.
7. She Q, Cheng Z, El-Chaar D, et al. Intraplacental choriocarcinoma coexisting with fetomaternal hemorrhage: case report, chemotherapy management, and literature review. Medicine. 2018;97:e9977.
8. Japan Council for Quality Health Care. 6th Report on prevention of recurrence, the Japan Obstetric Compensation System for Cerebral Palsy. Tokyo: Japan Council for Quality Health Care; 2016. Japanese.
9. Yamada T, Morikawa M, Yamada T, et al. Changes in hemoglobin F levels in pregnant women unaffected by clinical fetomaternal hemorrhage. Clin Chim Acta. 2013;415:124–7.
10. Tsuda H, Matsumoto M, Sutoh Y, et al. Massive fetomaternal hemorrhage. Int J Obstet Gynecol. 1995;50:47–9.
11. Maier JT, Schalinski E, Schneider W, et al. Fetomaternal hemorrhage, an update: review of the literature and an illustrative case. Arch Gynecol Obstet. 2015;292:595–602.
12. Hay DM, Forrester PI, Hancock RL, et al. Maternal serum alpha-fetoprotein in normal pregnancy. Br J Obstet Gynecol. 1976;83:534–8.
13. Khoo SK, Chang A, Mackay EV. A comparison of maternal serum levels of alpha-fetoprotein in normal and pre-eclamptic pregnancies. Br J Obstet Gynecol. 1978;85:914–20.
14. Mari G, Deter RL, Carpenter RL, et al. Noninvasive diagnosis by doppler ultrasonography of fetal anemia due to maternal red-cell alloimmunization. Collaborative group for doppler assessment of the blood velocity in anemic fetuses. N Engl J Med. 2000;342:9–14.
15. Bellussi F, Perolo A, Ghi T, et al. Diagnosis of severe fetomaternal hemorrhage with fetal cerebral doppler: case series and systematic review. Fetal Diag Ther. 2017;41:1–7.

16. Troia L, Al-Kouatly HB, McCurdy R, et al. The recurrence risk of fetomaternal hemorrhage. Fetal Diagn Ther. 2019;45:1–12.
17. Lindenburg ITM, van Kamp IL, Oepkes D. Intrauterine blood transfusion: current indications and associated risks. Fetal Diagn Ther. 2014;36:263–71.
18. Van Klink JMM, Koopman HM, Oepkes D, et al. Long-term neurodevelopmental outcome after intrauterine transfusion for fetal anemia. Early Hum Dev. 2011;87:589–93.
19. Korteweg FJ, Erwich JJHM, Timmer A, et al. Evaluation of 1025 fetal deaths: a proposed diagnostic workup. Am J Obstet Gynecol. 2012;206(53):e1–12.
20. O'Leary BD, Walsh CA, Fitzgerald JM, et al. The contribution of massive fetomaternal hemorrhage to antepartum stillbirth: a 25-year cross- sectional study. Acta Obstet Gynecol Scand. 2015;94:1354–8.
21. Rubod C, Deruele P, Goueff FL, et al. Long-term prognosis for infants after massive fetomaternal hemorrhage. Obstet Gynecol. 2007;110:256–60.
22. Tagaya M, Fujimaki H, Shimizu S, et al. Brain damage caused by severe fetomaternal hemorrhage. Pediatr Int. 2010;52:301–4.

Cases Associate with Umbilical Cord

Junichi Hasegawa and Chika Homma

Contents

Summary

- The etiology of cerebral palsy (CP) is often unknown, but one known cause is brain damage caused by hypoxia before and after birth.
- In particular, hypoxia during labor is often monitored by cardiotocogram (CTG) and is known to be closely related to abnormal findings on CTG.
- As for placental and umbilical cord abnormalities, they often elicit this CTG abnormality.

J. Hasegawa (✉) · C. Homma
Department of Obstetrics and Gynecology, St. Marianna University School of Medicine, Kawasaki, Kanagawa, Japan
e-mail: hasejun@marianna-u.ac.jp

Y. Matsuda (ed.), *Cerebral Palsy*, https://doi.org/10.1007/978-981-19-2217-6_19

- In the event of a highly hypoxic situation, such as placental abruption or umbilical cord prolapse, even if the baby is delivered quickly, there will be severe acidosis in the neonates.
- In fact, most cases of CP have a strong acidosis of less than 7 pH in the umbilical artery blood.

In this section, we describe the pathogenesis and problems of various cord factors associated with the development of cerebral palsy (CP) and discuss strategies to prevent CP using ultrasonography and cardiotocogram (CTG).

1 Problems with Umbilical Cord Problems

The umbilical cord is the only lifeline that transports the materials necessary to maintain life in utero. Because of its long and thin nature, the umbilical cord can cause problems. These include acute fetal heart rate abnormalities, non-reassuring fetal status (NRFS), and fetal death, as well as chronic fetal growth restriction (FGR).

In addition, there are two main causes of umbilical cord problems. One is that the normal umbilical cord accidentally suffers from inadequate blood flow, and the other is that it has a morphological abnormality (umbilical cord abnormality) caused by a problem in the development of the placenta or umbilical cord. The former includes umbilical cord prolapse, umbilical cord entanglement, true knot, etc. The latter includes velamentous cord insertion, hyper-coiled cord, and single umbilical artery.

2 Pathophysiology of Various Umbilical Cord Problems

2.1 Umbilical Cord Prolapse

Umbilical cord prolapse is a condition in which free loop of the umbilical cord prolapses beyond the presenting part of the fetus at the time of rupture of membrane, resulting in a rapid deterioration of umbilical cord circulation due to the narrow birth canal and the fetus. Therefore, the disease-free survival rate is only 87.5% even after 36 weeks of gestation [1]. If it occurs during delivery, the prognosis tends to be relatively good if it is recognized early by CTG and the baby is delivered rapidly. However, if it occurs at home and is recognized late, or if the time between the occurrence of cord prolapse and the delivery of the baby exceeds 25 min, the disease-free survival rate decreases [1].

It is less common in the cephalic position, where the space between the advanced part of the fetus and the birth canal is narrow, and more common in the transverse position, pelvic position, and multiple pregnancies, where there is more space between the advanced part and the birth canal. However, the CTG abnormality in the cephalic position is often more rapid and severe than that in the non-cephalic position because of the narrow space between the fetal head and the pelvis and the compression by the rigid fetal head.

In the case of amniotic fluid overload, the advanced part of the fetus floats in the amniotic cavity, and the umbilical cord is likely to enter the gap between the presenting part and the uterine wall. In cases of early preterm labor and cervical insufficiency, the amniotic cavity is relatively wide in relation to the fetus, and cord prolapse is likely to occur.

The decrease in fetal heart rate during umbilical cord prolapse is not only due to compression of the umbilical vessels but also due to vasoconstriction caused by a decrease in the temperature of the prolapsed umbilical cord, which worsens with time.

2.2 *Umbilical Cord Anomaly as a Developmental Abnormality*

2.2.1 Abnormality of the Umbilical Cord Attachment on the Placenta

The umbilical cord is usually attached to the center or slightly lateral side of the placenta, but in the case of velamentous cord insertion, the umbilical cord, which has normal Wharton's jelly, is attached to the membrane, and aberrant vessels (velamentous vessels), which lack Wharton's jelly, are seen connecting the placental parenchyma. When these velamentous vessels run near the inner uterine opening, it is called a vasa previa.

Abnormal polarity during implantation of the fertilized egg and trophotropism during formation of the placenta from the chorionic villus are thought to be involved in the development of umbilical cord placental insertion [2–5], which are often complicated by other placental anomalies because the placenta is formed from the chorionic villus at a distance from the site of the connecting stalk, which is the origin of the umbilical cord [6].

Velamentous cord insertion is the presence of portions of the omental vasculature that are not protected by Wharton's jelly, which can lead to abnormal pregnancy and delivery. The velamentous vessels are fragile and easily compressed by uterine contractions and fetal movements. In a study of delivered placentas, the frequency of NRFS is higher when the omental vessels are longer or when the placenta has greater structural abnormalities [7]. The rupture of the velamentous vessels when the rupture of membrane may result in sudden fetal death. The risk is especially high in vasa previa because the velamentous vessels are located near the inner uterine opening [8]. It is thought that anterior vessels and velamentous cord insertion located on the lower uterine segment are deeply related to NRFS and FGR not only because they are susceptible to the compression of the velamentous vessels by the advanced part of the fetus but also because of the structural abnormalities of the placenta.

2.2.2 Abnormalities of the Umbilical Cord Coiling (Hyper-coiled Cord and Hypo-coiled Cord)

The moderate coiling structure of the umbilical cord is thought to protect the umbilical vessels from external forces such as torsion, traction, and compression [9]. In the case of hyper-coiled cord and hypo-coiled cord, the umbilical cord is vulnerable to traction, compression, and torsion, and blood flow disturbance is likely to occur [10–12]. In hyper-coiled cord, congestion of blood flow is likely to occur. If congestion occurs in the umbilical cord blood flow, the fetus might fall into NRFS. It is also often seen in growth-restricted fetuses due to chronic congestion of the umbilical vessels. It is also thought that hypo-coiled cord can easily lead to a drop in umbilical venous pressure and blood flow insufficiency [9, 13]. It has been pointed out that such chronic congestion in the umbilical vein may cause microthrombi in the fetal thrombotic vasculopathy (FTV), which may affect the cerebral blood vessels and worsen the neurological prognosis [14].

Cases of FGR associated with hyper-coiled cord often result in fetal death. On the other hand, hyper-coiled cord and hypo-coiled cord often cause acute insufficiency of umbilical cord blood flow in a normally growing infant, leading to fetal death. In particular, in cases of fetal death due to hyper-coiled cord, constriction of the umbilical cord is often observed. Constriction of the umbilical ring due to hyper-coiled cord is a common finding in fetal death. Although most cases of hyper-coiled cord and hypo-coiled cord pass without any problems, they are often associated with abnormal fetal heart rate pattern at delivery.

3 Current Status of Cerebral Palsy Occurrence due to Umbilical Cord Problems

A study was conducted to clarify the causal relationship between maternal background, obstetric complications, abnormal deliveries, obstetric procedures, and other perinatal factors associated with the development of CP in cases approved for the Japan Obstetric Compensation System for Cerebral Palsy. A case-cohort study was conducted using 175 cases of CP and 17,475 cases of CP from the Japanese Society of Obstetrics and Gynecology (JSOG) Perinatal Database as controls. For comparison, we matched singleton births from 2009 to 2011, cases with 33 weeks or more of gestation and 2000 g or more of birth weight, hospital cases, and cases excluding congenital and neonatal factors [15].

The perinatal events considered to be the main cause of the development of CP in the cerebral palsy cases were placental abnormalities (31%), umbilical cord abnormalities (15%), maternal complications (10%), and neonatal complications (1%). Multivariate analysis showed that CP was associated with rapid delivery due to NRFS [risk ratio (RR) 37.182 [95% confidence interval (95% CI): 20.028–69.032]], uterine rupture [RR 24.770 (95% CI: 6.006–102.160)], and placental abruption [RR 20.891 (95%. The risk of rupture of the uterus [RR 24.770 (95% CI: 6.006–102.160)] and preterm labor [RR 3.153 (95% CI: 2.024–4.911)] was significantly higher. On the other hand, head presentation [RR 0.199 (95% CI: 0.088–0.450)] and scheduled cesarean section [RR 0.236 (95% CI: 0.067–0.828)] were reduced risk of CP [15].

Among the known causes of cerebral palsy, the risk of cerebral palsy is high in cases where rapid delivery is required, as in our results. As mentioned above, umbilical cord prolapse leading to rapid cord blood flow failure and the presence of cord abnormalities predispose to NRFS. The key is the use of appropriate CTG, their interpretation, and rapid and safe delivery when necessary.

During normal labor, placental perfusion is decreased due to strong uterine contractions. Therefore, the fetus is subjected to considerable stress just before delivery as it passes through the narrow pelvic cavity, and abnormal waveforms appear on CTG even in the normal course. This is especially true when there is an abnormal umbilical cord, but even in the absence of an abnormal umbilical cord abnormalities, abnormal waveforms often appear on CTG near the time of delivery due to compression of the umbilical cord and/or fetus. When the caregiver decides immediate delivery including vacuum extraction and/or uterine fundal pressure maneuver due to such CTG abnormalities in the delivery room, if the fetus cannot be delivered quickly after one or two such procedures, forceps delivery or cesarean section should be attempted. However, even in some cases when vacuum delivery and/or uterine fundal pressure maneuver fail, these procedure was continued to be performed strongly. In fact, there are not a few such cases in cerebral palsy cases applied to the Japan Obstetric Compensation System for Cerebral Palsy.

Uterine fundal pressure maneuver and continuous vacuum extraction of the fetal head worsen the uterus-placenta-fetal circulation. The intermittent phase of labor is a time to restore the uteroplacental circulation, but these inappropriate procedures that eliminate the intermittent phase may induce fetal hypoxia and acidosis. It is necessary to prepare in advance for NRFS, which requires rapid delivery, and to respond appropriately when it occurs.

4 The Prevention of CP due to Umbilical Cord Abnormalities

4.1 Limitations of CTG Management

Fetus is considered as normal condition when the fetal heart rate indicates nomocardia, with baseline variability and acceleration, without deceleration. On the other hand, persistent bradycardia, loss of variability, and recurrent (late or prolonged) deceleration are findings that strongly suggest acidosis. Although CTG is excellent in demonstrating fetal reassuring, it is difficult to predict the presence of acidosis based on abnormal findings. The actual diagnosis of NRFS and the decision for rapid delivery are left to the judgment of each physician.

In the twentieth century, the fetal Doppler was developed, and it became possible to measure the fetal heart rate in real time and to predict fetal hypoxia from the CTG, which was expected to improve the perinatal prognosis. However, there is an epidemiological report that not only the frequency of cerebral palsy remained unchanged but also the frequency of cesarean section increased due to false-positive CTG [16].

Eighty-eight percent of infants determined to have developed cerebral palsy due to hypoxia associated with an abnormal morphology of the umbilical cord have abnormal findings on CTG at delivery [17]. It is known that abnormal CTG waveforms in the presence of an abnormal umbilical cord are more likely to appear early in delivery [18, 19]. Although the onset of cerebral palsy is also associated with events that result in hypoxia during delivery, it is not uncommon for events to occur before delivery. There are limitations in reducing cerebral palsy related to umbilical cord anomalies by CTG only at the time of delivery.

4.2 Perinatal Management for Pregnant Women Using Ultrasound and CTG

Ultrasonography and CTG are the only established modalities that allow obstetricians to evaluate the condition of the fetus and its appendages in the management of pregnancy and delivery. We advocate screening for umbilical cord anomalies using ultrasonography and management of pregnancy and delivery according to the diagnosis of the umbilical cord abnormality so that we can respond promptly to NRFS due to acute umbilical cord problems at least at the time of delivery [20, 21].

It has been reported that the survival rate of infants with vasa previa diagnosed before delivery was 97%, whereas that of infants without preeclampsia was 44% [22]. Especially in the case of vasa previa, ultrasound diagnosis of them during pregnancy and scheduled cesarean section before the rupture of membrane can save fetuses with vasa previa. The same can be considered for other umbilical cord abnormalities.

If the fetus has an abnormal umbilical cord, it should be considered a high-risk delivery and treated with induction of labor, preparing cesarean section, and continuous CTG (Figs. 1 and 2, Table 1). As described in the "Guidelines for Obstetrics and Gynecology-Obstetrics Edition 2020" [23], early response to abnormal waveforms can be performed according to the situation of the institution in cases of ultrasound diagnosis of placental and umbilical cord abnormalities (Fig. 2, Table 1).

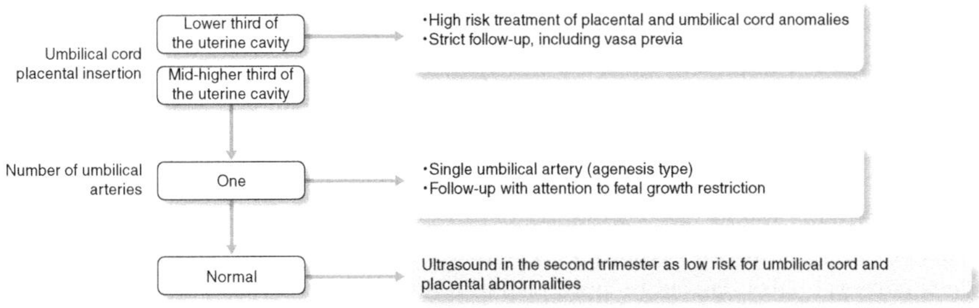

Fig. 1 Screening for umbilical cord abnormalities in early pregnancy [21]

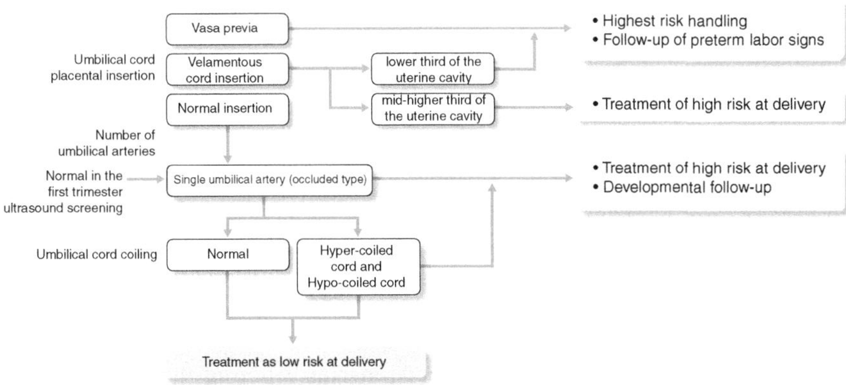

Fig. 2 Screening for umbilical cord abnormalities in mid-pregnancy [21]

Table 1 Ultrasound screening of the umbilical cord abnormalities before delivery [21]

Descending umbilical cord	Treat as highest risk
Nuchal cord	More than three times is treated as high risk at delivery
Reconfirmation of the hyper-coiled cord	Treatment of high risk at delivery
Reconfirmation of the single umbilical artery (occluded type)	Treatment of high risk at delivery

4.3 Avoidance of Umbilical Cord Prolapse During Delivery

As mentioned above, the occurrence of umbilical cord prolapse increases the likelihood of the development of cerebral palsy. We advocate preventing umbilical cord prolapse as much as possible and detecting it when the descending umbilical cord. We believe that this risk can be greatly reduced by detecting and responding to the prolapsed umbilical cord before the rupture of membrane. We recommend the practice of checking the position of the umbilical cord with transvaginal ultrasonography.

When medical treatment involves lifting the advanced part of the fetus upward, iatrogenic descending umbilical cord or prolapse may occur. Care should be taken during internal examinations, artificial rupture of the membranes, and the use of metroirintel to dilate the uterine cervix. Large-volume metroirintels are associated with much higher risk of cord prolapse, but even small-volume are not without risk [24]. Performing ultrasonography before and after these medical procedures may reduce cerebral palsy caused by cord prolapse during delivery. In addition, cervical ripening agents (dinoprostone vaginal tablet) are expected to reduce cord prolapse in the future, as they replace instrumental cervical ripening methods such as metroirintel [25].

4.4 Appropriate Response to Umbilical Cord Prolapse

If umbilical cord prolapse occurs, an emergency cesarean section should be performed because of the sudden compression of the umbilical cord between the advanced part of the fetus and the birth canal, resulting in NRFS. An emergency cesarean section (Grade A cesarean section) is indicated in facilities where this is possible. The longer the time between diagnosis and delivery of the infant (more than 20 min), the worse the prognosis becomes, so the baby should be delivered as soon as possible [1].

When an umbilical cord prolapse occurs, manual return of the umbilical cord back into the uterus is often performed, but this is counterproductive. Touching the umbilical cord not only causes umbilical cord compression but also induces vasoconstriction of the umbilical vessels [26]. The decrease in fetal heart rate at the time of umbilical cord prolapse is due to vasospasm caused by the decrease in temperature of the evacuated umbilical cord, in addition to the compression of the umbilical cord.

During the preparation and transfer of the cesarean section, the infant should be elevated by pushing up the advanced part of the fetus with the internal examination finger to make a gap without touching the umbilical cord, and the infant should be placed in the chest-knee position.

References

1. Hasegawa J, Sekizawa A, Ikeda T, et al. Clinical risk factors for poor neonatal outcomes in umbilical cord prolapse. J Matern Fetal Neonatal Med. 2016;29:1652–6.
2. Hasegawa J, Nakamura M, Sekizawa A, et al. Prediction of risk for vasa previa at 9–13 weeks' gestation. J Obstet Gynaecol Res. 2011;37:1346–51.
3. Hasegawa J, Matsuoka R, Ichizuka K, et al. Cord insertion into the lower third of the uterus in the first trimester is associated with placental and umbilical cord abnormalities. Ultrasound Obstet Gynecol. 2006;28:183–6.

4. Hasegawa J. Taiban/saitai ijyou no hassyou to byoutai mechanism no chouonpa hasseigakuteki kenkyuu [Ultrasonographic embryological study of the pathogenesis and pathological mechanisms of placental and umbilical cord anomalies]. Acta Obstet Gynaecol Japonica. 2014;66:2559–65. Japanese.
5. Hasegawa J. Sonoembryological evaluations of the development of placenta previa and velamentous cord insertion. J Obstet Gynaecol Res. 2015;41:1–5.
6. Monie IW. Velamentous insertion of the cord in early pregnancy. Am J Obstet Gynecol. 1965;93:276–81.
7. Hasegawa J, Matsuoka R, Ichizuka K, et al. Velamentous cord insertion and atypical variable decelerations with no accelerations. Int J Gynaecol Obstet. 2005;90:26–30.
8. Catanzarite V, Maida C, Thomas W, et al. Prenatal sonographic diagnosis of vasa previa: ultrasound findings and obstetric outcome in ten cases. Ultrasound Obstet Gynecol. 2001;18:109–15.
9. Degani S, Lewinsky RM, Berger H, et al. Sonographic estimation of umbilical coiling index and correlation with Doppler flow characteristics. Obstet Gynecol. 1995;86:990–3.
10. de Laat MW, Franx A, Bots ML, et al. Umbilical coiling index in normal and complicated pregnancies. Obstet Gynecol. 2006;107:1049–55.
11. Rana J, Ebert GA, Kappy KA. Adverse perinatal outcome in patients with an abnormal umbilical coiling index. Obstet Gynecol. 1995;85:573–7.
12. Strong TH Jr, Jarles DL, Vega JS, et al. The umbilical coiling index. Am J Obstet Gynecol. 1994;170:29–32.
13. Di Naro E, Ghezzi F, Raio L, et al. Umbilical cord morphology and pregnancy outcome. Eur J Obstet Gynecol Reprod Biol. 2001;96:150–7.
14. Redline RW, Boyd T, Campbell V, et al. Maternal vascular underperfusion: nosology and reproducibility of placental reaction patterns. Pediatr Dev Pathol. 2004;7:237–49.
15. Hasegawa J, Toyokawa S, Ikenoue T, et al. Relevant obstetric factors for cerebral palsy: from the nationwide obstetric compensation system in Japan. PLoS One. 2016;11:e0148122.
16. Nelson KB, Dambrosia JM, Ting TY, et al. Uncertain value of electronic fetal monitoring in predicting cerebral palsy. N Engl J Med. 1996;334:613–8.
17. Japan Council for Quality Health Care. 6th Report on prevention of recurrence, the Japan Obstetric Compensation System for Cerebral Palsy. Tokyo: Japan Council for Quality Health Care; 2016. Japanese.
18. Hasegawa J, Matsuoka R, Ichizuka K, et al. Do fetal heart rate deceleration patterns during labor differ between various umbilical cord. J Perinat Med. 2009;37:276–80.
19. Hasegawa J, Matsuoka R, Ichizuka K, et al. Atypical variable deceleration in the first stage of labor is a characteristic fetal heart-rate pattern for. J Obstet Gynaecol Res. 2009;35:35–9.
20. Takita H, Hasegawa J, Arakaki T, et al. Antenatal ultrasound screening using a check list before delivery for predicting a non-reassuring fetal status during labor. J Matern Fetal Neonatal Med. 2018;31:1–6.
21. Hasegawa J. Ultrasound screening of umbilical cord abnormalities and delivery management. Placenta. 2018;62:66–78.
22. Oyelese Y, Catanzarite V, Prefumo F, et al. Vasa previa: the impact of prenatal diagnosis on outcomes. Obstet Gynecol. 2004;103:937–42.
23. Japan Society of Obstetrics and Gynecology, editor/supervised. Sanfujinka Shinryou Guideline Sankahen [Guidelines for obstetrics and gynecology—obstetrics]. 2020 ed. Tokyo: Japan Society of Obstetrics and Gynecology Secretariat; 2020. Japanese.
24. Hasegawa J, Sekizawa A, Ikeda T, et al. The use of balloons for uterine cervical ripening is associated with an increased risk of umbilical cord prolapse: population based questionnaire survey in Japan. BMC Pregnancy Childbirth. 2015;15:4.
25. Hasegawa J, Sekizawa A, Arakaki T, et al. Declined use of cervical ripening balloon did not reduce the incidence of umbilical cord prolapse in Japan. Obstet Gynaecol Res. 2020;46:1349–54.
26. Barrett JM. Funic reduction for the management of umbilical cord prolapse. Am J Obstet Gynecol. 1991;165:654–7.

Intrapartum Hypoxia

Koichiro Shimoya and Mika Sugihara

Contents

K. Shimoya (✉) · M. Sugihara
Department of Obstetrics and Gynecology 1, Kawasaki Medical School, Kurashiki, Okayama, Japan
e-mail: shimoya@med.kawasaki-m.ac.jp

Y. Matsuda (ed.), *Cerebral Palsy*, https://doi.org/10.1007/978-981-19-2217-6_20

Summary

- In both fetuses and neonates, hypoxia progressively exacerbates respiratory and metabolic acidemia and tissue acidosis. This tissue acidosis is associated with multiple organ failure and, although rare, leads to hypoxic-ischemic encephalopathy with subsequent neurologic damage.
- In the past, it was thought that most cerebral palsy was caused by hypoxia during delivery, but now it is thought that only about 1/5 of cerebral palsy is caused by hypoxia during delivery. However, it is still one of the most important causes of cerebral palsy, and it is necessary to reduce the number of cases of cerebral palsy by appropriate delivery management and neonatal resuscitation.

1 An Overview of Parturient Hypoxia

Due to advances in perinatal care, our country has one of the lowest perinatal mortality rates in the world. Cerebral palsy is defined as "permanent but changeable motor and postural abnormalities based on non-progressive lesions of the brain occurring between conception and the neonatal period (within 4 weeks of birth), excluding progressive disease, transient movement disorders, and motor developmental delay that is expected to normalize in the future." Table 1 shows the names of diagnoses in the neonatal period in the "10th Report on Prevention of Recurrence, The Japan Obstetric Compensation System for Cerebral Palsy" [1]. 41.4% of the 2457 cases examined were diagnosed as hypoxic-ischemic encephalopathy. This system covers cerebral palsy equivalent to Level 1 or 2 of the Physical Disability Certificate, which is not caused by congenital or neonatal factors, for children who meet certain weight and gestational weeks, and the scope of application has been further expanded for children born after January 2015. Although not all cerebral palsy cases were examined, hypoxia is one of the causes of cerebral palsy in children.

The incidence of cerebral palsy was reported to be 1.7 per 1000 live births according to the "Report of Epidemiological Survey on the Actual Condition of Children with Cerebral Palsy" in October 2018 [2]. According to this report, hypoxic-ischemic encephalopathy accounted for 18.2% of the cases, as shown in Table 1. Although neonatal pseudoparalysis was observed in 50.2% of cases, not all neonatal pseudoparalysis is considered to be caused by hypoxia, because it is caused by various factors. In the past, it was believed that cerebral palsy was caused during delivery, which led to medical trials and contributed to the exhaustion of perinatal care, but hypoxia during delivery is thought to be the cause of only about 1/5 of all cases. These reports are consistent with Nelson et al.'s report that the prevalence of cerebral palsy in the United States was 2 per 1000 and that perinatal paralysis occurred in only 1/5 of children with cerebral palsy [3].

Table 1 Diseases and other conditions considered to be risk factors for cerebral palsy (231 cases) [2]

	Diseases considered to be risk factors, etc.	Number of events (e.g., accidents, crimes, meetings, housing starts, hits on a web page)	Percentage (%)
Prepartum	Cerebral malformation	31	13.4
	Chromosomal abnormality	15	6.5
	Genetic abnormality	10	4.3
	Inborn errors of metabolism	1	0.4
	Other congenital anomalies	24	10.4
	Intrauterine infection	16	6.9
(In the) birthing process	Neonatal paralysis	116	50.2
	Fetal aspiration syndrome	7	3.0
	Intracranial hemorrhage	41	17.7
	Hypoxic-ischemic encephalopathy (brain damage from lack of oxygen)	42	18.2
	Periventricular leukomalacia (leucomalacia)	66	28.6
	Cerebral infarction	10	4.3
	Respiratory distress syndrome	61	26.4
	Neonatal transient hyperventilation	20	8.7
Postpartum	Meningitis	4	1.7
	Encephalitis	3	1.3
	ALTE	10	4.3
	Abuse	1	0.4
	Other trauma	1	0.4
	Other diseases, etc.	24	10.4

ALTE apparent life-threatening event

Table 2 Conditions causing fetal hypoxia during delivery

- Umbilical cord prolapse (umbilical cord ptosis)
- Hypertonic contraction
- Uterine rupture
- Placental abruption
- Supine hypotension syndrome
- Maternal convulsions, cardiac arrest
- Hypotension due to epidural or spinal subarachnoid anesthesia
- Amniotic fluid embolism
- Placental insufficiency

Hypoxia, which can lead to hypoxic-ischemic encephalopathy, can occur during pregnancy, labor, or the postpartum period (neonatal period). Table 2 lists the conditions that may cause hypoxia during delivery. Many of these conditions occur acutely or suddenly, and it is often difficult to deal with them.

2 Pathophysiology Associated with Cerebral Palsy

The exchange of substances in utero takes place between the mother and the body via the placenta. Oxygen is also supplied transplacentally and diffuses into the fetal blood. Gas exchange is carried out by maternal blood flowing into the uterine arteries, spiral arteries, and intervillous spaces on the maternal side and by umbilical cord blood flow from the fetal side into the umbilical arteries and intravillous capillaries.

In the fetal period, the majority of hemoglobin is composed of hemoglobin F, which has a higher affinity for oxygen than in the adult, and thus higher oxygen saturation can be obtained even at lower partial pressures of oxygen than in maternal blood. The fetal hemoglobin has a higher oxygen saturation and hemoglobin concentration than the maternal hemoglobin, so that the fetal arterial oxygen content and oxygen supply to peripheral tissues are maintained. The fetus removes carbon dioxide by placental circulation, but when the ability to remove carbon dioxide is reduced, H_2CO_3 accumulates, causing respiratory acidemia with no increase in organic acids. Organic acids, such as lactic acid, increase due to impaired gas exchange and anaerobic glycolysis in the placenta. The accumulation of these organic acids is called metabolic acidemia. In metabolic acidemia, HCO_3^- is decreased because bicarbonate is used to buffer organic acids; the increase in carbonic acid accompanied by the increase in organic acids due to the decrease in HCO_3^- is a factor in mixed acidemia. Hypoxia during parturition leads to a gradual exacerbation of respiratory to metabolic acidemia and then tissue acidosis. This tissue acidosis leads to hypoxic-ischemic encephalopathy, which is associated with multiple organ failure and subsequent neurologic damage.

3 Conditions That Can Cause Fetal Hypoxia During Delivery

The conditions that cause parturient hypoxia listed in Table 2 are outlined below.

3.1 Umbilical Cord Compression

Compression of the umbilical cord causes hypoxia in the fetus. Variable deceleration of cardiotocogram (CTG) may be observed due to vagal reflex caused by the interruption of blood flow. When cord compression (pressure change) occurs frequently, prolonged transient bradycardia appears because recovery of heart rate is delayed because it takes time to restore blood flow even after the compression is released.

3.2 Prolapse of the Umbilical Cord and Forelying of the Umbilical Cord

Prolapse of the umbilical cord is defined as the prolapse of the umbilical cord after rupture of the membranes prior to the advanced part of the fetus, passing through the uterine opening and suspending in the vaginal or interpubic space. It is more likely to occur in the breech presentation, especially in the footling presentation, when there is a wide gap between the advanced part of the fetus and the lower part of the uterus. It is also more likely to occur in cases of spontaneous or artificial rupture of the membranes before the baby's head has entered the pelvis, when the metreurynter (obstetrical balloon) used for cervical dilation has prolapsed. After spontaneous water or artificial rupture of the membranes, it is necessary to perform an internal examination to check for prolapse of the umbilical cord. When cord prolapse occurs, the mother may be asymptomatic, but the CTG show a sudden deceleration or bradycardia unrelated to labor pain. When such an abnormal fetal heart rate pattern is observed, it is important to first check for the presence of an umbilical cord in the cervical canal or vagina by speculum examination and then to check for the palpable pulsation of the umbilical cord by internal examination. In addition, if necessary, ultrasonography should be used to confirm the presence or absence of umbilical cord prolapse. (For details, see the chapter on "Umbilical Cord Factors.")

3.3 Hypertonic Contractions

Hypertonic contraction is a condition of excessive contractions of the uterine muscles. It can also occur in spontaneous labor, but is most often seen with the administration of uterotonics. It is relatively easy to diagnose by checking the CTG and the complaint of the pregnant woman. Maternal blood flow to the placenta through the spiral artery is obstructed by uterine contractions, resulting in fetal hypoplasia. If a uterine contractile drug is being administered, it should be discontinued or halved, and if necessary, an inhibitor of uterine contractions should be considered.

3.4 Uterine Rupture

Rupture of the uterus is a relatively uncommon but critical condition for both mother and fetus. It rarely occurs during pregnancy and most often during delivery. It is classified as either non-scarring or scarring rupture. The most common risk factor is rupture of a scarred uterus with a previous cesarean section. Risk factors for non-scarring uterine rupture are multiple and often difficult to predict, including high fertility, macrosomia, dystocia, and trauma (e.g., rapid labor, hypertonic contraction, uterine fundal pressure). In order to predict uterine rupture, it is important to comprehensively evaluate the symptoms, clinical findings, and findings of the CTG. Although it is difficult to predict uterine rupture in patients with sudden onset of uterine rupture, uterine rupture should be suspected and responded to when several types of deceleration, such as late or variable deceleration, precede the appearance of prolonged deceleration. When fetal bradycardia or maternal shock symptoms appear with sudden and persistent abdominal pain, or when fetal heart rate suddenly fails and labor pain disappears, rupture of the uterus should be suspected and treated. Prepare for cesarean section while performing systemic management of the mother, such as transfusion of fluids and blood.

3.5 Placental Abruption

Placental abruption is defined as the separation of the placenta from its normal position, i.e., attached to the uterine body, from the uterine wall before the delivery of the fetus during pregnancy or during the course of labor. Risk factors include a previous history of placental abruption, gestational hypertension, and trauma. Symptoms include genital bleeding, uterine contractions, lower abdominal pain, hardening of the abdominal wall called plate-like hardness, and bloody amniotic fluid. However, symptoms such as genital hemorrhage, uterine contractions, and lower abdominal pain are nonspecific and are also seen in imminent preterm labor, making diagnosis based on symptoms difficult. The most useful diagnostic tool is the CTG. Because of acute placental insufficiency, a decrease in baseline variability, deceleration, and prolonged bradycardia may occur. If we suspect placental abruption based on the CTG and clinical symptoms, we consider emergency cesarean section or rapid delivery by suction or forceps depending on the progress of delivery.

See the chapter on "Premature Separation of the Normal Placenta" for more information.

3.6 Maternal Respiratory and Circulatory Abnormalities (Supine Hypotension Syndrome, Cardiac Arrest)

One of the most common abnormalities of maternal respiratory circulation is supine hypotension. In this syndrome, the inferior vena cava is compressed by the enlarged pregnant uterus and spine, causing a decrease in venous return. In addition, it is said that this causes a decrease in cardiac output, resulting in a decrease in blood pressure. This supine hypotension syndrome causes a decrease in uterine placental blood flow, which may result in abnormal fetal heart rate and appear on the CTG. The initial symptoms include nausea, vomiting, coldness, pallor, cyanosis, and hyperpnea, and the possibility of supine hypotension syndrome should be considered in conjunction with CTG.

First, the mother should be repositioned. The side lying position is recommended instead of the supine position. In addition, the left lateral recumbency is most recommended from the viewpoint of preventing a decrease in fetal blood oxygen saturation. If positional change is difficult, it is also effective to manually shift the uterus to the left.

In addition, amniotic fluid embolization, which is known as a rapid anaphylactic-like reaction, or other conditions that lead to maternal cardiac arrest may cause acute placental insufficiency due to maternal circulatory failure, which may manifest as fetal heart rate abnormalities. There are various conditions that can cause maternal cardiac arrest, including cardiac and macrovascular diseases, cerebral hemorrhage, and uterine rupture. Although it is necessary to search for the cause of cardiac arrest, it is important to save the mother's life first. The cause of the cardiac arrest should be investigated by calling for help, preparing resuscitation equipment, moving the uterus to the left, performing chest compressions, and securing the airway.

3.7 *Maternal Convulsions (Eclampsia, Epileptic Seizures)*

A convulsive seizure is a seizure in which a muscle contracts involuntarily and independent of the patient's will. Convulsive seizures are caused by a variety of factors including epilepsy, stroke, brain tumor, meningitis, cardiogenic shock, electrolyte abnormalities, and hysteria. Most maternal convulsions are caused by eclampsia. When a pregnant woman has a seizure, maternal first aid (checking vitals, securing the airway, administering oxygen, and securing the intravenous route) should be given first priority, followed by appropriate anticonvulsant therapy. Once the seizures have resolved, differentiate between eclampsia and other diseases including stroke. It is difficult to differentiate between eclampsia and stroke based on clinical symptoms alone, and a brain CT or MRI is necessary for accurate diagnosis.

In addition, it is important to check the CTG because fetal dysfunction (NRFS) is likely to occur after a seizure. Transient bradycardia often resolves within a short time after the seizure disappears. Once the convulsions have disappeared and the mother's condition is stable, early delivery of the baby should be considered.

3.8 *Epidural and Spinal Anesthesia*

Spinal subarachnoid anesthesia dilates arteries and veins by sympathetic nerve block. Dilation of arteries decreases vascular resistance, and dilation of veins decreases cardiac preload, resulting in post-spinal hypotension [4]. This causes a sudden decrease in blood pressure in the mother, resulting in symptoms such as nausea and vomiting, as well as a decrease in placental blood flow, which may lead to hypoxemia and acidosis. This sequence of events may appear as prolonged bradycardia on the CTG. In addition, transient bradycardia is also said to appear when the analgesic effect of spinal subarachnoid anesthesia causes a rapid decrease in blood epinephrine, resulting in a decrease in β-activity, and the effect of norepinephrine causes contraction of uterine blood vessels and uterine tone [5]. Since transient bradycardia often subsides within 5 to 10 min, careful observation of the CTG is necessary. Epidural anesthesia used in painless labor and delivery is effective in decreasing uterine arterial vascular resistance and increasing placental blood flow, but like spinal subarachnoid anesthesia, it may cause a rapid decrease in maternal blood pressure by causing sympathetic nerve block. As a result, prolonged bradycardia may be observed on the fetal heart rate labor diagram. Both spinal subarachnoid anesthesia and epidural anesthesia cause abnormal fetal heart rate by decreasing maternal blood pressure. Since hypotension due to anesthesia can be expected, it is important to prevent it by increasing the circulating plasma volume by loading extracellular fluid in advance.

4 Toward Prevention

It must be said that measures to prevent the occurrence of hypoxia during delivery itself are limited. It is critical not to administer inappropriate uterotonics and to perform appropriate fetal monitoring and maternal management, but it is important to provide appropriate medical care with reference to the recommendations in the "Guidelines for Obstetrics and Gynecology 2020" jointly prepared by the Japanese Society of Obstetrics and Gynecology and the Japanese Society of Obstetricians and Gynecologists. In addition, it is important to be prepared to respond to a sudden change in the mother's condition or abnormal waveforms in the CTG and to learn neonatal cardiopulmonary resuscitation (NCPR). Furthermore, the recommendations of the Committee for the Prevention of Recurrence of the Japan Obstetric Compensation System for Cerebral Palsy should be shared among the staff.

Prevention will be divided into prepartum care, response to hypoxia during delivery, and response to the newborn.

4.1 Prepartum Care

Before delivery, it is important to obtain accurate information on the pregnant woman's medical history, pregnancy history, and family history and to identify risk factors. It is also necessary to know the obstetric complications in the course of pregnancy, fetal growth, and amniotic fluid volume by ultrasonography. The World Health Organization (WHO) recommends the administration of magnesium sulfate hydrate in preterm births of less than 32 weeks of gestation, because there is a report on the brain protection of infants by magnesium sulfate hydrate [6]. In the Obstetrics and Gynecology Clinical Practice Guidelines 2017, magnesium sulfate hydrate administration for brain protection was described only as an explanation, but in the Obstetrics and Gynecology Clinical Practice Guidelines 2020, it is stated that "magnesium sulfate hydrate is administered for the purpose of fetal brain protection" and that magnesium sulfate administration is "Level C."

4.2 Response to Delivery (Intrapartum Resuscitation)

If severe fetal heart rate abnormalities persist, severe sequelae such as cerebral palsy may occur in the newborn, resulting in fetal or neonatal death. The mother's general condition should be checked, and the cause of the prolonged bradycardia should be investigated, and effective fetal resuscitation should be performed. Figure 1 summarizes the measures to be taken when an abnormal fetal heart rate pattern appears.

4.2.1 Maternal Positioning

It may be effective for supine hypotension syndrome and abnormal heart rate associated with umbilical cord compression. In supine hypotension syndrome, the enlarged uterus causes compression of the inferior vena cava and inferior aorta, which results in decreased cardiac output and inadequate uteroplacental circulation, leading to abnormal heart rate. Therefore, the lateral supine position is preferable,

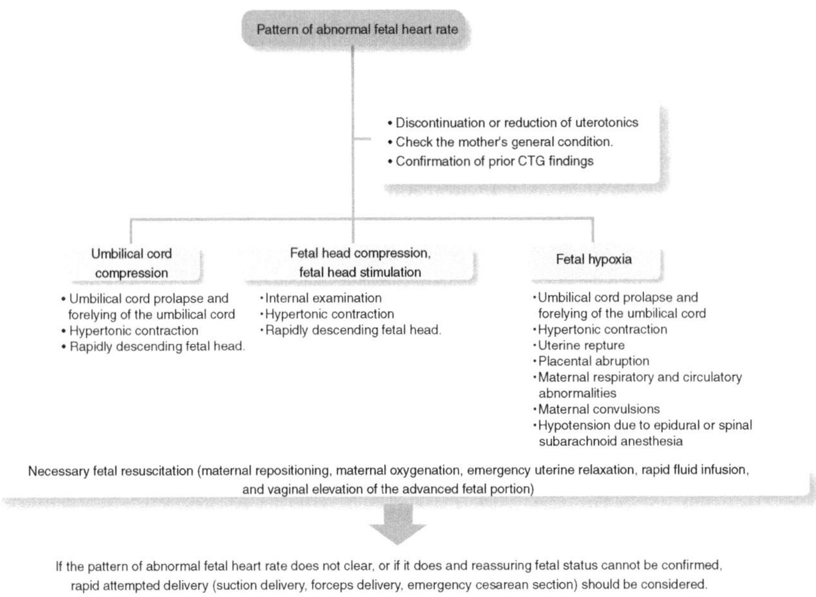

Fig. 1 Response to the appearance of abnormal fetal heart rate patterns

and the left lateral supine position has been reported to be the best from the viewpoint of fetal blood oxygen saturation [7–9]. Also, in the case of umbilical cord compression, maternal repositioning may relieve the compression. If the left lateral lying position is not effective, the right lateral lying position may be effective.

4.2.2 Oxygen Administration to the Mother

Fetal resuscitation is often performed because of its simplicity, but it cannot be expected to be effective unless the administration method is appropriate. Inhalation oxygen concentration is important. When administered in a circuit with an inspiratory oxygen concentration of less than 50%, the efficacy is not consistent, and when administered in a circuit with an inspiratory oxygen concentration of approximately 80–100%, an increase in fetal blood oxygen saturation has been confirmed [10]. A non-rebreather mask (reservoir mask with one-way valve) can be used to ensure 80–100% oxygenation at an oxygen flow rate of 10 L/min or higher [7]. An oxygen inhalation concentration of about 50% can also be maintained by flowing 10–15 L/min of oxygen through a simple mask. However, there is no clear evidence that maternal oxygenation was effective in avoiding cesarean section or prevented a decrease in umbilical artery blood pH in the neonate [11].

4.2.3 Emergency Uterine Relaxation

It is effective in cases of abnormal fetal heart rate due to uterine contractions such as hypertonic contraction. Currently, the most commonly used drugs are nitroglycerin and ritodrine hydrochloride. Nitroglycerin is administered intravenously at a dose of 60–90 μg (maximum 100 μg) slowly. Ritodrine hydrochloride is familiar and easy to use, but it is not indicated for use in full-term labor. 1/10 to 1/5 ampule of utemerin injection® (Kissei Pharmaceutical Co., Ltd.) (50 mg/5 mL per ampule) administered intravenously over several minutes is another option.

4.2.4 Rapid Infusion

Rapid infusion of lactated Ringer's solution has been reported to increase fetal blood oxygen saturation [9]. 500 to 1000 mL/20 min is recommended, but pulmonary edema may occur in some cases.

4.2.5 Transvaginal Elevation of the Advanced Fetal Portion

This is a method of vaginally elevating the advanced part of the fetus with an internal finger to relieve pressure in the case of prolonged bradycardia due to prolapse of the umbilical cord after spontaneous or artificial water rupture or sudden descent of the baby's head [12]. Although it is simple, there is little evidence that it is effective.

4.2.6 Handling the Neonatal Period

It is necessary to perform accurate neonatal resuscitation for neonatal death, and all medical staff should be familiar with neonatal resuscitation techniques. For this purpose, all medical staffs should be familiar with neonatal resuscitation, and they should always be prepared for neonatal resuscitation. In the case of hypoxemia requiring advanced neonatal resuscitation including tracheal intubation, cerebral hypothermia can be expected to prevent brain damage including cerebral palsy if certain conditions are met, such as an Apgar score of 5 points or less at 10 min. For details, please refer to the chapter of "Neonatal Hypothermia." If hypothermia (33.5–34.5 °C) is started within 6 h after birth for moderate to severe hypoxic-ischemic encephalopathy after 36 weeks of gestation, the neurological prognosis can be improved.

4.3 CTG Patterns Directly Related to Cerebral Palsy

The CTG corresponding to Level 5 [abnormal waveform (high level)] of the level classification is considered to be the CTG pattern directly related to cerebral palsy [13]. In other words, the waveform is considered to be as shown below.

1. Repeated late deceleration with loss of baseline variability
2. Repeated variable deceleration with loss of baseline variability
3. Prolonged deceleration with loss of baseline variability
4. Severe bradycardia (<80 bpm) with decreased baseline variability or loss of baseline variability
5. Sinusoidal pattern

Cerebral palsy caused by hypoxia during labor is still a critical issue for perinatal care providers. Although it is impossible to prevent all cases of hypoxia due to various factors, it is important to correctly understand the occurrence of hypoxia by reading the CTG; to share emergency responses with all staff involved in perinatal care, including simulation education; and to appropriately use neonatal resuscitation. By doing so, we hope to reduce the incidence of cerebral palsy caused by hypoxia during delivery.

References

1. Japan Council for Quality Health Care. 10th Report on prevention of recurrence, The Japan Obstetric Compensation System for Cerebral Palsy. Tokyo: Japan Council for Quality Health Care; 2020. Japanese. Available from: http://www.sanka-hp.jcqhc.or.jp/documents/prevention/report/pdf/Saihatsu_Report_10_All.pdf. Accessed 14 Sept 2020.
2. Japan Council for Quality Health Care, Project Team for Epidemiological Survey on the Actual Condition of Children with Cerebral Palsy. Report of epidemiological survey on the actual condition of children with cerebral palsy, Oct 2018. Japanese. Available from:

http://www.sanka-hp.jcqhc.or.jp/documents/report/pdf/nouseimahijinojittaihaakunikansuruekigakuchousahoukokusyo.pdf. Accessed 14 Sept 2020.
3. Nelson KB, Blair E, Nelson KB, et al. Prenatal factors in singletons with cerebral palsy born at or near term. N Engl J Med. 2015;373:946–53. https://doi.org/10.1056/NEJMra1505261.
4. Ando Y. Teiousekkaiji no sekizui kumomakuka masuigo teiketsuatsu nitaisuru shouatsuyaku touyo no taiji saitaiketsuheno eikyou [Effect of pressure-raising drug administration on fetal cord blood for hypotension after spinal subarachnoid anesthesia during cesarean section]. Anesthesia. 2012;61:875–9. Japanese.
5. Friedlander JD, Fox HE, Cain CF, et al. Fetal bradycardia and uterine hyperactivity following subarachnoid administration of fentanyl during labor. Reg Anesth Pain Med. 1997;22:378–81.
6. Jayaram PM, Mohan MK, Farid I, et al. Antenatal magnesium sulfate for fetal neuroprotection: a critical appraisal and systematic review of clinical practice guidelines. J Perinat Med. 2019;47:262–9. https://doi.org/10.1515/jpm-2018-0174.
7. Aldrich CJ, D'Antona D, Spencer JA, et al. The effect of maternal posture on fetal cerebral oxygenation during labor. Br J Obstet Gynaecol. 1995;102:14–9.
8. Carbonne B, Benachi A, Lévèque ML, et al. Maternal position during labor: effects on fetal oxygen saturation measured by pulse oximetry. Obstet Gynecol. 1996;88:797–800.
9. Simpson KR, James DC. Efficacy of intrauterine resuscitation techniques in improving fetal oxygen status during labor. Obstet Gynecol. 2005;105(105):1362–8.
10. Simpson KR. Intrauterine resuscitation during labor: should maternal oxygen administration be a first-line measure? Semin Fetal Neonatal Med. 2008;13:362–7.
11. Raghuraman N, Wan L, Temming LA, et al. Effect of oxygen vs room air on intrauterine fetal resuscitation: a randomized noninferiority clinical trial. JAMA Pediatr. 2018;172:818–23.
12. Sayed Ahmed WA, Hamdy MA. Optimal management of umbilical cord prolapse. Int J Women's Health. 2018;10:459–65.
13. Japan Society of Obstetrics and Gynecology/Japan Society of Obstetricians and Gynecologists. CQ411 Taiji shinpakusuu jintsuuzu no hyoukahou to sono taiouha? [CQ411 How to evaluate fetal heart rate labor charts and what to do about it?]. In: Sanfujinka shinryo Guideline, Sanka hen [Guidelines for obstetrics and gynecology, obstetrics edition]. 2020 ed. Tokyo; Japan Society of Obstetrics and Gynecology; 2020. p. 228–32. Japanese.

Uterotonic Agents

Sho Fujiwara and Kazuhide Ogita

Contents

S. Fujiwara · K. Ogita (✉)
Department of Obstetrics and Gynecology, Rinku General Medical Center, Izumisano, Osaka, Japan
e-mail: k-ogita@rgmc.izumisano.osaka.jp

Y. Matsuda (ed.), *Cerebral Palsy*, https://doi.org/10.1007/978-981-19-2217-6_21

Summary

- Contractile drugs are used to stimulate uterine contractions to achieve delivery before spontaneous contractions occur or when spontaneous labor is diminished.
- Labor induction tends to take longer than natural childbirth.
- Contractile drugs may be associated with the development of cerebral palsy when used inappropriately.

1 Types of Uterine Contractions and How to Use Them

From 1990 to 2018, the overall frequency of labor induction nearly tripled in the United States, rising from 9.5% in 1990 to 27.1% in 2018 [1].

Delivery before the onset of spontaneous labor should be underwent when the risk of continued pregnancy is considered to be equivalent to the perinatal risk on delivery [2]. The relative risks of continued pregnancy and delivery are influenced primarily by gestational age, and the severity of the maternal/fetal condition and are rarely precisely determined.

The interventions for delivery before the onset of spontaneous labor are induction of labor or cesarean delivery. Considering the increased maternal risks associated with cesarean delivery, including maternal mortality, deep vein thrombosis, hysterectomy, postpartum fever, and wound infection, as well as the increased frequency of uterine rupture, placenta previa, and placenta accreta in the next pregnancy, and the added risk of complications from anesthesia, induction of labor is generally preferred in the absence of contraindications to labor or vaginal delivery. Induction of labor is generally preferred when there is no contraindication to labor or vaginal delivery.

2 Involvement of Bishop Score

Bishop score is the most used cervical assessment system in clinical practice in the United States [3]. There is no universally accepted threshold that is considered appropriate for induction and promotion of labor. However, a higher Bishop score increases the likelihood of vaginal delivery [3, 5–7], whereas a lower Bishop score increases the possibility of cesarean delivery [4]. Therefore, when the cervix is favorable, oxytocin is administered without cervical ripening procedure. When cervical ripening is unfavorable, a drug or mechanical cervical ripening devices are recommended before administration of uterotonic agents.

3 Indications for Induction of Labor/Augmentation of Labor

Examples of common conditions for which induction is often medically/clinically indicated include, but are not limited to, those listed in Table 1 [2]. Other social indications include the wishes of the expectant mother.

The multicenter ARRIVE trial [8] evaluated the perinatal and maternal effects of planned induction of labor at 39 weeks 0 days to 39 weeks 4 days' gestation compared with expectant management in more than 6100 women in a low-risk labor waiting group in the United States. The results of this large study are as follows:

- The risk of cesarean delivery was reduced [18.6% vs. 22.2%, relative risk (RR) 0.84 [95% confidence interval (CI): 0.76–0.93]].
- Reduced the risk of gestational hypertension [9.1% vs. 14.1%, RR 0.64 (95% CI: 0.56–0.74)].
- The risk of neonatal respiratory support was reduced [3.0% vs. 4.2%, RR 0.71 (95% CI: 0.55–0.93)].
- There was a slight reduction in the frequency of the combined outcome of perinatal death or severe neonatal complications (not statistically significant) [4.3% vs. 5.4%, RR 0.80 (95% CI: 0.64–1.00)].
- Increased median time spent in the labor room (20 h vs. 14 h).

However, this study dose not show the advantage for induction of labor before 39 weeks gestation compared with waiting for spontaneous labor.

4 Uterotonic Agents Used in Japan

There are three types of uterine contractile drugs used in Japan: (1) oxytocin, (2) prostaglandin $F_{2\alpha}(PGF)_{2\alpha}$, and (3) prostaglandin $E_2(PGE)_2$.

Table 1 Common conditions for which induction of labor is indicated

Fetal factor	• When neonatal care is required to save a child's life • Chorioamnionitis • Perimenopause and its prevention • Excessive amniotic fluid • Pregnancy with diabetes mellitus • If a giant baby is expected • Fetal death in utero • In addition, when it is judged that early delivery of the baby is necessary
Maternal factors	• Slight contractions • Early water breaking • Pregnancy hypertension • Prevention of sudden birth • If the continuation of the pregnancy is likely to cause danger to the mother

4.1 Oxytocin

Oxytocin administration is the most common and proven method of labor induction; according from a network meta-analysis of methods of labor induction in 2016, the use of intravenous oxytocin administration plus amniotomy and the use of vaginal PGE_1 were the two approaches most likely to achieve vaginal delivery within 24 h [9]. It has been approved in 2020 in Japan.

4.1.1 Pharmacological Action

Administration of oxytocin is effective for periodic uterine contractions from approximately 20 weeks of gestation. Myometrial reactivity increases with increasing gestational age up to 34 weeks of gestation [10]. The increase in myometrial reactivity is mainly due to an increase in myometrial oxytocin receptor binding sites [11]. Activation of the receptor triggers signaling events that stimulate contraction, mainly by increasing intracellular calcium levels [12].

Oxytocin is polypeptide thus cannot be administered orally because the is degraded by gastrointestinal enzymes into a small, inactive form. Therefore, oxytocin should administer intravenously (by this route, its half-life has been estimated to be 3–6 min [13]).

Progression during spontaneous labor is not related to increased oxytocin levels. Uterine contractions are also unrelated to changes in plasma oxytocin levels, and hypotonic contractions does not appear to be the result of oxytocin deficiency [14]. However, mutations in oxytocin receptors related genes appear to be associated with the amount of required oxytocin during induction of labor and the duration of labor [15].

4.1.2 Instructions for Use (Monitoring Uterine Contraction and Fetal Heart Rate)

When oxytocin is given, continuous monitoring of uterine contraction and fetal heart rate (FHR) should be performed so that the dose can be adjusted based on uterine contraction and FHR patterns.

Before using oxytocin, confirm the fetus is not severe fetal distress (Category 3 fetal heart rate pattern) [16].

4.1.3 Regarding Dosage and Administration (Low-Dose Method) [16]

Dissolve 5 units in 500 mL of 5% sugar solution, Ringer's solution, or saline solution (10 milliunits/mL).

Starting volume: 1–2 mm units/min (6–12 mL/h)
Maintenance dose: 5–15 mm units/min (30–90 mL/h)
Maximum dosage: 20 mm units/min (120 mL/h)
Increasing dose: Increase by 1–2 mm units/min (6–12 mL/h) after at least 30 min

If oxytocin is being administered at the time of uterine tachysystole, the dose should be reduced or discontinued until resolution of tachysystole, even if the FHR is not suggestive of fetal hypoxia or acidosis. If there are adverse changes in FHR, standard interventions, such as cesarean section, vacuum delivery, or forceps delivery, should be performed [17, 18].

No studies have evaluated the optimal approach to restarting after oxytocin is discontinued; one approach is to restart at 1/2 of previous dose when oxytocin is discontinued within less than 30 min, or at the first dose ordered if it is discontinued for more than 30 min [19–21].

4.1.4 Side Effect

Arrhythmia (VT), cardiac arrest, shock, dyspnea, tachyystole, signs of fetal hypoxemia, cloudy meconium staining, etc.

4.1.5 Contraindications and Cautious Administration [16]

Contraindications and cautions for $PGF_{2\alpha}$ administration are listed in Table 2.

4.2 PGE_2

4.2.1 How to Use

Confirm that there is no fetal dysfunction (Category 2–3 fetal heart rate waveform) prior to use [16].

4.2.2 Dosage and Administration

There are oral and vaginal usage.

The first oral dose is 1 tablet (0.5 mg), and the next dose should be taken at least 1 h later, up to a maximum of 6 tablets (3 mg) per day [16].

The vaginal formulation was approved in Japan in January 2020 and became available in April 2020. It is a vaginal insert containing 10 mg of dinoprostone and is a timed-release formulation (the drug is released at a rate of 0.3 mg/h). The insert should be left in place until labor begins or for 12 h.

Table 2 Contraindications and cautious administration

	Oxytocin	$PGF_{2\alpha}$	PGE_2
Taboo	• Within 1 h of the last dose of PGE_2 • Severe fetal dysfunction • Impending uterine rupture • More than two previous cesarean sections	• Abnormalities in the position of the placenta such as pelvic position • Severe fetal dysfunction • Bronchial asthma and its history • Previous cesarean section • Within 1 h of PGE_2 administration	• Abnormalities in the position of the placenta such as pelvic position • Severe fetal dysfunction • Previous hysterectomy • Previous cesarean section • Within 1 h of uterine contraction
	• Hypersensitivity to the drug in question • Previous cesarean section with an incision in the uterine body (classic cesarean section, T-shaped incision, bottom incision, etc.) • Hysteroscopic myomectomy (including hysteroscopic myomectomy) • Concurrent use with other uterine contractile drugs • Not enough time has passed during or after prasteronic acid administration • Within an hour of Metro Intel insertion • Simultaneous use with hygroscopic cervical dilators (Laminaria, etc.) • Placenta previa • In the case of apparent infant-head pelvis imbalance • Pelvic stenosis • Horizontal position • Premature detachment of the normal placenta (fetal presence) • Hypersystole		
Cautious administration	• Fetal insufficiency • Pregnancy • Cardiac, renal, and vascular disorders • Dystocia due to anomalous fetal position • Soft canal sclerosis • One previous cesarean section • Uterine incisions other than those listed in the contraindications • Older first-time mothers • Premature separation of normal placenta (in case of fetal death)	• Glaucoma • Heart disease • Hypertension • Fetal insufficiency • Premature separation of normal placenta (in case of fetal death) • Acute pelvic cavity infection and its history	• Glaucoma • Bronchial asthma and its history
	• Pelvic disproportion of the head is suspected • Multiple pregnancies • Fertile woman		

4.2.3 Side Effects

Maternal adverse effects are including nausea and vomiting, facial flushing, hyperemesis gravidarum, and diarrhea; fetal adverse effects are meconium staining of amniotic fluid, fetal bradycardia, fetal tachycardia, and fetal dysfunction.

Vaginal suppository, there were relatively few systemic adverse effects such as maternal fever, nausea, and vomiting.

4.2.4 Contraindications and Cautious Administration [16]

Contraindications and cautions for PGE_2 administration are listed in Table 2.

5 Association with Cerebral Palsy

As for the quantitative and epidemiological analysis of cerebral palsy (CP), the "10th Report on Prevention of Recurrence, The Japan Obstetric Compensation System for Cerebral Palsy" (2020) [22] is the most recent, and it contains statistics on 2457 cases for which causal analysis reports were published by then. Of these, 346 (14.1%) were classified as having induction of labor and 524 (21.3%) as having augmentation of labor, which is not a particularly large number compared with the general case. In 870 cases, oxytocin administration was the most common (515 cases, 21%), followed by $PGF_{2\alpha}$ (79 cases, 3.2%) and PGE_2 (132 cases, 5.4%). As for other procedures, artificial rupture of membranes was performed in 473 cases (19.3%), genital bleeding in 148 cases (6.0%), and cervical dilators such as laminaria in 44 cases (1.8%), which were not uncommon.

Each series of "Report on Prevention of Recurrence of the Japan Obstetric Compensation System for Cerebral Palsy" has thematic analyses, and there are analyses on uterotonic agents in the first (2011) and third (2013) reports. According to the tenth report [22], out of the 999 cases analyzed, 257 cases were uterotonic agents were used. Of the 257 cases in which uterotonic agents were used, the cases in which only oxytocin was used by year of birth is as follows: 34 cases (77.3%) in 2009, 26 cases (60.5%) in 2010, 26 cases (70.3%) in 2011, 33 cases (67.3%) in 2012, 33 cases (80.5%) in 2013, and 25 cases (58.5%) in 2014. In 2014, there were 25 (58.1%) cases. In 209 (81.3%) cases, a single uterotonic agent was used, and in 48 (18.7%) cases, multiple uterotonic agents were used. There were no case in which pluriel uterotonic agents were used. Of the 220 cases in which oxytocin was used, 9 (22.0%) were in 2009, 8 (23.5%) in 2010, 8 (26.7%) in 2011, 19 (47.5%) in 2012, 22 (55.0%) in 2013, and 18 (51.0%) in 2014. In 2014, 18 cases (51.4%) were reported, and the rate has been around 50% since 2013. The details by year of birth of cases in which the method of continuous fetal heart rate monitoring by cardiotocogram was 26 (63.4%) in 2009, 26 (765%) in 2010, 20 (66.7%) in 2011, 31 (77.5%) in 2012, 34 (85.0%) in 2013, and 27 (77.1%) in 2014. In 2014, however, there were 8 cases (22.9%) in which fetal heart rate monitoring was intermittent. According to "Points to keep in mind when inducing or promoting labor with uterine contractions" (revised 2011 edition), when multiple drugs are used in the same case, the administration of the next drug should be started after a certain period of time from the end of the first drug administration and should not be used simultaneously. Although there were no cases of simultaneous administration in the analyzed cases, there were cases in which oxytocin was immediately switched without an interval after the use of $PGF_{2\alpha}$, and cases in which the time between the oral administration of PGE_2 and the start of oxytocin was short.

In the 56 cases analyzed, cervical ripening agents (e.g., prasterone sulfate sodium hydrate) were used in 9 cases, hygroscopic cervical dilation devices (e.g., laminaria) were used in 2 cases, metreurynter were inserted in 13 cases, and amniotomy was performed in 26 cases. (There were duplicates.)

In the cases analysis, cervical ripening device was administered at the same time as oxytocin administration, a hygroscopic cervical dilator was left in place when oxytocin was initiated, and cervical ripening devices and oxytocin administration were initiated at the same time as the insertion of metroirintel. The report pointed that "Prasterone sulfate sodium hydrate preparation was administered at the same time as oxytocin administration, and the fact that the administration was not performed according to the package inserts is a deviation from the standard." In addition, there was a case in which an artificial rupture of membranes was performed while oxytocin was being administered without continuous monitoring. According to "Guidelines for Obstetrics and Gynecology, Obstetrics Edition 2020," "Q415-1 What should be confirmed before starting administration of uterine contractile drugs (oxytocin, $PGF_{2\alpha}$, and prostaglandin E_2 tablets)?" In section [16], "Do not administer contractions during insertion of hygroscopic cervical dilators (e.g., laminaria), intravenous administration of prasterone sulfate sodium (e.g., Levospa®), or not long enough after administration, or during administration of other contractions" is listed as recommendation level A. "The Report on the Prevention of Recurrence of the Japan Obstetric Compensation System for Cerebral Palsy" also states that "administration of oxytocin is started at the same time as insertion of metroirintel. Therefore, it is necessary to use the drug in accordance with the content of the package insert" and "It is necessary to leave an appropriate interval when shifting from the dinoprost drug to the oxytocin."

From the above, it can be concluded that the reported incorrect using of uterotonic agents in cases of cerebral palsy were listed as follows:

1. When the dose (starting dose, increasing dose, maximum dose) is higher dose than the standard dose
2. Inappropriate FHR monitoring while using uterotonic agents
3. If the administration of the next drug is started within a certain period after the completion of the first drug administration

4. If oxytocin is started while a hygroscopic cervical dilator has been inserted
5. When cervical ripening agents or oxytocin are started at the same time as the use of metreurynter
6. Use of a uterotonic agents despite an FHR waveform suggestive of nonreassuring fetal status
7. Use of oxytocin despite not being a diagnosis of prolonged labor or labor arrest (inappropriate indication)

6 Pathophysiology

According to the "Causes of the Onset of Cerebral Palsy" of the "Third Report on the Prevention of Recurrence of the Japan Obstetric Compensation System for Cerebral Palsy" the following information was described in relation to the use of uterotonic agents [23].

Of the 56 cases subjected to analysis, there was one case in which the main cause of the onset of cerebral palsy was considered to be hypersystole caused by the use of uterotonic agents, such as follows: "The cause of the onset of cerebral palsy is considered to be the persistent hypoxia for 80 min before the delivery, and the possibility of hypersystole caused by oxytocin is considered to be a factor." There were 36 cases in which the main cause of the onset of cerebral palsy was other than the use of uterine contractions, and 19 cases in which the cause of the onset of cerebral palsy was "not clear" or "difficult to identify." However, even in these cases, as shown below, there were 6 cases in which the use of uterine contractile drugs "may have affected," "cannot be denied to have affected," or "may have been an aggravating factor" in some way.

It may be due to a combination of factors such as administration of uterotonic agents, decrease in placental blood flow due to epidural anesthesia, and direct effect of local anesthetics on the fetus.

Although it does not meet the definition of hypersystole, the possibility that the use of oxytocin affected the fetus cannot be ruled out.

The use of oxytocin to augment uterine contractions and the time required for neonatal resuscitation may have contributed to the worsening of hypoxia.

Vacuum delivery with fundal pressure was undergone 11 times, and the administration of uterotonic agents in the presence of fetal distress may have been aggravating factors.

The administration of oxytocin was continued when Category 2 to Category 3 FHR pattern appeared, which may have affected the fetal hypoxia.

It is unclear whether hypersystole/tachysystole existed because of inappropriate tocogram measurement; abnormal uterine contraction induced by oxytocin may have exacerbated fetal hypoxemia and acidosis.

In those cases, there is a possibility of inducing hypersystole and nonreassuring fetal status due to fetal hypoxia caused by uterine contractions.

However, most of the uterine contractions are measured using external pressure gauges, and it is thought that there are cases in which hypersystole and tachysystole are not accurately measured.

7 Toward Prevention

The recommendations from the Committee for the Prevention of Recurrence published in 2013 are shown in Table 3. Adherence to these recommendations in the use of uterotonic agents, neonatal resuscitation, and confirming for signs of fetal hypoxemia may prevent the onset of CP.

Table 3 Recommendations from the Recurrence Prevention Committee published in 2013 (modified from Ref. [23])

1. About the use of uterine contraction medicine
(a) Indications, conditions, and contraindications should be thoroughly reviewed, and the drug should be used only after obtaining written explanation and consent. When verbal consent is obtained, such as in case of emergency, it should be written in the medical record
(b) The well-being of the fetus should be assessed before the use of uterine contractions is started
(c) The use of uterine contractions and cervical ripening device may cause hypersystole. Therefore, during induction and promotion of labor, cardiotocogram should be worn appropriately, fetal well-being and labor should be constantly evaluated, and labor should be carefully monitored. If an abnormal fetal heart rate pattern appears, it should be considered that continue uterotonic agents or not
(d) Follow the dosage and administration for proper use
2. The use of multiple uterine contraction drugs
(a) If oxytocin or $PGF_{2\alpha}$ is used, it should be used at least 1 h after the last dose of PGE_2
(b) If PGE_2 is used, it should be used at least 1 h after the last dose of oxytocin or $PGF_{2\alpha}$, and not use at the same time
3. Other measures to induce or promote labor while using uterotonic agents
(a) If cervical ripening is inadequate, cervical ripening should be followed by induction and promotion of labor
(b) Do not use cervical ripening agents or hygroscopic cervical dilators at the same time as uterine contractions
In the case of concomitant use of metreurynter and uterotonic agents, uterotonic agents should be started at least 1 h after the insertion of metrethrinsel and after observation with a delivery monitoring device
The following points are important for use • Follow the dosage • Continue to monitor fetal heart rate during use to detect nonreassuring fetal status • Do not use in combination with or in a manner that may lead to excessive labor or uterine rupture

References

1. Martin JA, Hamilton BE, Osterman MJK, et al. Births: final data for 2018. Natl Vital Stat Rep. 2019;68:1.
2. ACOG Committee on Practice Bulletins. Obstetrics. ACOG Practice Bulletin No. 107: induction of labor. Obstet Gynecol. 2009;114:386. Reaffirmed 2019.
3. Bishop EH. Pelvic scoring for elective induction. Obstet Gynecol. 1964;24:266.
4. Gibson KS, Waters TP. Measures of success: prediction of successful labor induction. Semin Perinatol. 2015;39:475.
5. Vrouenraets FP, Roumen FJ, Dehing CJ, et al. Bishop score and risk of cesarean delivery after induction of labor in nulliparous women. Obstet Gynecol. 2005;105:690.
6. Kolkman DG, Verhoeven CJ, Brinkhorst SJ, et al. The Bishop score as a predictor of labor induction success: a systematic review. Am J Perinatol. 2013;30:625.
7. Teixeira C, Lunet N, Rodrigues T, et al. The Bishop score as a determinant of labour induction success: a systematic review and meta-analysis. Arch Gynecol Obstet. 2012;286:739.
8. Grobman WA, Caughey AB. Elective induction of labor at 39 weeks compared with expectant management: a meta-analysis of cohort studies. Am J Obstet Gynecol. 2019;221:304.
9. Alfirevic Z, Keeney E, Dowswell T, et al. Methods to induce labour: a systematic review, network meta-analysis and cost-effectiveness analysis. BJOG. 2016;123:1462.
10. Calderyro-Barcia R, Sereno JA. The response of human uterus to oxytocin throughout pregnancy. In: Oxytocin. London: Pergamon Press; 1959.
11. Fuchs AR, Fuchs F, Husslein P, et al. Oxytocin receptors in the human uterus during pregnancy and parturition. Am J Obstet Gynecol. 1984;150:734.
12. Arrowsmith S, Wray S. Oxytocin: its mechanism of action and receptor signalling in the myometrium. J Neuroendocrinol. 2014;26:356.
13. Rydén G, Sjöholm I. The metabolism of oxytocin in pregnant and non-pregnant women. Acta Obstet Gynecol Scand Suppl. 1971;9(Suppl 9):37.
14. Thornton S, Davison JM, Baylis PH. Plasma oxytocin during the first and second stages of spontaneous human labour. Acta Endocrinol (Copenhagen). 1992;126:425.
15. Grotegut CA, Ngan E, Garrett ME, et al. The association of single-nucleotide polymorphisms in the oxytocin receptor and G protein-coupled receptor kinase 6 (GRK6) genes with oxytocin dosing requirements and labor outcomes. Am J Obstet Gynecol. 2017;217:367.e1.
16. Japanese Society of Obstetrics and Gynecology/Japan Society of Obstetricians and Gynecologists, supervised/editor. CQ415-1 Shikyushushukuyaku (oxytocin, prostaglandin F2α, narabini prostaglandin E2 jyou no sansha) touyomae ni kakuninnsubekikotoha? [CQ415-1 What should be confirmed before starting administration of uterine contractile drugs (oxytocin, prostaglandin F2α, and prostaglandin E2 tablets)?]. In: Sanfujinka shinryou Guideline, Sankahen [Guidelines for obstetrics and gynecology, obstetrics]. Tokyo: Japan Society of Obstetrics and Gynecology; 2020. p. 245–9. Japanese.
17. Sharma SK, Gajraj NM, Sidawi JE. Prevention of hypotension during spinal anesthesia: a comparison of intravascular administration of hetastarch versus lactated Ringer's solution. Anesth Analg. 1997;84:111.
18. Pullen KM, Riley ET, Waller SA, et al. Randomized comparison of intravenous terbutaline vs nitroglycerin for acute intrapartum fetal resuscitation. Am J Obstet Gynecol. 2007;197:414.e1.
19. https://www.ihs.gov/medicalprograms/mch/f/documents/Tachysystole2.pdf. Accessed 24 May 2012.
20. Care of the patient receiving oxytocin for labor induction or augmentation. University of Michigan Hospital. Nov 2010. obgyn.med.umich.edu/sites/obgyn.med.... edu/.../ind-aug_labor.pdf. Accessed 24 May 2012.

21. mail.ny.acog.org/website/OxytocinForInduction.pdf. Accessed 24 May 2012.
22. Japan Council for Quality Health Care. 10th Report on prevention of recurrence, the Japan Obstetric Compensation System for Cerebral Palsy. Tokyo: Japan Council for Quality Health Care; 2020. p. 88–9. Japanese.
23. Japan Council for Quality Health Care. 3rd Report on prevention of recurrence, the Japan Obstetric Compensation System for Cerebral Palsy. Tokyo: Japan Council for Quality Health Care; 2013. p. 106–34. Japanese.

Assisted Vaginal Delivery (Including Kristeller Maneuver)

Hiroshi Ishikawa

Contents

Summary

- One of the goals of assisted vaginal delivery (instrumental delivery: vacuum device or forceps) is to prevent the progression of fetal hypoxia and acidosis.
- Unfortunately, some instrumental delivery cases are suggested to be an aggravating factor of cerebral palsy.

H. Ishikawa (✉)
Department of Obstetrics and Gynecology, Kanagawa Children's Medical Center, Yokohama, Kanagawa, Japan
e-mail: hishikawa@kcmc.jp

Y. Matsuda (ed.), *Cerebral Palsy*, https://doi.org/10.1007/978-981-19-2217-6_22

- Both vacuum and forceps deliveries should be started after confirming that the maximum circumference of the fetal head sufficiently moves down into the pelvis and that the fetal head is at +2 station or below.
- Uterine fundal pressure (Kristeller maneuver) should be carefully performed because it may aggravate the uteroplacental circulation.
- Call for help should be performed before instrumental delivery to prepare for situations, such as cesarean section in case of unsuccessful vaginal birth or shoulder dystocia.
- A practitioner should evaluate whether the fetal head is descending after the first or second traction. If there is no progress, they should prepare for forceps delivery or cesarean section.
- A practitioner should carefully observe the newborn baby after birth to detect complications, such as subgaleal hematoma.
- Indications, summaries, and methods of childbirth should be appropriately recorded at the time of each treatment.

1 Assisted Vaginal Delivery and Cerebral palsy

According to the "10th Report on Prevention of Recurrence, The Japan Obstetric Compensation System for Cerebral Palsy," of the 2457 cases of cerebral palsy covered by this system (for which cause analysis reports were completed by the end of September 2019), 260 were vacuum deliveries, 21 were forceps deliveries, 12 were combined vacuum and forceps deliveries, and 87 were cesarean sections after assisted vaginal deliveries. In summary, an assisted vaginal delivery (vacuum or/and forceps delivery) was performed for 380 (15%) of the 2457 cases of cerebral palsy.

Most of these cases unfortunately resulted in cerebral palsy due to hypoxic-ischemic encephalopathy (HIE) despite the best efforts of the obstetrician to treat nonreassuring fetal status (NRFS). One of the goals of assisted vaginal delivery (instrumental delivery: vacuum device or forceps) is to prevent the progression of fetal hypoxia and acidosis during labor. Appropriate assisted vaginal delivery prevents cerebral palsy. An assisted vaginal delivery basically should not result in cerebral palsy.

However, some instrumental delivery cases are suggested to be an aggravating factor of cerebral palsy. I analyzed 41 cases of the cause analysis reports, which were performed vacuum or/and forceps delivery in 2015–2016 and covered by the Japan Obstetric Compensation System for Cerebral Palsy, and 18 cases (44%) were pointed out that assisted vaginal delivery or Kristeller maneuver may have been an "aggravating factor" of cerebral palsy [1]. In some cases, although assisted vaginal delivery was appropriately performed, cerebral palsy occurred due to its complications such as subgaleal hematoma.

In this section, I will introduce typical cases which assisted vaginal delivery was suggested to be the cause of cerebral palsy and a summary of cause analysis report was officially published by the Japan Obstetric Compensation System for Cerebral Palsy. I will also discuss the points and preventive measures for each case. I will not discuss the conditions of application for assisted vaginal delivery or the timing of implementation, because cardiotocography (CTG) has not been officially published.

2 Summary of Assisted Vaginal Delivery

[Case 1] Unsuccessful Vacuum Delivery from Sp ± 0 cm (Primipara)
40 weeks and 1 day pregnant

At 11:45: Spontaneous rupture of membranes occurred. Administration of oral antibiotics was started.

40 weeks and 2 days pregnant

At 9:00: Blood test = white blood cell 19,700/μL, CRP 5.73 mg/dL.
At 15:00: Patient was diagnosed with inadequate uterine contractions. Labor was augmented with oxytocin infusion.
At 20:10: Sacral epidural anesthesia was performed.
At 22:10: Vacuum delivery with Kristeller maneuver was performed. CTG showed that the fetal heart rate became bradycardia of less than 80 beats/min and it lasted for about 15 min.
Unknown time: A cesarean section was decided due to severe fetal bradycardia.
At 22:45: Childbirth by cesarean.

Findings in a newborn baby

Birth weight was 3370 g, Apgar score was 0 points for 1 min and 4 points for 5 min. Baby was diagnosed with hypoxic-ischemic encephalopathy after birth.

Umbilical cord blood gas analysis

pH 7.44, BE −4.8 mmol/L (sic).

2.1 Causes of Cerebral Palsy in the Cause Analysis Report

The report says "The cause of cerebral palsy is suggested to be fetal hypoxia and acidosis occurred during delivery" and "The cause of fetal hypoxia and acidosis is suggested to be uteroplacental insufficiency which was induced by combining vacuum delivery with Kristeller maneuver and other factors such as umbilical cord compression."

2.2 Medical Assessment in the Cause Analysis Report

The report says "It is common to perform a vacuum delivery when the fetal head at 0 station and the head does not descend any more, but it is not common to continue traction when the fetal bradycardia is not recovered."

2.3 Author's Discussion

We should consider what is the summary (criteria) of vacuum extraction delivery from this case. Guideline for Obstetrical Practice in Japan 2020 says its criteria are "cervix fully dilated and the rupture of membranes" and "engagement of fetal head (it means that the fetal head at 0 station or more)." However, the guidelines also say that "it is better to wait traction until the fetal head position is sufficiently descending (lower than +2 station) or to perform a cesarean section rather than performing vacuum extraction at a higher station." So, it does not mean that they unconditionally recommend vacuum delivery at 0 station or +1.

For forceps delivery, guideline says that "as a general rule, its criteria are a lower middle position and the sagittal suture should be in the midline and straight," and the commentary recommends +2 station or lower. From the standpoint of the author, who has preferentially learned forceps assisted delivery, I feel that vacuum delivery should not be performed at a position higher than the appropriate forceps position, because vacuum delivery has less traction power than forceps. "Assessment of fetal head descent and forceps assisted delivery" written by Takeda and Seki [2] shows details how to assess the fetal head position. I also would like to recommend this book to doctors who do not perform forceps delivery. In the book, Takeda says that "the criteria for vacuum delivery should be +2 station or lower the same as forceps delivery," and I agree with him.

Furthermore, what is truly important is that the maximum circumference of the fetal head is fully engaged into pelvis, and the descent of the fetal head is just one of the materials used to estimate the fetal engagement (Fig. 1). Especially in cases of abnormal rotation, the largest circumference of the fetal head may not be sufficiently engaged in the pelvis even if the lowest part of the head seems to be descended (Fig. 2). During internal examinations, it is important to make a habit of comprehensively assessing the descent of the fetal head not only from the descent of the lowest part of the head but also from the fetal head rotation and palpation of the pubic bone.

In addition, what is interesting in this case is that the fetal heart rate became bradycardic during vacuum delivery with uterine fundal pressure. It is known that the fetal heart rate has problem during assisted vaginal delivery due to decreased oxygen supply to fetus caused by deterioration of uteroplacental circulation and the umbilical cord compression by fetal descent. The addition of uterine fundal pressure (Kristeller maneuver) may increase the intrauterine pressure and aggravate the uteroplacental circulation. Although the uterine fundal pressure was usually

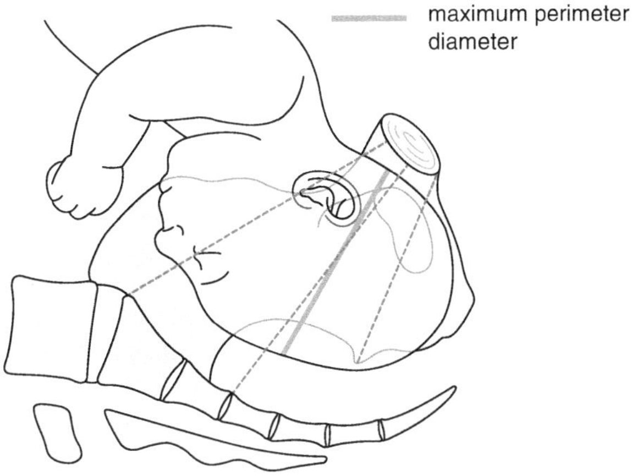

Fig. 1 Relationship between the lowest part and largest circumference of the fetal head with normal rotation [2]. If the lowest part of the fetal head is at +3 station, the largest circumference of fetal head (suboccipitobregmatic circumference) is sufficiently engaged in the pelvis and is about to reach the lower space

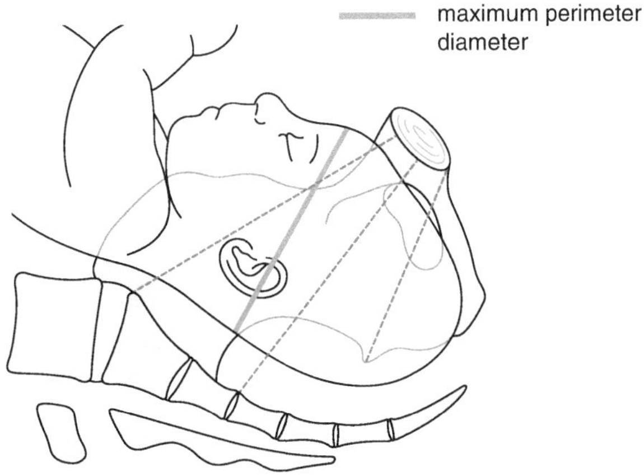

Fig. 2 Relationship between the lowest part and the largest circumference of the fetal head with abnormal rotation (fronto-anterior position) [2]. The lowest part of the fetal head is at +3 station, the same as in Fig. 1, but the largest circumference (occipitofrontal circumference) is in the pelvic inlet. The baby must be pulled for longer distance before birth

performed for the quick child birth, there was no obvious effect of uterine fundal pressure on shortening the second stage of labor according to Cochrane review [3] (but the evidence level was low). We should recognize that the uteroplacental circulation is obstructed during assisted vaginal delivery or uterine fundal pressure, so that the uterine fundal pressure should be performed only as an adjunct to assisted vaginal delivery, and it should be done in the shortest possible time.

3 Method of Assisted Vaginal Delivery

[Case 2] Unsuccessful Vacuum Delivery After 10 Pulls (Primipara)
41 weeks and 1 day pregnant

At 2:20: Patient was admitted to the hospital due to onset of labor.

41 weeks and 2 days pregnant

At around 20:00: Mild to severe prolonged decelerations appeared on CTG.
At around 21:50: Tachycardia, reduced variability or loss of variability, absence of acceleration, repetitive late decelerations appeared on CTG.
At 23:56: Oxytocin augmentation was started due to prolonged labor with inadequate uterine activities after cervix fully dilated.

41 weeks and 3 days pregnant

At around 0:02: Bradycardia of less than 80 beats/min appeared on CTG.
At 0:33: Vacuum-assisted birth (total 10 pulls) with Kristeller maneuver was performed due to absence of labor pains.

Findings in a newborn baby

Birth weight was 3119 g, and Apgar score was 1 point for 1 min and 0 points for 5 min. Baby was diagnosed with hypoxic-ischemic encephalopathy after birth.

Umbilical cord blood gas analysis

Not implemented.

3.1 *Causes of Cerebral Palsy in the Cause Analysis Report*

The report says that "The cause of cerebral palsy is suggested to be fetal hypoxic and acidosis during delivery," and "the fetus became hypoxic due to umbilical cord compression against a background of placental dysfunction with late-term pregnancy, and the hypoxic condition was aggravated by vacuum delivery combined with Kristeller Maneuver."

3.2 *Medical Assessment in the Cause Analysis Report*

The report says that "It was medically appropriate to select the vacuum-assisted delivery under the conditions of fetal bradycardia, fully dilated cervix and fetal head at +2 station at around 0:02 a.m. on 41 weeks and 3 days of gestation, but it is uncommon to pull the fetus 10 times."

3.3 *Author's Discussion*

Although I think it was inappropriate to augment labor with oxytocin when the CTG showed reduced to loss of variability, the conditions of "fully opened cervix and fetal head Sp +2 cm" were appropriate to apply the vacuum-assisted delivery.

Nevertheless, the fact that more than 10 pulls were required may show the difficulty of vacuum-assisted delivery. The Guidelines for Obstetrical Practice has always stated that "there is no method to predict the success of vacuum assisted delivery with certainty" since the first edition. This case makes us keenly aware of this fact.

If there is no way to predict success, the important thing is to assess the process of vacuum-assisted delivery. We must properly assess whether the fetal head is descending or not. If it is going to be unsuccessful, we must switch to another method. When should we consider switching, for example, after how many tractions had done or how many minutes have passed?

The Guidelines for Obstetrical Practice in Japan 2020 answered that "the total traction time (time from the cup attachment to the end of all the pulls) exceed 20 minutes" or "the total number of pulls (including slip-off) is five" to this question. But it does not mean that "we should switch to another method after 20 minutes or 5 pulls." These criteria are not based on a high level of evidence but on guidelines and consensus from other countries, so the time and frequency should be as low as possible. In a cohort study in the United Kingdom, more than 3 pulls and 10 min of pulls were associated with newborn adverse events [4], and other studies have reported an increase in head hematoma and fracture [5] and an increase in unsuccessful delivery with more than 3 pulls [4]. Based on these findings, the Royal College of Obstetricians and Gynaecologists (RCOG) guidelines [6] clearly state that "pulls should be stopped if delivery is not imminent even after 3 pulls." So, it is better to reconsider before "five pulls" or "20 minutes."

It is important to assess whether the fetal head has descended after the first or second pull. If there is no progress in delivery, for example, there is no response, or the fetal head does not move, we should switch to forceps delivery or speed up the preparation for cesarean section as soon as possible. If the fetal head does not descend by pulls, it will not descend by repetition. In the meantime, the fetal circulation failure will be worser.

In some cases, the cup slips off and it is not possible to assess the fetal head descent. The causes of slip-off include following.

1. The center of the cup is not correctly placed at the flexion point (3 cm anterior to the posterior fontanelle on the sagittal suture).
2. The direction of traction does not follow the pelvic line.
3. Insufficient negative pressure due to defective equipment.
4. Excessive fetal caput succedaneum.

Simulation training for proper vacuum-assisted delivery is also available through Advanced Life Support in Obstetrics ALSO®.

If the baby still slips out, there may be an abnormality in the size of fetal head or rotation of the fetal head. In the book, "Assessment of fetal head descent and forceps assisted delivery" [2], Seki wrote, "if the baby slips off two or three times, we should change from vacuum delivery to forceps or cesarean section, and if the baby slips off even once, we should be cautious enough and consider switching to another method of delivery." A slip-off may cause the practitioner to lose his composure. It is necessary to reexamine whether the cause of slip-off is inappropriate technique or dystocia.

It is rare for a forceps delivery practitioners to experience slip-off. However, even with forceps, it is necessary to assess the descent of the fetal head during the delivery. I feel that forceps delivery does not require multiple pulls and strong traction like vacuum delivery, because forceps strongly grasp the fetal head. When strong tractions are needed, excessively large fetus or abnormal fetal rotation may be suspected. These assessment and switching are more important than vacuum-assisted delivery.

4 Shoulder Dystocia After Assisted Vaginal Delivery

[Case 3] A Case of Shoulder Dystocia After Forceps Delivery (Primipara)
39 weeks and 5 days pregnant

Balloon catheter was inserted due to no progress in labor.

39 weeks and 6 days pregnant

At 8:30: Dinoprostone injection was started for induction of labor.
At 5:10 p.m.: Prolonged deceleration and uterine hyperstimulation were seen on CTG, and then administration of dinoprostone injection was stopped.
At 18:18: Reduced variability, severe prolonged deceleration, and repeated severe late deceleration were seen on CTG.
At 18:49: Administration of dinoprostone injection was resumed.
At 19:20: A forcep-assisted delivery was performed due to fetal distress. When the fetal head was delivered, bloody amniotic fluid was seen in a fetal nose. Long time and strong traction were needed for delivering shoulders due to shoulder dystocia.

Findings in a newborn baby

Birth weight was 3440 g, Apgar score was 3 points for 1 min and 5 points for 5 min. Baby was diagnosed with hypoxic-ischemic encephalopathy after birth.

Umbilical cord blood gas analysis value

pH 6.784, BE −22 mmol/L.

4.1 Causes of Cerebral Palsy in the Cause Analysis Report

The report says that "we believe that the cause of cerebral palsy is fetal hypoxia and acidosis caused by placental abruption."

4.2 *Medical Evaluation in the Cause Analysis Report*

The report says that "resuming administration of dinoprostone injection and performing forceps delivery were one of the options after the practitioner decided the quick child birth" and "the process of forceps delivery (it was done after confirming the fetal head position) is common."

4.3 *Author's Discussion*

The cause of cerebral palsy in this case was regarded as placental abruption, and shoulder dystocia after forceps delivery was not mentioned as a cause. However, it is common that shoulder dystocia occurs after vacuum or forceps deliveries.

In the "Guidelines for Obstetrical Practice in Japan 2020," the treatment of shoulder dystocia is described in the section of large fetus, but in reality, shoulder dystocia also occurs in non-large fetus. One of the factors of shoulder dystocia is assisted-vaginal delivery. In the published summary of the cause analysis report, shoulder dystocia occurred in seven cases, five of which were non-large fetus and four of which were assisted vaginal births.

Why does shoulder dystocia occur after assisted vaginal delivery? I have heard the theory that it is because the traction of the fetal head widens the fetal shoulder. Personally, I feel that it may be related to the fact that only the fetal head is rapidly delivered without the maximum circumference of the shoulder sufficiently descent into the birth canal. There may also be a bias that a fetus with shoulder dystocia has a wide shoulder and it is more likely to need an assisted vaginal delivery because of the prolonged second stage of labor.

Now, what should we do if shoulder dystocia occurs? The "Guidelines for Obstetrical Practice in Japan 2020" and other books describe several methods for the management of shoulder dystocia, and ALSO® provides systematic practical training. I will not go into the details in this section, but my personal opinion is that the most important thing is the number of personnel. We need one person for manual perineal protection, one for the right leg of the McRoberts maneuver, one for the left leg, and one for neonatal cardiopulmonary resuscitation (NCPR). In addition to the surgeon, four other people are needed. Also, we should consider other supporters to push the upper pubic margin and to raise the fetal head when performing the Rubin or Wood's screw maneuver. However, with the exception of the surgeon and NCPR practitioner, all of these procedures are relatively easy, so it is only necessary to have a sufficient number of personnel. It doesn't matter if that is a medical assistant, a patient husband, or even the head nurse on duty.

When applying an assisted vaginal birth, mobilize all available personnel. You may have to prepare for emergency cesarean section or shoulder dystocia, so you should make a habit of calling for help anyway.

5 Neonatal Complications of Assisted Vaginal Delivery, Importance of Documentation

[Case 4] A Case of Subgaleal Hematoma After Vacuum Delivery (Primipara)
38 weeks and 3 days pregnant

At 9:30: Patient was admitted due to premature rupture of membrane.
At 10:10: Oxytocin induction was started.
At 15:43: Vacuum-assisted delivery with uterine fundal pressure was performed. Fetus was in occiput posterior presentation.

Findings in a newborn baby

Birth weight was 3005 g, Apgar score was 9 points for 1 min and 10 points for 5 min. Baby was diagnosed with subgaleal hematoma, DIC (disseminated intravascular coagulation), hemorrhagic shock, and hypoxic-ischemic encephalopathy after birth.

Umbilical cord blood gas analysis

Not implemented.

5.1 Causes of Cerebral Palsy in the Cause Analysis Report

The report says that "we believe that the cause of the cerebral palsy is circulatory disturbance due to massive hemorrhage of the baby," "the cause of circulatory disturbance is likely to be subgaleal hematoma," and "vacuum delivery is an associated factor in the development of subgaleal hematoma."

5.2 Medical Evaluation in the Cause Analysis Report

The report says that "it is not common that the application and summary of vacuum assisted delivery with uterine fundal pressure were not written in the medical record. In addition, it is not common to perform vacuum assisted delivery and uterine fundal pressure without any findings of distress or prolonged second stage of labor from the medical record and CTG."

5.3 *Author's Discussion*

This is a case of cerebral palsy due to subgaleal hematoma after birth, despite successful vacuum delivery and no asphyxia. As far as I have searched the summary on the cause analysis report of the Japan Obstetric Compensation System for Cerebral Palsy, among 494 published cases, 23 newborns had subgaleal hematoma, and 19 were delivered by vacuum and 3 by both vacuum and forceps. Most of them (20 cases) had obvious hypoxia and acidosis in the peripartum period, and the direct cause of cerebral palsy was hypoxic-ischemic encephalopathy. However, there are a few cases, such as this case, which has no neonatal asphyxia and diagnosed as cerebral palsy due to subgaleal hematoma alone. The Japan Society of Obstetricians and Gynecology has reported several cases of neonatal death due to subgaleal hematoma after vacuum-assisted delivery [7].

In 1998, the US Food and Drug Administration (FDA) issued a warning about subgaleal hematomas associated with vacuum-assisted deliveries. The space between the galea aponeurotica and the periosteum of the skull is large, so that it can contain a lot of blood to cause hemorrhagic shock in newborn babies. The frequency increases with cases, which were switched from vacuum to forceps or cesarean delivery, but it can also occur with vacuum delivery alone.

How we can prevent a subgaleal hematoma? The FDA recommends "to avoid shaking or actively rotating baby head during traction." In addition, we believe that it is important to carefully monitor the newborn baby after vacuum-assisted delivery. Neonatal findings of a subgaleal hematoma include an enlarged head (which moves following the head movement and dents when pressed with a finger), and it often happened that the infant has already in hemorrhagic shock, when such findings are detected. It is important to recognize the signs of circulatory disturbance by vital signs as soon as possible.

Another concern in this case is the problem of recording in the medical record. This case was evaluated as "it is not common that the medical record does not contain the application and summary of the vacuum assisted delivery with uterine fundal pressure. In addition, since there were no findings of fetal distress or prolonged second stage of labor from the medical record and CTG, it is not common to perform vacuum delivery with uterine fundal pressure." As a member of the cause analysis committee, I had a lot of opportunities to read medical records, and I found most of them does not have an information of applications, summaries, and methods of assisted vaginal delivery. I can find many medical records, which do not have even what time the vacuum delivery was started. In this condition, it is impossible to validate the medical treatment when an adverse event occurs.

In fact, there is a civil trial which the medical side lost, because a summary of the vacuum delivery was not recorded (Yamaguchi District Court, adjudgment on July 8, 2015) [8]. In this case, after two times unsuccessful vacuum deliveries and three times unsuccessful forcep deliveries were performed at a small clinic, a cesarean section was done at a bigger medical center, and the newborn baby died due to subgaleal hematoma. There was no documentation of the degree of fetal head descent in the medical records of the clinic, and the doctor claimed in the court that it was station +2 to +3. However, the court found the clinic guilty of negligence based on preoperative findings at the medical center, which clearly documented the degree of fetal head descent as ±0 station. If the sufficient information was documented in the medical record, the result of judgment might have been different.

For the reasons stated above, medical records are important. Even if it is impossible to simultaneously document a complete record, it is desirable to record as soon as possible (if the record is made on another day, the date and time should be added). At a minimum, the following items should be recorded.

1. Time of decision to attempt rapid delivery
2. Applications for rapid delivery
3. Summary (cervix fully dilated, rupture of membranes already occurred, degree of fetal head descent, fetal presentation, etc.)
4. Method and time (start time of pulls and frequency of pulls)
5. Findings of the neonatal follow-up

I outlined four cases, which may have been associated with the development of cerebral palsy, and considered its mechanisms and preventive measures. Although most instrumental-assisted deliveries are performed without any adverse effects on the child, it is important to recognize that a few cases had adverse events, so that we should take preventive measures for all instrumental deliveries.

References

1. Ishikawa H. Anzenna kyukyuu suibenhou; tokushu-nouseimahi wo ikani yobousuruka? [Safe rapid delivery method, Special issue on how to prevent cerebral palsy?]. Perinat Med. 2018;48:309–12. Japanese.
2. Takeda S, Seki H, editors. Jitoukakoudo no hyouka to kanshi suibenjyutsu [Assessment of fetal head descent and forceps assisted delivery]. Medical View: Tokyo; 2015. Japanese.
3. Hofmeyr GJ, Vogel JP, Cuthbert A, et al. Fundal pressure during the second stage of labour. Cochrane Databse Syst Rev. 2017;3:CD006067.
4. Murphy DJ, Liebling RE, Patel R, et al. Cohort study of operative delivery in the second stage of labour and the standard of obstetric care. BJOG. 2003;110:610–5.
5. Simonson C, Barlow P, Dehennin N, et al. Neonatal complications of vacuum-assisted delivery. Obstet Gynecol. 2007;109:626–33.
6. Royal College of Obstetricians and Gynaecologists. Operative vaginal delivery. Green-top Guideline No. 26. 2011. Available from: https://www.rcog.org.uk/globalassets/documents/guidelines/gtg_26.pdf. Accessed 4 Aug 2020.
7. Japan Association of Obstetricians and Gynecologists. Kyuin bunben to shinseiji boujyoukenmakuka kesshu [Vacuum delivery and neonatal subgaleal hematoma]. JAOG News. 2015;67(3). Japanese. Series ijifunsou [Series of medical disputes].
8. Kasama T. Mutsuubunbenka de okonatta kyuuin kanshibunbentou niyotte boujyoukenmakukesshu wo hasshou si koga shiboushita jirei nitsuki tekiou no kakuninbusoku wo kashitsu toshite soungaibaishou wo mitometa saibanrei [A case of death of a child due to a subcapillary hematoma caused by suction and forceps delivery under painless delivery, in which damages were awarded on the basis of negligence and lack of confirmation of indications]. Obstet Gynecol. 2018;75:578–82. Japanese.

Prolonged Labor

Kiyotake Ichizuka

Contents

Summary

- If there is no intrauterine infection and the fetus is healthy, there is no need to intervene in the fetal adaptation, even in cases of prolonged labor. However, if the delivery is prolonged, intrauterine infection occurs, or fetal heart rate monitoring shows abnormalities, appropriate medical intervention should be considered, even if the fetal heart rate improves.

1 Overview of Prolonged Labor/Arrest of Labor

1.1 Definition

According to the definition of the Japanese Society of Obstetrics and Gynecology, prolonged labor is "one that does not lead to the delivery of a fetus even after 30 h in nulliparous women and more than 15 h in multiparous who has given birth."

K. Ichizuka (✉)
Department of Obstetrics and Gynecology, Showa University Northern Yokohama Hospital, Yokohama, Kanagawa, Japan
e-mail: ichizuka@med.showa-u.ac.jp

Y. Matsuda (ed.), *Cerebral Palsy*, https://doi.org/10.1007/978-981-19-2217-6_23

Arrest of labor is defined as "a case in which labor pains started and delivery progressed at one time, but after the uterine cervix was almost fully opened, labor pains continued as before, but progress of delivery was not observed for more than 2 h."

In contrast, the American College of Obstetricians and Gynecologists (ACOG) defines the arrest of labor as "the absence of uterine cervical dilation for 2 h or the cessation of fetal head descent for 1 hour in both nulliparous and multiparous after the active phase of the first stage of labor (uterine cervical dilation of 3–4 cm) based on the Friedman curve" [1]. However, the Friedman curve was developed in the 1950s based on the course of deliveries in 500 nulliparous women at a single institution [2], and recently there have been many controversial reports concerning the Friedman curve.

Spong et al. [3], in a workshop held by the American Society of Maternal and Fetal Medicine (SMFM), the National Institute of Child Health and Development (NICHD), and the ACOG, defined the active phase of the first stage of labor as the stage starting at 6 cm of uterine cervical dilation. In the first stage of labor, cessation of uterine cervical dilatation with proper uterine contractions for 4 h or more or improper uterine contractions for 6 h or more was defined as arrest of labor. In the second stage of labor, they proposed that the cessation of labor be defined as the failure of the head to descend after more than 3 h in nulliparous women and after more than 2 h in multiparous women [3]. However, some reports suggest that this recommendation is not evidence-based and that this proposal is premature [4, 5], so the definition of prolonged labor or arrest of labor remains controversial.

Suzuki et al. [6] reported that the curve of labor in Japanese nulliparous women is slower than that of the Friedman curve, so racial differences should be kept in mind when making a diagnosis.

1.2 Causes of Prolonged Labor

For labor to be completed smoothly, all three elements (i.e., a deliverable fetus, appropriate birth canal status, and labor pain as delivery force) must be present. If any of these elements is not present, labor may be prolonged.

Fetal abnormalities include abnormal fetal presentation, position, synclitism, and rotation. In cases of malrotation, the progression is often slow after the fetal head enters the pelvis. Such cases tend to prolong the first stage of labor, especially after the uterine cervical dilation has reached 4–5 cm.

Abnormalities of the birth canal include pelvic contraction and rigidity of soft tissue in the birth canal. The progression tends to be slow when the maximum circumference of the fetal head is level with the minimum anteroposterior pelvic diameter.

Abnormal uterine contractions include primary and secondary weak labor pain.

1.3 Management of Prolonged Labor

Internal and external examinations are used to evaluate the fetal position, synclitism, and rotation. Recently, there have been many reports citing the utility of ultrasonography in evaluating the progress of labor and prolonged labor, so ultrasonography should be actively utilized [7–9]. If no maternal or fetal abnormalities or a non-reassuring fetal status (NRFS) on fetal heart rate monitoring are noted, the patient can be followed-up. However, if weak labor is diagnosed, labor augmentation should be considered. Instrumental delivery or Caesarean section should not be performed when prolonged labor is the sole indication [3]. If the uterine cervix does not open for more than 2 h despite effective labor, Caesarean section may be considered. If the second stage of labor is prolonged, instrumental delivery is possible.

1.4 The Prolonged Labor Prognosis

Prolonged labor affects both the mother and child. In the second stage of labor, it is often accompanied by perineal edema, leading to vulvar hematoma and aggravation of laceration of the birth canal during delivery. Furthermore, the risk of postpartum urinary incontinence is said to increase in such cases [10].

However, while there is a consensus concerning the adverse effects of such prolonged labor on the mother, there is reportedly no association between a prolonged second stage of labor and the neonatal prognosis, such as a low Apgar score, neonatal seizures, or neonatal intensive care unit (NICU) admission without additional findings indicating an NRFS on fetal heart rate monitoring [11–13], although there are some reports that neonatal asphyxia and brain hemorrhaging are increased [14–16]. Therefore, at present, there is no consensus concerning the effects on the child.

The benefits of increased vaginal delivery by avoiding Caesarean section need to be compared with the increased risk of maternal and neonatal adverse effects in the second stage of labor [16].

1.5 Association with Cerebral Palsy

Prolonged labor itself has not been reported to be directly associated with cerebral palsy. However, prolonged labor has been associated with chorioamnionitis (CAM), and prolonged labor after rupture of membrane is associated with exacerbation of CAM, and the transition from CAM to fetal inflammatory response syndrome (FIRS) causes excessive production of inflammatory cytokines in the fetus, which damages neurons and leads to the development of fetal periventricular leukomalacia (PVL), the cause of cerebral palsy. Although fetal PVL caused by FIRS is more likely to occur in preterm infants than in full-term ones, the cord blood cytokine levels are also high in full-term infants with cerebral palsy, suggesting that fetal inflammation may cause brain cell damage, as in preterm infants [17].

However, the pathogenesis of cerebral palsy in full-term infants may differ from that in preterm infants, as the pathogenesis of cerebral palsy in full-term infants is based on a decreased cerebral blood flow and microthrombus formation due to circulatory failure caused by septic shock [18]. The pathological mechanism of "prolonged delivery → (rupture of membrane) → CAM → FIRS → cerebral palsy" seems likely.

2 Case Control Study

Torbenson et al. [19] conducted a case-control study (control 104) on 26 cases of ischemic encephalopathy due to events during delivery (singleton, >35 weeks' gestation) and reported that, among various factors during delivery, a prolonged seconds stage of labor increased the risk of developing ischemic encephalopathy on a multivariate analysis (adjusted odds ratio [AOR] 9.49 [95% confidence interval: 1.06–135.3, $P = 0.042$]). They concluded that the causes of ischemic encephalopathy in prolonged labor may be multifactorial, as it was difficult to deliver the fetus by Caesarean section after prolonged labor in 4 of the 26 cases.

3 Current Situation in Japan/Report from the Recurrence Prevention Committee (Toward the Prevention of Recurrence)

In the eighth Annual Report on the Prevention of Recurrence by the Recurrence Prevention Committee of the Japan Obstetric Compensation System for Cerebral Palsy (JOCSC), prolonged labor was taken up in the analysis in line with the theme. According to the report, of the 1606 cases of cerebral palsy diagnosed, 104 (6.5%) were singleton deliveries that met the definition of prolonged labor as defined by the Japanese Society of Obstetrics and Gynecology and resulted in vaginal delivery. Fetal heart rate abnormalities were observed in 103 of the 104 cases. Regardless of the pattern and duration of fetal heart rate abnormalities, and whether or not the fetal well-being was judged to be healthy after the appearance of abnormal waveforms, the longer the time between the appearance of an abnormal fetal heart rate and the delivery of the baby, the lower the Apgar score and the higher the rate of severe neonatal asphyxia (Fig. 1). Furthermore, the percentage of cases with an umbilical artery blood gas pH value of ≥7.2 tended to decrease in same 103 cases (Fig. 2) [20]. Therefore, when delivery time is expected to be prolonged, the causes of prolonged delivery should be investigated for each of the three elements of labor

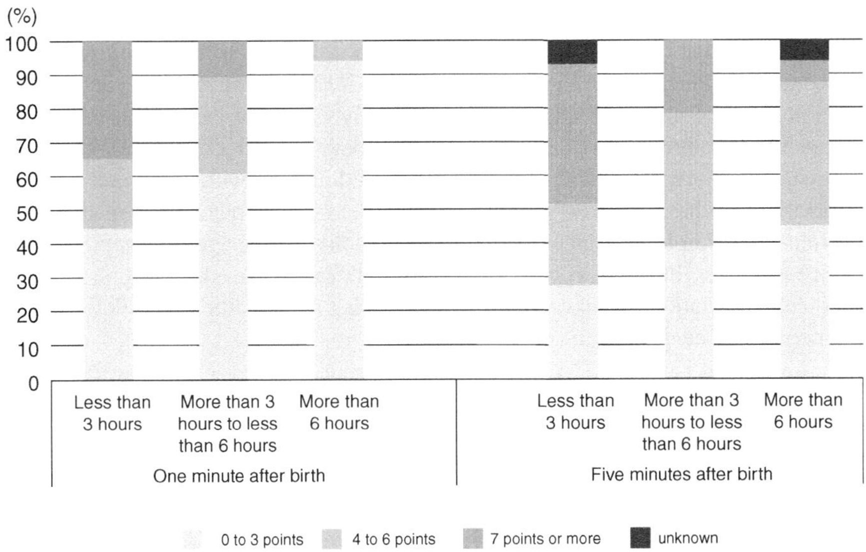

Fig. 1 Time from the appearance of abnormal fetal heart rate findings to delivery of the baby and Apgar score (Reproduced from Ref. [20])

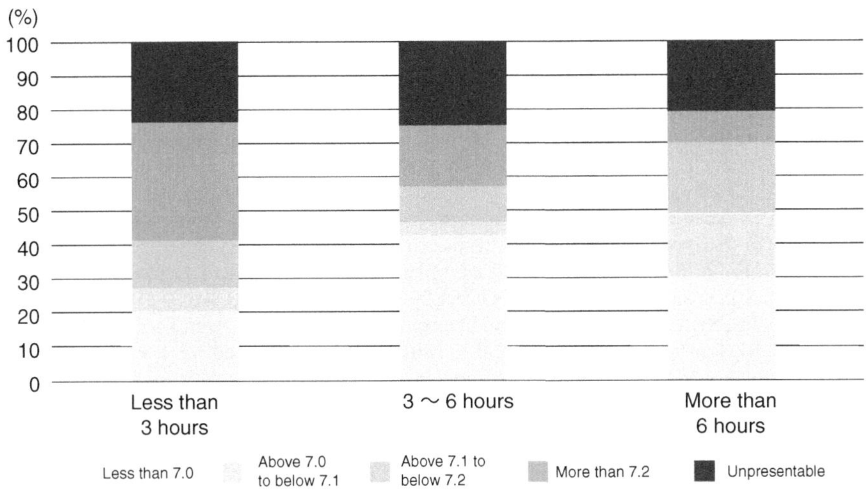

Fig. 2 Time from the appearance of abnormal fetal heart rate findings to delivery of the baby and umbilical artery blood gas analysis (pH) [20]

mentioned above, and appropriate interventions should be performed, tailored to each element.

Prolonged labor was also shown to be associated with CAM. In this eighth Annual report, intrauterine infections were observed in 21 (21.2%) of 99 cases of cerebral palsy with prolonged labor and 63 (12.5%) of 503 cases of cerebral palsy without prolonged labor, and intrauterine infections tended to be more frequent in cases with prolonged labor than in those without it [20]. However, a placental histopathological examination was performed in only 24.4% of cases with prolonged labor; it is recommended that placental histopathological examinations be performed when severe neonatal asphyxia is observed in cases with prolonged labor. In 34 (35.1%) of the 97 cases of prolonged labor, the medical record was inadequate.

In cases of prolonged labor, the duration of delivery management is prolonged, which increases the frequency of complaints and events. The adequate collection of medical information is important for understanding the condition after delivery and for reviewing the delivery management.

References

1. American College of Obstetricians and Gynecologists. Dystocia and augmentation of labor. Practice Bulletin. 2003;49.
2. Friedman EA. The graphic analysis of labor. Am J Obstet Gynecol. 1954;68:1568–75.
3. Spong CY, Berghella V, Wenstrom KD, et al. Preventing the first cesarean delivery: summary of a joint Eunice Kennedy Shriver National Institute of Child Health and Human Development, Society for Maternal-Fetal Medicine, and American College of Obstetricians and Gynecologists Workshop. Obstet Gynecol. 2012;120:1181–93.
4. Cohen WR, Friedman EA. Perils of the new labor management guidelines. Am J Obstet Gynecol. 2015;212:420–7.
5. Cohen WR, Friedman EA. Guidelines for labor assessment: failure to progress? Am J Obstet Gynecol. 2020;222:342.e1–4.
6. Suzuki R, Horiuchi S, Ohtsu H. Evaluation of the labor curve in nulliparous Japanese women. Am J Obstet Gynecol. 2010;203:226.e1–6.
7. Dall'Asta A, Angeli L, Masturzo B, et al. Prediction of spontaneous vaginal delivery in nulliparous women with a prolonged second stage of labor: the value of intrapartum ultrasound. Am J Obstet Gynecol. 2019;221:642.e1–642.e13.
8. Bellussi F, Ghi T, Youssef A, et al. The use of intrapartum ultrasound to diagnose malpositions and cephalic malpresentations. Am J Obstet Gynecol. 2017;217:633–41.
9. Molina FS, Nicolaides KH. Ultrasound in labor and delivery. Fetal Diagn Ther. 2010;27:61–7.
10. Brown SJ, Gartland D, Donath S, et al. Effects of prolonged second stage, method of birth, timing of caesarean section and other obstetric risk factors on postnatal urinary incontinence: an Australian nulliparous cohort study. Br J Obstet Gynaecol. 2011;118:991–1000.
11. Saunders NS, Paterson CM, Wadsworth J. Neonatal and maternal morbidity in relation to the length of the second stage of labour. Br J Obstet Gynaecol. 1992;99:381–5.
12. Menticoglou SM, Manning F, Harman C, et al. Perinatal outcome in relation to second-stage duration. Am J Obstet Gynecol. 1995;173:906–12.
13. Myles TD, Santolaya J. Maternal and neonatal outcomes in patients with a prolonged second stage of labor. Obstet Gynecol. 2003;102:52–8.
14. Cheng YW, Hopkins LM, Caughey AB. How long is too long: does a prolonged second stage of labor in nulliparous women affect maternal and neonatal outcomes? Am J Obstet Gynecol. 2004;191:933–8.
15. Allen VM, Baskett TF, O'Connell CM, et al. Maternal and perinatal outcomes with increasing duration of the second stage of labor. Obstet Gynecol. 2009;113:1248–58.

16. Laughon SK, Berghella V, Reddy UM, et al. Neonatal and maternal outcomes with prolonged second stage of labor. Obstet Gynecol. 2014;124:57–67.
17. Shalak LF, Laptook AR, Jafri HS, et al. Clinical chorioamnionitis, elevated cytokines, and brain injury in term infants. Pediatrics. 2002;110:673–80.
18. Romero R, Espinoza J, Gonçalves LF, et al. Fetal cardiac dysfunction in preterm premature rupture of membranes. J Matern Fetal Neonatal Med. 2004;16:146–57.
19. Torbenson VE, Tolcher MC, Nesbitt KM, et al. Intrapartum factors associated with neonatal hypoxic ischemic encephalopathy: a case-controlled study. BMC Pregnancy Childbirth. 2017;17:415.
20. Japan Council for Quality Health Care. About prolonged delivery. 8th report on prevention of recurrence, the Japan obstetric compensation system for cerebral palsy—toward the improvement of obstetric care. Tokyo: Japan Council for Quality Health Care. 2018. Japanese.

Maternal Respiratory and Circulatory Failure

Jun Yoshimatsu

Contents

Summary

- Maternal respiratory circulatory failure causes cerebral palsy from decreased perfusion and oxygenation of the interchorionic space.
- Chronic maternal respiratory and circulatory failure can cause fetal growth retardation (FGR) but does not actively cause cerebral palsy.
- In acute maternal respiratory and circulatory failure, cerebral palsy can be avoided by rapid recovery by resuscitation or early delivery.
- In the case of maternal cardiopulmonary arrest, classical delivery within 4–5 min is expected to result in uninjured survival. In addition, cerebral palsy is rather rare and often results in death or uninjured survival.
- Amniotic fluid embolism and group A streptococcus (GAS) infection are aggravated by persistent strong uterine contractions in addition to decreased perfusion and oxygenation of the intervillous spaces due to acute maternal respiratory circulatory failure.
- The purpose of a perimortem cesarean section is to resuscitate the mother, but it is also beneficial to the fetus.

J. Yoshimatsu (✉)
Department of Obstetrics and Gynecology, National Cerebral and Cardiovascular Center, Suita, Osaka, Japan
e-mail: yoshimatsu.jun.hp@ncvc.go.jp

Y. Matsuda (ed.), *Cerebral Palsy*, https://doi.org/10.1007/978-981-19-2217-6_24

1 Overview of Respiratory and Circulatory Failure

The condition in which the partial pressure of oxygen in arterial blood falls below 60 mmHg is called respiratory failure [1]. There are various causes of respiratory failure, but many of them are serious, such as acute respiratory distress syndrome and pulmonary thromboembolism. Circulatory failure is a condition in which the effective blood flow to vital organs is reduced for some reason and the organs are unable to maintain their functions. Acute causes include hemorrhage, infection, heart failure, and anaphylaxis.

During pregnancy, the diaphragm is elevated, but the respiratory rate remains almost unchanged, and preinspiratory volume, minute ventilation, and lung capacity increase, while preexpiratory volume and residual air volume decrease. As a result, minute ventilation increases and oxygenation is enhanced. In terms of circulation, circulating blood volume increases, and cardiac output (the amount of blood pumped from the heart per minute) increases due to increases in stroke volume and heart rate. The increase in minute ventilation and cardiac output are both physiological changes that occur to increase the oxygen supply to the intervillous spaces per unit time. In respiratory failure, oxygenation is impaired, and the partial pressure of oxygen in the maternal arterial blood is decreased. In circulatory failure, the blood flow of the maternal blood to the intervillous space is decreased. In other words, the physiological increase in oxygen delivery to the intervillous space is inhibited, and the oxygenation of the placenta is impaired. In other words, the oxygenation of the fetus is impaired, and an environment that causes damage to the central nervous system emerges.

Acute respiratory and circulatory failure, if severe, can lead to shock and cardiopulmonary arrest. In the report of the Japan Obstetric Compensation System for Cerebral Palsy in 2020 [2], we found that 13 cases (0.5%) of maternal respiratory and circulatory failure due to amniotic fluid embolism were the main cause of cerebral palsy (CP) and 24 cases (0.5%) of maternal respiratory and circulatory failure other than amniotic fluid embolism were the main cause of CP (0.5%) and maternal respiratory and circulatory failure other than amniotic fluid embolism in 24 cases (1.0%). In addition, in the 2019 report, maternal respiratory and circulatory failure was taken up as a theme, and three cases of amniotic fluid embolism and one case of GAS infection were introduced, suggesting that it is also important to pay attention to and manage sudden changes in maternal respiratory and circulatory status when fetal heart rate abnormalities appear [3].

In this section, in order to decipher the relationship between maternal respiratory insufficiency and cerebral palsy, we will first outline chronic hypoperfusion of the intervillous spaces and then describe the relationship between maternal cardiopulmonary arrest, the most common cause of respiratory insufficiency, and cerebral palsy in each disease that causes respiratory insufficiency.

2 Chronic Reduction of Circulation and Its Relation to Fetal Growth

Bamfo et al. [4] reported that when pregnant women with normal cardiac structures underwent echocardiography within 10 days before delivery, the cardiac output of mothers born with fetal growth retardation (FGR) was lower than that of mothers born with normal newborns. This decrease in cardiac output was due to a decrease in single beat volume, not heart rate. Vasapollo et al. [5] compared various parameters of echocardiography, heart rate, and blood pressure between mothers with normal fetuses and fetuses of mothers with fetal growth retardation (FGR). This report also shows that cardiac output is lower than normal in FGR mothers and that systemic vascular resistance is more elevated. This report also indicates that the decrease in cardiac output is mainly due to a decrease in single-beat output. Even in the presence of maternal cardiac disease, there are many reports showing an association between cardiac output and fetal growth.

Chronic impaired perfusion of the intervillous spaces affects fetal growth but has not been associated with cerebral palsy. This may be because the degree of hypoperfusion of the intervillous spaces is mild in chronic respiratory insufficiency, and compensatory changes such as placental vascularization are observed in response to the chronic process.

3 Acute Respiratory and Circulatory Failure and Cerebral Palsy

The most extreme form of acute respiratory and circulatory failure is maternal cardiopulmonary arrest. In this case, the new oxygen supply to the intervillous spaces ceases.

In 1986, Katz et al. [6] reviewed articles from the past 20 years and found that 70% of surviving infants were delivered within 5 min and 95% were delivered within 15 minutes, indicating that neonatal survival increases within 4–5 min of maternal cardiopulmonary arrest. Katz et al. [7] reviewed again 20 years later the subsequent review of 1985–2004 as a follow-up and reported that 34 neonates out of 38 cases of maternal cardiopulmonary arrest survived and 75% were delivered within 15 min.

In 2012, Einavas et al. [8] compared the time from cardiopulmonary arrest to birth in surviving and non-surviving neonates and reported that it was 14 ± 11 min and 22 ± 13 min, respectively. These data are basically about survival and non-survival. But what about intact survival?

In a review by Benson et al. [9], they found that the time from cardiopulmonary arrest to birth increases the number of cases with poor neurological prognosis and

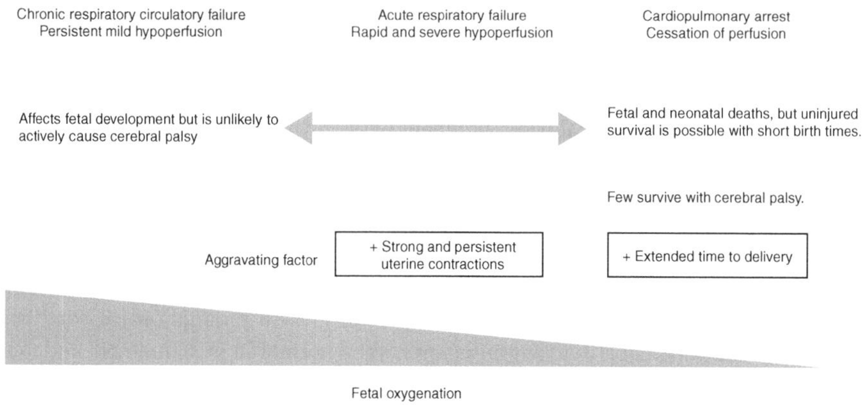

Fig. 1 Degree of fetal oxygenation, maternal events, and cerebral palsy. Maternal respiratory insufficiency can range from chronic respiratory and circulatory failure to cardiopulmonary arrest, and in each situation, there is a varying degree of fetal oxygenation and consequently a varying prognosis for the child. Affects fetal development but is unlikely to actively cause cerebral palsy. Fetal and neonatal deaths, but uninjured survival is possible with short birth times

that 50% intact survival is achieved in 26 min. When the oxygen supply to the intervillous spaces is interrupted by maternal cardiopulmonary arrest, the oxygenation of the fetus is rapidly interrupted, and the prognosis is determined by the duration of the interruption: intact survival, cerebral palsy, or death. However, there are not many cases of survival with cerebral palsy. Most of them either die or survive without neurological damage (Fig. 1).

In perimortem cesarean delivery reported to Confidential Enquiries into Maternal Deaths (CEMD) from 1970 to 1996, none of the surviving cases had a child with neurological damage [10]. The timing of survival with cerebral palsy in maternal cardiopulmonary arrest is considered to be very narrow. In addition, there is no report that there is a difference according to the disease leading to cardiopulmonary arrest.

4 Amniotic Fluid Embolism and Cerebral Palsy

Amniotic fluid embolism is a condition that presents with acute respiratory failure and disseminated intravascular coagulation (DIC) caused by the inflow of amniotic fluid components into the maternal bloodstream. The prognosis for both mother and infant are poor. Anaphylactic reaction is considered to be the main cause of the condition and respiratory failure occurs very rapidly. Amniotic fluid embolism with cardiopulmonary collapse accounts for 12% of maternal deaths in Japan [11]. Although there is no report on the incidence of cerebral palsy, amniotic fluid embolism accounts for 0.5% of the cerebral palsy cases analyzed in the Japan Obstetric Compensation System for Cerebral Palsy, as mentioned above.

In a report on 44 of 66 cases of amniotic fluid embolism registered in the United Kingdom between 1997 and 2004 for which information was available for analysis, seven of the infants born to 13 deceased mothers were present, four of whom had acidosis, two of whom developed hypoxic-ischemic encephalopathy, and finally one of whom developed cerebral palsy. In one case, cerebral palsy developed. Of the 18 surviving mothers whose infants were alive in utero at the time of acute respiratory and circulatory failure, 14 had surviving infants. Four of the surviving infants developed hypoxic-ischemic encephalopathy, and one of them developed cerebral palsy [12], according to the authors.

The development of cardiopulmonary collapse amniotic fluid embolism leads to acute respiratory circulatory failure and decreased perfusion to the interchorionic space. In the case presented in the report from the Obstetric Medical Compensation System, strong uterine contractions were observed after the onset of amniotic fluid embolism, and hypertrophic labor was recorded [3]. Hyperemesis gravidarum further decreases perfusion to the intervillous space, which further inhibits oxygen delivery to the fetus and accelerates cerebral palsy and death.

5 GAS Infection and Cerebral Palsy

When toxic shock occurs in GAS infection, rapid and strong uterine contractions are also observed. In the case presented in the Ninth Report on the Prevention of Recurrence of the Japan Obstetric Compensation System for Cerebral Palsy, hyperemesis gravidarum was also recorded by cardiotocography (CTG) [3]. Obstruction of blood flow to the uterus due to strong and sustained uterine contractions and septic shock prior to acute cardiopulmonary collapse can cause significant impairment of fetal oxygenation. As a result, intrauterine fetal death occurs. In the analysis of maternal deaths in Japan, 90% of cases of fetal death in utero occurred during pregnancy. Although the incidence of cerebral palsy is not clear, Crum et al. [13] showed from a review that four out of five cases of cerebral palsy occurring between 29 and 34 weeks of gestation resulted in intrauterine fetal death.

6 Total Spinal Subarachnoid Anesthesia and Cerebral Palsy

Total spinal subarachnoid anesthesia (total spinal anesthesia) is a condition in which the anesthetic high extends beyond the upper cervical cord into the brainstem, causing respiratory arrest, loss of consciousness, and hypotension. In obstetrics, it may occur during anesthesia for cesarean section or labor analgesia. Respiratory arrest and hypotension decrease perfusion of the interchorionic space. Oxygenation of the fetus can be maintained by administering 100% oxygen for respiratory arrest and by administering a hypotensive agent for hypotension. If this is not done properly, fetal death from cerebral palsy may result. In a US study, 93% of unnoticed subarachnoid stray epidural catheter tubes were found during labor analgesia [14]. Although the frequency of cerebral palsy is not clear, in Japan, cerebral palsy was reported in 1 of 4 cases of total paraplegia from 2008 to 2017 in which the mother survived. Of the three cases in which the mother died, two died and one survived without injury.

7 If the Mother Has Acute Respiratory and Circulatory Failure

If the mother is in a critical condition, priority is given to maternal rescue. Resuscitation is given priority regardless of the condition of the fetus. The purpose of this procedure is to save the life of the mother in case of cardiopulmonary arrest. It is advantageous for resuscitation to deliver the baby and relieve the pressure on the great vessels. On the other hand, if the infant can be delivered as early as possible after cardiopulmonary arrest, the infant can survive without sequelae. Katz et al. [6], cited earlier in this review, focused on the prognosis of the infant after maternal cardiopulmonary arrest and found that the success rate of maternal resuscitation improved, confirming the usefulness of cesarean section for maternal resuscitation. The current concept of cesarean section in the perimortem stages is based on the findings from cesarean sections performed for the purpose of saving the mother and not for the fetus. In any case, there are only two ways to ensure fetal survival without sequelae in the setting of acute maternal respiratory failure. Either the acute respiratory failure must be corrected early to restore oxygen to the fetus or the child's oxygen source must be transferred from the placenta to its own lungs, i.e., delivery. Again, in the case of acute maternal respiratory and circulatory failure, the focus is on maternal resuscitation. However, these resuscitative procedures, including cesarean section at term, are also beneficial to the survival of the child.

References

1. Yokoyama T. Kouseisyou Tokuteishikkann "Kokyufuzen" Cyousakenkyu Gyouseki [Results of research on respiratory failure, a specific disease of the Ministry of Health and Welfare]. 1982. Japanese.
2. Japan Council for Quality Health Care. 10th report on prevention of recurrence, the Japan obstetric compensation system for cerebral palsy. Tokyo: Japan Council for Quality Health Care. 2020. Japanese.
3. Japan Council for Quality Health Care. 9th report on prevention of recurrence, the Japan obstetric compensation system for cerebral palsy. Tokyo: Japan Council for Quality Health Care. 2019. Japanese.
4. Bamfo JE, Kametas NA, Turan O, et al. Maternal cardiac function in fetal growth restriction. BJOG. 2006;113:784–91.
5. Vasapollo B, Valensise H, Novelli GP, et al. Abnormal maternal cardiac function precedes the clinical manifestation of fetal growth restriction. Ultrasound Obstet Gynecol. 2004;24:23–9.

6. Katz VL, Dotters DJ, Droegemueller W. Perimortem cesarean delivery. Obstet Gynecol. 1986;68:571–6.
7. Katz V, Balderston K, DeFreest M. Perimortem cesarean delivery: were our assumptions correct? Am J Obstet Gynecol. 2005;192:1916–21.
8. Einav S, Kaufman N, Sela HY. Maternal cardiac arrest and perimortem cesarean delivery: evidence or expert-based? Resuscitation. 2012;83:1191–200.
9. Benson MD, Padovano A, Bourjeily G, et al. Maternal collapse: challenging the four-minute rule. EBioMedicine. 2016;6:253–7.
10. Whitten M, Irvine LM. Postmortem and perimortem caesarean section: what are the indications? J R Soc Med. 2000;93:6–9.
11. Committee for Review and Evaluation of Cases of Maternal Death. Botaianzenheno teigen 2019, vol. 10 [Recommendations for maternal safety in 2019, vol. 10]. Tokyo: Japan Society of Obstetricians and Gynecologists. 2020. Japanese.
12. Tuffnell DJ. United Kingdom amniotic fluid embolism register. BJOG. 2005;112:1625–9.
13. Crum NF, Chun HM, Gaylord TG, et al. Group A streptococcal toxic shock syndrome developing in the third trimester of pregnancy. Infect Dis Obstet Gynecol. 2002;10:209–16.
14. D'Angelo R, Smiley RM, Riley ET, et al. Serious complications related to obstetric anesthesia: the serious complication repository project of the Society for Obstetric Anesthesia and Perinatology. Anesthesiology. 2014;120:1505–12.

GBS Infection

Katsumi Mizuno

Contents

Summary

- Group B streptococcus (GBS) is the most frequent causative agent of neonatal infections, causing sepsis and meningitis in neonates and often leaving them with visual disturbances and cerebral palsy (CP). Therefore, prevention of neonatal GBS infection is also important to prevent CP.
- The measures described in "Guidelines for Obstetrics and Gynecology 2020" have reduced early-onset GBS infections to about one-third. However, the number of delayed GBS infections has not decreased, and it is necessary to review the measures against GBS infections once again to prevent CP.

K. Mizuno (✉)
Department of Pediatrics, Showa University School of Medicine, Tokyo, Japan
e-mail: katsuorobi@med.showa-u.ac.jp

Y. Matsuda (ed.), *Cerebral Palsy*, https://doi.org/10.1007/978-981-19-2217-6_25

1 Neonates and Group B Streptococcal Infections

Group B streptococcus (GBS) is currently the most frequent causative agent of neonatal infections. Ten to thirty percent of pregnant women carry GBS, and if prophylactic measures are not taken, GBS becomes established in 50% of the babies born to carriers, and about 1% of these babies will develop the disease [1]. In other words, 0.5–1.5 newborns per 1000 will develop GBS infection. According to a nationwide questionnaire survey by Matsubara et al. [2], sepsis and meningitis accounted for 73% and 26%, respectively, of early-onset GBS infections. The mortality rate is 4.5% in early-onset GBS infections, and the sequelae rate is about 30% in those who develop meningitis, so it is still an important neonatal infection.

Infection progresses rapidly in neonates, leading to sepsis and meningitis, and the prognosis is extremely poor. Meningitis in neonates often causes visual disturbance and cerebral palsy (CP), and prevention of neonatal GBS infection is also important to prevent CP.

The administration of antimicrobial agents described in the "Guidelines for Obstetrics and Gynecology 2020" (see below) reduced early-onset GBS infections to about one-third. However, delayed-onset GBS infections have not decreased, and because they are an important cause of meningitis, it is necessary to review measures against GBS infections once again to prevent CP.

2 Neonatal Meningitis and the Pathogenesis of Brain Damage

When a neonate develops meningitis, the pathogen reaches the brain-blood barrier and is recognized by antigen-presenting cells by binding to Toll-like receptors (TLRs). As a result, nuclear factor-kappa B (NF-kappa B) and mitogen-activated protein kinase (MAPK) pathways are activated, followed by the expression of proteins involved in the inflammatory response. Many brain cells produce cytokines, chemokines, and other inflammatory molecules in response to bacterial stimuli. Polymorphonuclear leukocytes accumulate in these cells and release superoxide and nitric oxide, resulting in peroxynitrite production and oxidative stress. This cascade leads to lipid peroxidation, mitochondrial damage, and disruption of the blood-brain barrier, resulting in cellular damage [3].

3 A Case in Which the Main Cause of Cerebral Palsy Was Considered to Be Group B Streptococcal Infection [4]

Among the 43 cases in which the main cause of CP onset was considered to be GBS infection, 18 cases had early-onset GBS infection and 25 cases had late-onset GBS infection. Table 1 shows the status of GBS screening by mode of delivery, its results, and antimicrobial administration in early-onset and late-onset GBS infections.

Table 1 Group B streptococcus (GBS) screening practices and antimicrobial administration during pregnancy (Modified from Ref. [4])

	Early-onset GBS infection (18)		Delayed-onset GBS infection (25)	
	Vaginal delivery	Caesarean section	Vaginal delivery	Caesarean section
	Number of cases (%)		Number of cases (%)	
Screening available	18 (100)	0 (zero)	18 (72)	5 (20)
Positive	5[a] (27.8)	–	5 (20)	1 (4)
(With antibiotics[b])	0 (0)	–	4 (16)	0 (0)
Negative	13[c] (72.2)	–	13 (52)	4 (16)
(With antimicrobial therapy) Within 5 weeks from last screening to delivery of baby	9 (50)	–	10 (40)	2 (8)
Unscreened	0 (0)	0 (0)	0 (0)	2[d] (8)

[a] Of the 5 cases of early-onset GBS infection with positive GBS screening, four were negative after the second or subsequent screening, and one was delivered within 20 min of admission
[b] "With antimicrobial agents" refers only to those administered in the manner recommended for the prevention of early-onset GBS infection in the Obstetrics and Gynecology Clinical Practice Guidelines, Obstetrics Edition 2020, and excludes those administered for impending preterm labor or preterm water breaking
[c] Of the 13 cases of early-onset GBS infection with negative screening, there were 4 cases of full-term birth that were more than 6 weeks after negative screening
[d] Two cases of late-onset GBS infection without screening were cases of scheduled cesarean section

4 Early-Onset Group B Streptococcal Infection

Among the cases in which the main cause of CP was considered to be early-onset GBS infection, there were four cases of full-term births in which more than 6 weeks had passed since the GBS screening was negative. According to "Guidelines for Obstetrics and Gynecology 2020," the timing of GBS culture test, incorrect specimen collection method (especially, the specimen should be collected by inserting the swab into the anus after wiping the area around the vaginal entrance with the swab), selection of culture medium, and culture method are related to the prevention of GBS infection. The CQ 603 is cited in part below.

However, even if the infant is screened appropriately and the result is negative for GBS, the newborn should be observed with consideration that early-onset GBS infection can still occur. If any of the symptoms or risk factors listed in Table 2 are observed, blood count, CRP, X-ray, urine, and other tests should be performed. Antimicrobial therapy should be initiated based on a comprehensive evaluation of the test results. Since meningitis may occur in neonates from the early stage of the disease, a spinal fluid test should be performed if it is suspected. If respiratory distress is observed in a neonate undergoing follow-up at a delivery institution, it should be noted that even if the results of GBS screening during pregnancy are negative, it does not mean that the neonate will not develop early-onset GBS infection and that neonates often present with respiratory distress as one of the systemic

Table 2 Symptoms and risk factors seen in neonatal infections (Modified from Ref. [1])

Symptoms seen in neonatal infections	• Not doing well • Poor skin color • Poor suckling performance • Apnea • Unstable body temperature (fever, hypothermia) • Abdominal distention, vomiting • Jaundice • Irritability
Risk factors for neonatal infections	• Premature rupture of membrane (more than 18 or 24 h) • Premature rupture of membrane of preterm delivery

symptoms of non-respiratory diseases. In addition, neonates often present with respiratory distress as one of the systemic symptoms of non-respiratory diseases, so it is necessary to observe the development of symptoms and the presence or absence of symptoms suspected of neonatal infection, such as fever, hypothermia, and poor skin color, and to understand the general condition of the infant to differentiate it from respiratory diseases.

5 CQ603 How Can We Prevent Early-Onset Group B Streptococcus (GBS) Infection in Full-Term Neonates?

5.1 Answer

1. Confirm the presence of GBS by the following methods.
   (a) GBS culture test at 35–37 weeks of pregnancy (B).
   (b) Specimens should be collected from the entrance of the vagina and anus (C).
   (A) Intravenous penicillin and other antimicrobial agents to prevent infection of the newborn during vaginal delivery or after the premature rupture of the membrane in pregnant women with the following conditions (B).
   (a) GBS identified in Answer 1.
   (b) The older infant has GBS infection.
   (c) GBS detected in urine culture during this pregnancy.
   (d) Patients with unknown GBS status, 18 h or more have passed since the water broke, or have fever of 38.0° or higher.
   (Reprinted from [5])

6 Delayed-Onset Group B Streptococcal Infection

Delayed-onset GBS infections that occur after 7 days of age are more likely to occur at home or elsewhere after hospital discharge. In a report by Berardi et al. on 100 cases of late-onset GBS infection, 57 were diagnosed as sepsis and 36 as meningitis; 15 had severe brain lesions at discharge, 14 of which were complicated by

Table 3 25 eligible cases that led to cerebral palsy (CP) (Created based on Ref. [4])

Cases	Number of cases (%)
Poor feeding (poor swallowing, no feeding)	14 (56)
Lack of vitality (lack of energy, no crying, limp, sleeping)	11 (44)
Fever (body temperature 38.0 °C or higher, feeling of warmth)	9 (36)
Grumpy (bad mood, won't stop crying)	6 (24)
Poor complexion and skin color (pallor, flushing)	5 (20)
Vomiting	4 (16)
Change in respiratory status (grunting, sputum-like breathing)	4 (16)
Convulsions (twitching, staring)	2 (8)

meningitis. Of these, 14 were complicated by meningitis. In other words, 14% of late-onset GBS infections may cause brain damage, and it is important to take measures against late-onset GBS infections to prevent CP.

Among the 2457 cases for which causal analysis reports were sent to parents of infants with CP and delivery institutions by the end of September 2019, 43 cases were determined that the main cause of CP was GBS infection, and among them, 25 cases were diagnosed as delayed-onset GBS infection [4]. Delayed-onset GBS infection develops as septicemia and meningitis, and the most common symptoms are fever, feeding difficulties, and convulsions [1].

There is no established method for prevention of delayed-onset GBS infection, and its clinical symptoms are nonspecific, so it is important to understand the vague symptoms of "somewhat listlessness." For this reason, it is desirable to provide health guidance to parents at the time of discharge from the hospital and at the time of post-discharge checkups, so that they will immediately consult with medical institutions if they feel "somewhat listless." In addition, when the guardians are consulted about the complaint that the child is "somewhat listless," it is necessary to immediately recommend that the guardians visit a medical institution for a thorough examination. Table 3 shows the results of a detailed analysis of 25 cases that later led to CP.

7 Future Challenges in Delayed-Onset Group B Streptococcal Infections

As mentioned earlier, antimicrobial administration during delivery reduced early-onset GBS infections, but Berardi et al. [6] reported that acquired GBS infections were 0.32 per 1000 newborns, almost unchanged from the value before antimicrobial administration during delivery, 0.35 per 1000. Inode et al. [7] reported that maternal carriage of GBS was maintained in half of the cases even after maternal antimicrobial administration. Since the incidence of GBS infection is higher in preterm infants (1.4 per 1000 live births) compared with full-term infants (0.24 per 1000 live births) [6], it is necessary to consider the possibility of late-onset GBS infection in preterm infants with nonspecific symptoms.

The route of infection is an issue to be addressed. Previous case reports have identified breast milk as one of the routes of transmission of delayed-onset GBS infection [8–13]. In the report by Berardi et al. breast milk samples were collected from 44 of 45 lactating women whose infants were diagnosed as GBS infections, and 11 of the samples were positive for GBS. Bacterial counts were performed on 6 samples, and 3 samples obtained from women with mastitis were above 1000,000 CFU/mL, and the remaining 3 samples were below 100,000 CFU/mL. In Japan, there have been many case reports in which breast milk was considered to be the cause of delayed GBS infection, and repeated infections have been observed [14]. In addition, Filleron et al. [15] reported that 18 of 21 reported cases of delayed GBS infection suspected to be caused by breast milk were GBS type III, but it is unclear how many mothers' breast milk detects GBS type III. Furthermore, the mechanism by which GBS is transferred to breast milk has not been clarified, although it has been suggested that GBS may be present in the mother's milk ducts or transferred to milk from the intestinal microflora.

8 Prevention: Delayed-Onset Group B Streptococcal Infection

As can be seen from Table 3, delayed GBS infection occurs even if the GBS screening test in the second half of pregnancy is negative, so it might be argued if the culture test of breast milk of all mothers is performed. If the GBS positive rate in breast milk is much higher than the incidence of late-onset GBS infection (0.32 out of 1000), there must be some mechanism that prevents late-onset GBS infection, even if GBS is detected in breast milk. In addition, in full-term infants who are diagnosed as late-onset GBS infection, breastfeeding may be stopped and be changed to formula feed, but in special circumstances, breastfeeding may be continued while pasteurization of breast milk is performed [16].

What to do about breastfeeding when a diagnosis of delayed GBS infection is made will have to be discussed in the future. In any case, it is important to suspect GBS infection at an early stage based on the child's symptoms and to provide treatment as soon as possible.

References

1. Takahashi N. B gun youketsusei rensakyukin [Group B Streptococcus]. In: Committee on Neonates, Japanese Society of Pediatrics, editor. Shinseiji no primary care [Primary care of the newborn]. Tokyo: Shindan to chiryou sha. 2016. p. 57–9. Japanese.
2. Matsubara K. Shinseiji niokeru B gun rensakyukin (GBS) shinshusei kansenshou no kinnen no tokuchou [Recent features of group B Streptococcus (GBS) invasive infections in neonates]. Japanese. [Internet]. http://medical.radionikkei.jp/kansenshotoday_pdf/kansenshotoday-170118.pdf. Accessed 12 May 2020.

3. Koedel Uwe. Toll-Like receptors in bacterial meningitis. Curr Top Microbiol Immunolo. 2009;336:15–40.
4. Japan Council for Quality Health Care. Chapter 3 Thematic analysis IV neonatal management. In: Japan Council for Quality Health Care. The 10th report on the prevention of recurrence of the obstetric medical compensation system. Tokyo: Japan Council for Quality Health Care. 2020. p. 27. Japanese.
5. Japanese Society of Obstetrics and Gynecology/Japan Society of Obstetricians and Gynecologists. Guidelines for obstetrics and gynecology 2020 [Sanfujinka Shinryo guideline Sankahen 2020]. Tokyo: The Japanese Society of Obstetrics and Gynecology. 2020. p. 297. Japanese.
6. Berardi A, Rossi C, Lugli L, et al. Group B streptococcus late-onset disease: 2003-2010. Pediatrics. 2013;131:e361–8.
7. Inode Y. B gun youketsusei rensakyuukin youseibotai niokeru bunbenji no yobouteki koukinzai no soutouyoryou to shinseiji ikouritsu tono kanren [Association between total dose of prophylactic antimicrobial agents at delivery and neonatal transfer rate in group B streptococcus-positive mothers]. J Japan Soc Perinatal Neonatal Med. 2010;46:567. Japanese.
8. Bingen E, Denamur E, Lambert-Zechovsky N, et al. Analysis of DNA restriction fragment length polymorphism extends the evidence for breast milk transmission in Streptococcus agalactiae late-onset neonatal infection. J Infect Dis. 1992;165:569–73.
9. Kotlw M, Zhang GW, Daggard G, et al. Late-onset and recurrent neonatal group B streptococcal disease associated with breast-milk transmission. Pediatr Dev Pathol. 2003;6:251–6.
10. Olver WJ, Bond DW, Boswell TC, et al. Nonatal group B streptococcal disease associated with infected breast milk. Arch Dis Child Fetal Neonatal Ed. 2000;83:f48–9.
11. Dinger J, Muller D, Pargac N, et al. Breast milk transmission of group B streptococcal infection. Pediatr Infect Dis J. 2002;21:567–8.
12. Godambe S, Shah PS, Shah V. Breast milk as a source of late onset neonatal sepsis. Pediatr Infect Dis J. 2005;24:381–2.
13. Dillon HC Jr, Khare S, Gray BM. Group B streptococcal carriage and disease: a 6-year prospective study. J Pediatr. 1987;110:31–6.
14. Kenny JF. Recurrent group B streptococcal disease in an infant associated with the ingestion of infected mother's milk. J Pediatr. 1977;91:158–9.
15. Filleron A, Lombard F, Jacquot A, et al. Group B streptococci in milk and late neonatal infections: an analysis of cases in the literature. Arch Dis Child Fetal Neonatal Ed. 2014;99:F41–7.
16. Kohata N, Yamaguchi N, Shibasaki A et al. Keibonyuu GBS kansenshou wo kurikaeshita chouteishusseitaijyuuji ni pasteur sakkinn de bonyuuikuji wo keizokudekita ichirei [A case of very low birth weight infant with repeated GBS infection who could continue breastfeeding with pasteurization]. J Japan Soc Premature Infants Newborns. 2012;24:700. Japanese.

Birth Asphyxia

Koya Kawase and Osuke Iwata

Contents

Summary

- Birth asphyxia is a condition caused by impaired gas exchange in the placenta before and during delivery, or in the newborn's lungs after delivery.
- Birth asphyxia is a major cause of cerebral palsy.
- Hypoxic-ischemic encephalopathy is a severe brain injury that occurs secondary to birth asphyxia. Spatial patterns of brain injury depend on several factors, such as the degree and duration of hypoxia and ischemia.
- In mature infants, severe but transient hypoxic-ischemic events cause basal ganglia and thalamic injuries, leading to athetoid cerebral palsy. By contrast, mild but prolonged hypoxic-ischemic events cause cortical and subcortical white matter injury, leading to upper limb-dominant spastic diplegia.
- Appropriate delivery management and neonatal resuscitation are important to prevent hypoxic-ischemic encephalopathy arising from birth asphyxia.

K. Kawase (✉) · O. Iwata
Department of Pediatrics and Neonatology, Nagoya City University Graduate School of Medical Sciences, Nagoya, Japan
e-mail: kkawase@med.nagoya-cu.ac.jp

Y. Matsuda (ed.), *Cerebral Palsy*, https://doi.org/10.1007/978-981-19-2217-6_26

1 Underlying Disease (Concept of Perinatal Complications)

Birth asphyxia is a condition in which the respiratory and circulatory transition from the intrauterine to the extrauterine environment is disturbed. Birth asphyxia was classically defined based on the Apgar score. Recently, however, the definition of birth asphyxia is considered to be neonatal hypoxia caused by impaired gas exchange in the placenta before and during delivery, or in the newborn's lungs after delivery. In approximately 90% of all cases, birth asphyxia arises secondary to fetal distress before or during delivery [1]. These factors include maternal shock, preterm labor, placental abruption, uterine rupture, fetomaternal transfusion syndrome, fetal growth restriction, placenta previa, abnormal fetal position, cephalopelvic disproportion, cord prolapse, and cord compression. By contrast, risk factors for postnatal birth asphyxia without fetal distress include congenital anomalies, congenital diaphragmatic hernia, severe respiratory failure, total anomalous pulmonary venous return, and congenital neuromuscular disease. Birth asphyxia causes hypoxic-ischemic injuries to organs, including hypoxic-ischemic encephalopathy (HIE).

2 Pathophysiology Associated with Cerebral Palsy

When the fetus or neonate is hypoxic, bradycardia may occur; however, cerebral blood flow is maintained by lowering cerebral vascular resistance. However, when hypoxia is severe or prolonged, cerebral blood flow is reduced, resulting in ischemia. As a result, anaerobic metabolism increases due to decreased oxygen supply, leading to a reduction in ATP production at the cellular level [2]. In most severe cases, when the membrane potential cannot be maintained due to the lack of ATP, ischemic depolarization occurs, leading to impaired active transport of virtually all substances indispensable to maintain homeostasis. Next, glutamate, an excitatory neurotransmitter, is released from the axon terminals. Excessive glutamate binding to N-methyl-D-aspartate (NMDA) receptors in neurons allows the entry of Ca^{++} ions into the postsynaptic neuron, causing damage to the mitochondria and endoplasmic reticulum [3]. Furthermore, activation of nitric oxide synthase releases free radicals, leading to cell apoptosis and irreversible cell injury [4]. Subsequently, free radicals and inflammatory cytokines are generated by postischemic reperfusion, and irreversible damage spreads to the entire brain [5].

In HIE, neuronal death or tissue necrosis in specific regions of the brain occur alone or in combination, depending on the degree and duration of hypoxia and ischemia. HIE in mature infants can be classified into two major types based on the spatial patterns of brain injury on magnetic resonance imaging (MRI) [6]. One type is basal ganglia and thalamic injury. The other type is watershed injury, which is characterized by cortical and subcortical white matter injuries.

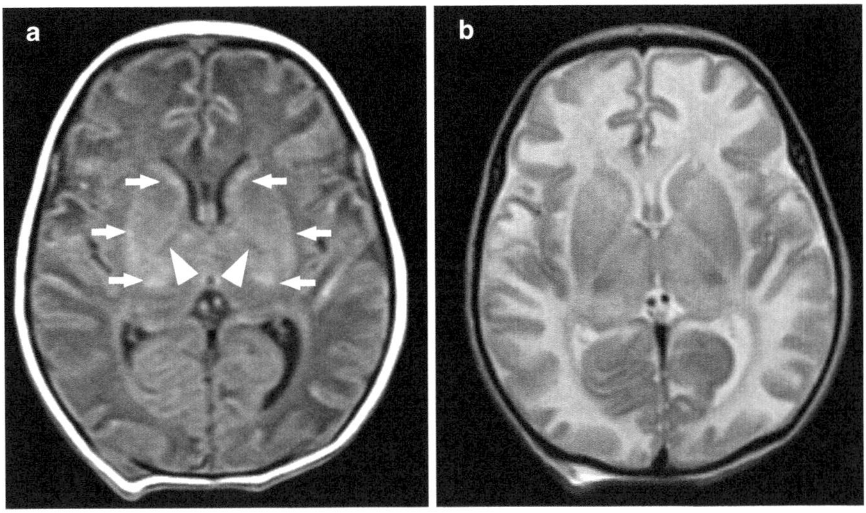

Fig. 1 Head MRI image of an infant with basal ganglia and thalamic injury. This is a day 10 post-birth head MRI image of an infant born at 39 weeks of gestation. Apgar scores at 1 and 5 min were 1 and 2, respectively. On admission, the blood pH was 7.00, and the base excess was −26.6 mmol/L. T1-weighted images show hyperintensity of the bilateral caudate nuclei, the lateral part of the putamen, and the thalamus (white arrows). T1-weighted images also show hypointensity of the posterior limb of the internal capsule (white arrowheads). (**a**) T1-weighted image. (**b**) T2-weighted image

Basal ganglia and thalamic injury (Fig. 1) is caused by a brief (less than 10 min) but rapid and very intense hypoxic-ischemic event called total (profound) asphyxia [7, 8], such as placental abruption, uterine rupture, or umbilical cord prolapse. The basal ganglia, thalamus, and brainstem are vulnerable to injury, because of their high oxygen and energy demands during the neonatal period.

However, extremely intense hypoxic-ischemic events lasting longer than 10 min can cause extensive damage to the cortex, white matter, basal ganglia, and thalamus (Fig. 2). This type of injury is called total brain injury [9].

Watershed injury is caused by a relatively mild but prolonged (>30 min) hypoxic-ischemic event called prolonged partial asphyxia [7]. In this type of injury, ischemia occurs at the border zones in the terminal fields of the anterior, middle, and posterior cerebral arteries (watershed areas), while cerebral blood flow is redistributed to the brainstem and basal ganglia (Fig. 3). This type of injury is also called "border-zone injury" or "parasagittal cerebral injury" because of their lesions [10].

In preterm infants born after less than 32 weeks of gestation, hypoxic-ischemic injury to the periventricular white matter often results in periventricular leukomalacia (PVL); see "Intraventricular hemorrhage and periventricular leukomalacia" for PVL.

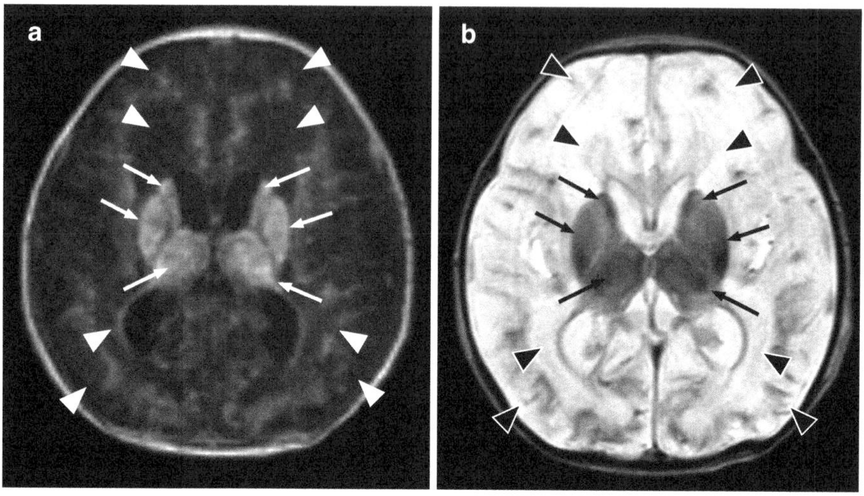

Fig. 2 Head MRI image of an infant with basal ganglia and thalamic injury with extensive cortical and white matter damage. This is a day 12 post-birth head MRI image of an infant born at 39 weeks of gestation with an unknown Apgar score. T1-weighted images show hyperintensity of the bilateral caudate nuclei, putamen, and thalamus (white arrows). T2-weighted images show hypointensity of these lesions (black arrows). T1-weighted images show hypointensity of the extensive cortex and white matter (white arrowheads). T2-weighted images show hyperintensity of these lesions (black arrowheads). (**a**) T1-weighted image. (**b**) T2-weighted image

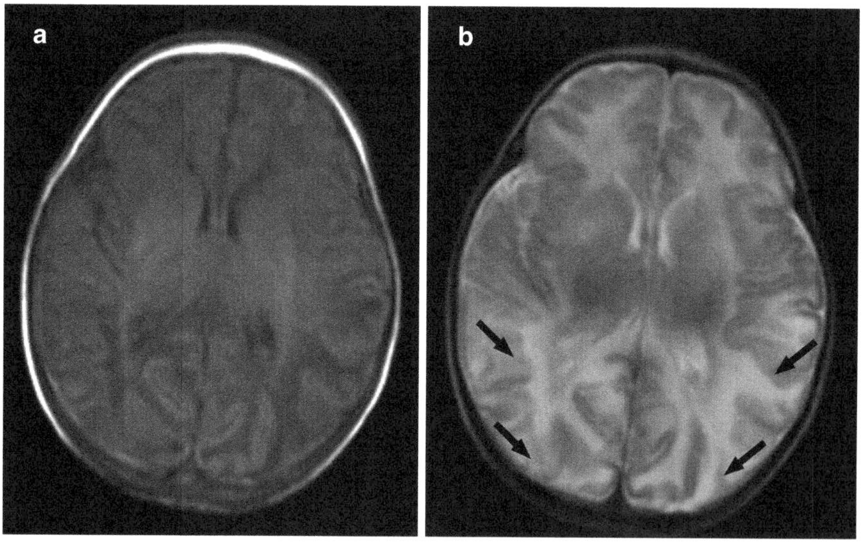

Fig. 3 Head MRI image of an infant with watershed injury. This is a day 12 post-birth head MRI image of an infant born by forceps delivery at 40 weeks of gestation. The Apgar scores at 1 and 5 min were 5 and 8, respectively. T2-weighted image shows hyperintensity of the bilateral watershed area with occipital predominance (black arrows). (**a**) T1-weighted image. (**b**) T2-weighted image

3 Current Status of Underlying Diseases in Cerebral Palsy

According to the "Survey Report on Understanding the Actual Condition of Children with Cerebral Palsy" reported by the Japan Council for Quality Health Care in 2018, birth asphyxia was present in 50%, and HIE was observed in 18% of cases with cerebral palsy [11]. Birth asphyxia and HIE are the most common causes of cerebral palsy. According to a report that examined head MRI findings, basal ganglia and thalamic injuries were found in 13% of cases with cerebral palsy, and watershed injuries were found in 3% of cases [12]. In general, cases with basal ganglia and thalamic injury have a more severe clinical presentation at birth than those with watershed injury, and the outcome for subsequent motor development is poorer [6]. In basal ganglia and thalamic injury, the motor centers and pathways of the extrapyramidal tract are injured, resulting in athetoid cerebral palsy, characterized by fluctuating muscle tone, postural instability, and involuntary movements. In this type of HIE, abnormal signal intensities in the posterior limb of the internal capsule (PLIC) on MRI are associated with neurodevelopmental outcomes, including cerebral palsy. Under normal conditions, PLIC, where bundles of myelinated axons pass, shows high signal on T1-weighted images and low signal on T2-weighted images. If the signal of PLIC is lost on T1-weighted images in association with basal ganglia and thalamic injury, more than 70% of infants may develop cerebral palsy [13]. By contrast, in watershed injury, intelligence and language impairment are the main symptoms [14], but upper limb-dominant spastic paraplegia may also occur [15].

4 Towards Prevention

4.1 Delivery Management

As noted in the introduction, in approximately 90% of all cases, birth asphyxia arises secondary to fetal distress before or during delivery [1]. Fetal hypoxia presents as abnormal fetal heart rate on monitoring. As of January 2022, the Perinatal Committee of the Japan Society of Obstetrics and Gynecology proposed a classification of fetal heart rate patterns and recommended responses and procedures based on the classification [16]. For details, please refer to the references [16]. Fetal heart rate patterns were classified into five levels based on the combination of the heart rate at baseline, type of deceleration, and baseline variability. Rapid delivery, such as vacuum or forceps delivery, and emergency cesarean section are recommended for levels 4 and 5. It is desirable for medical staff involved in the delivery to accurately judge the timing of rapid delivery based on fetal heart rate monitoring. Additionally, it is necessary to prepare for neonatal resuscitation before delivery in cases of birth asphyxia.

4.2 Neonatal Resuscitation

As mentioned above, birth asphyxia can occur even in cases without fetal distress. In Japan, relatively more infants are born at small birth centers than in Europe and the United States. In most cases wherein fetal abnormalities are not detected before delivery, pediatricians usually do not attend delivery procedures. It is necessary that not only pediatricians but also obstetricians, midwives, and other staff involved in the delivery should be able to perform standardized resuscitation based on neonatal cardiopulmonary resuscitation (NCPR).

The Japan Society of Perinatal and Neonatal Medicine has developed the "Japanese NCPR Guidelines and Resuscitation Algorithm" and is conducting a nationwide training program [17]. After birth, if there is no spontaneous breathing or the heart rate of the newborn is less than 100 beats per minute (bpm), positive pressure ventilation should be started within 60 s at the latest according to the NCPR algorithm. If the heart rate is less than 60 bpm even with effective ventilation, chest compressions in conjunction with ventilation are required. If the heart rate persists at less than 60 bpm even with resuscitation, adrenaline administration should be considered. For more information, see references [17].

Acknowledgments We thank Dr. Mari Sugimoto, Department of Pediatrics, Toyohashi Municipal Hospital, for providing the head MRI images.

References

1. Ferriero DM. Neonatal brain injury. N Engl J Med. 2004;351:1985–95.
2. Lai MC, Yang SN. Perinatal hypoxic-ischemic encephalopathy. J Biomed Biotechnol. 2011;2011:609813.
3. Johnston MV, Trescher WH, Ishida A, et al. Neurobiology of hypoxic-ischemic injury in the developing brain. Pediatr Res. 2001;49:735–41.
4. Zhao M, Zhu P, Fujino M, et al. Oxidative stress in hypoxic-ischemic encephalopathy: molecular mechanisms and therapeutic strategies. Int J Mol Sci. 2016;17:2078.
5. Solevåg AL, Schmölzer GM, Cheung PY. Novel interventions to reduce oxidative-stress related brain injury in neonatal asphyxia. Free Radic Biol Med. 2019;142:113–22.
6. Miller SP, Ramaswamy V, Michelson D, et al. Patterns of brain injury in term neonatal encephalopathy. J Pediatr. 2005;146:453–60.
7. Myers RE. Four patterns of perinatal brain damage and their conditions of occurrence in primates. Adv Neurol. 1975;10:223–34.
8. Barkovich AJ. MR and CT evaluation of profound neonatal and infantile asphyxia. Am J Neuroradiol. 1992;13:959–72; discussion 973.
9. Ghei SK, Zan E, Nathan JE, et al. MR imaging of hypoxic-ischemic injury in term neonates: pearls and pitfalls. Radiographics. 2014;34:1047–61.
10. Volpe JJ, Pasternak JF. Parasagittal cerebral injury in neonatal hypoxic-ischemic encephalopathy: clinical and neuroradiologic features. J Pediatr. 1977;91:472–6.
11. Japan Council for Quality Health Care, Project Team for Epidemiological Survey on the Actual Condition of Children with Cerebral Palsy. Report of epidemiological survey on the actual condition of children with cerebral palsy, 2018. Japanese. [Internet]. http://www.sanka-

hp.jcqhc.or.jp/documents/report/pdf/nouseimahijinojittaihaakunikansuruekigakuchousahou-kokusyo.pdf. Accessed 14 Sept 2020.
12. Bax M, Tydeman C, Flodmark O. Clinical and MRI correlates of cerebral palsy: the European cerebral palsy study. JAMA. 2006;296:1602–8.
13. Martinez-Biarge M, Diez-Sebastian J, Rutherford MA, et al. Outcomes after central grey matter injury in term perinatal hypoxic-ischaemic encephalopathy. Early Hum Dev. 2010;86:675–82.
14. Steinman KJ, Gorno-Tempini ML, Glidden DV, et al. Neonatal watershed brain injury on magnetic resonance imaging correlates with verbal IQ at 4 years. Pediatrics. 2009;123:1025–30.
15. Yokochi K. Nouseimahi no kangaekata [Cerebral palsy]. No To Hattatsu. 2009;41:327–33. Japanese.
16. Okai T, Ikeda T, Kawarabayashi T et al. Iinkaiteian—Taijishinpakusuuhakei no bunrui nimotozuku bunbenjikanri no shishin 2010 ed. [Intrapartum management guidelines based on fetal heart rate pattern classification 2010 ed]. J Obstet Gynaecol Res. 2010;36:925–8. Japanese.
17. Hosono M. Nihon kyuukyuusosei guideline 2020 ni motozuku shinseiji soseihou text [Textbook of neonatal resuscitation based on the Japanese guidelines for emergency resuscitation]. 4th ed. Tokyo: Medical View. 2021. Japanese.

Prematurity

Hiroko Horie-Ota and Kazushige Ikeda

Contents

Summary

- Prematurity is a term commonly used to describe preterm infants born at less than 37 weeks of age. Preterm infants are born in the middle of the organ maturation process and are therefore "immature." Premature infants have many difficulties adapting to the extrauterine environment and suffer from various complications. Cerebral palsy is one such condition. The risk of cerebral palsy increases as the gestational weeks progress and the birth weight decreases; therefore, immaturity is a risk factor for cerebral palsy.
- Understanding the characteristics of preterm infants and managing them in a way that prevents hypoxemia, blood pressure fluctuations, and infections will help prevent cerebral palsy.

H. Horie-Ota · K. Ikeda (✉)
Division of Neonatology, Department of Pediatrics, Saitama City Hospital, Saitama City, Saitama, Japan
e-mail: kazuiked@keio.jp

Y. Matsuda (ed.), *Cerebral Palsy*, https://doi.org/10.1007/978-981-19-2217-6_27

1 Prematurity as a Risk Factor for Cerebral Palsy

The etiology of cerebral palsy is multifactorial. According to UpToDate, the most common reasons for cerebral palsy are prematurity (78%), intrauterine growth restriction (34%), intrauterine infection (28%), maternal hemorrhage before delivery (27%), severe placental pathology such as placental abruption or placenta previa (21%), and multiple births (20%). Considering that background factors other than prematurity can also be linked to preterm birth, premature infants are therefore at a higher risk of cerebral palsy.

Prematurity is a term used to describe preterm births occurring at less than 37 weeks of age. Preterm infants are born during the organ maturation process and often have difficulties adapting to the extrauterine environment. Therefore, they suffer from various complications, including cerebral palsy. In previous reports on the incidence of prematurity and cerebral palsy, many have included low-birth-weight infants in the definition of the term "prematurity," probably because in some countries the birth weight may be a more objective indicator than gestational weeks at birth.

2 Report on Prematurity and Cerebral Palsy

As is well-known, the risk of cerebral palsy increases with decreasing weeks of gestation and birth weight. In Japan, Kono et al. [1] reported on the prevalence of cerebral palsy at gestational weeks and birth weight (Table 1).

In this section, "prematurity" is defined as preterm birth or low birth weight. The most frequently cited English-written articles on prematurity and risk of cerebral palsy reported since 2013 are shown in Table 2.

Table 1 Prevalence of cerebral palsy in 3-year-olds born at various weeks of gestation and with different birth weights (created based on ref. [1, 2])

By gestational weeks [1]						
Gestational weeks	22 weeks	23 weeks	24 weeks	25 weeks	26 weeks	27 weeks
Prevalence % (CP/no CP)	20% (28/110)	16% (100/507)	11% (108/895)	12% (157/1111)	9% (143/1422)	9% (162/1572)

By birth weight [2]		
Birth weight	<1000 g	1000 ~ 1500 g
Prevalence %	9.2% (885/9608)	4.8% (574/11,938)

Table 2 Most frequently cited reports on immaturity and risk of cerebral palsy

Ishii et al. [3] (2013)	They compared the neurological outcomes of 22- to 23-week preterm infants born between January 1, 2003, and December 31, 2005, in Japan at 22–25 weeks of gestation with those of other weeks at 3–3.5 years of age. (Cohort study)	22 weeks gestation = 21.7%, 23 weeks gestation = 17.8%, 24 weeks gestation = 8.1%, 25 weeks gestation = 15.0%
Oskoui et al. [4]	They conducted a systematic review and meta-analysis of 49 studies (1985–2011) to examine the association between the prevalence of cerebral palsy and weeks of live birth and birth weight. (Cohort study)	Less than 28 weeks gestation = 111.80/1000 After 36 weeks gestation = 1.35/1000 Less than 1000 g = 56.64/1000 1000–1499 g = 59.18/1000 1500–2499 g = 10.17/1000 2500 g or more = 1.33/1000
Marke et al. [5] (2013)	They investigated the association between neurological outcome at 8 years of age and the number of weeks of gestational age in preterm infants born at less than 33 weeks of age in France in 1997–1998. (Cohort study)	24–26 weeks gestation = 7.3% 27–28 weeks gestation = 4.6% 29–30 weeks gestation = 3.4% 31–32 weeks gestation = 2.0%
Synnes et al. [6] (2016)	They studied the neurological outcome at 21 modified weeks in preterm infants born at less than 29 weeks between 2009 and 2011 in 28 Canadian neonatal intensive care units. (Cohort study)	Less than 23 weeks gestation = 13.1% 24 weeks gestation = 12.2% 25 weeks gestation = 8.4% 26 weeks gestation = 6.7% 27 weeks gestation = 4.0% 28 weeks gestation = 4.8%
Serenius et al. [7] (2016)	They examined the neurological outcome at 2.5 years of corrected age in preterm infants born at less than 27 weeks of gestation in Sweden between April 1, 2004, and March 31, 2007. (Cohort study)	Less than 27 weeks gestation = 7.0%
Pierrat et al. [8] (2017)	They investigated the neurological outcome at 2 years of corrected age in preterm infants born at less than 34 weeks' gestation in France in 2011. (Cohort study)	24–26 weeks gestation = 6.9% 27–31 weeks gestation = 4.3% 32–34 weeks gestation = 1.0%
Kono et al. [9] (2018)	They researched the neurological prognosis of preterm infants born at 22–24 weeks of age in Japan between 2003 and 2007 and between 2008 and 2012. (Retrospective study)	• 2003–2007: 22 weeks gestation = 24.4%, 23 weeks gestation = 24.4%, 24 weeks gestation = 11.8% • 2008–2012: 22 weeks gestation = 13.3%, 23 weeks gestation = 9.8%, 24 weeks gestation = 8.7%

3 Type of Cerebral Palsy

Cerebral palsy is mainly classified as spastic (spastic paraplegia, hemiplegia, and quadriplegia), dyskinetic (including dystonia and athetosis), and ataxic.

Spastic paraplegia is caused by periventricular leukomalacia (PVL), which is often observed in preterm infants. Severe hyperbilirubinemia and hypoxemia are the major causes of dyskinetic cerebral palsy.

In contrast, spastic hemiplegia is more common in full-term neonatal stroke and fetal blood flow disorders, and spastic quadriplegia is more common in full-term small-for-gestational-age infants owing to intrauterine infections or fetal growth restriction. Ataxic paralysis occurs in infants with cerebellar hypoplasia, but the cause is often unknown.

4 Pathogenesis of Prematurity

When prematurity is associated with cerebral palsy other than PVL and intraventricular hemorrhage, the pathogenesis is assumed to be complex.

4.1 Immaturity of the Central Nervous System

Compared with full-term infants, preterm infants have less blood flow to the cerebral white matter. In addition, the autoregulation of cerebral blood flow is immature. Therefore, the brain of preterm infants is prone to ischemia.

4.2 Immaturity of Respiration

Although many preterm infants require ventilator management owing to respiratory immaturity, the effects of medical procedures such as ventilators (e.g., hypocapnia due to hyperventilation) and those of bronchopulmonary dysplasia have been described as risk factors for cerebral palsy.

4.3 Immaturity of Circulatory Dynamics

It is presumed that preterm infants have more episodes of cerebral ischemia associated with blood pressure fluctuations than full-term infants because of circulatory instability such as patent ductus arteriosus (PDA), late-onset circulatory collapse, and sepsis.

4.4 *Immaturity of the Gastrointestinal Tract and Liver Function*

Delayed enteral feeding, increased enterohepatic circulation, and decreased bilirubin excretion associated with immature liver function are possible causes.

4.5 *Other Causes*

Surgery owing to PDA or gastrointestinal perforation, postnatal steroid administration, sepsis, and hypoglycemia may contribute to cerebral palsy associated with immaturity.

5 Prevention

Appropriate management of premature delivery can reduce the risk of preterm labor. The Guidelines of the Japan Society of Obstetrics and Gynecology, Obstetrics Edition 2020 [10], states tocolytic agents and maternal steroids for the management of impending preterm labor.

Magnesium sulfate has been reported to be effective not only in inhibiting uterine contractions but also in protecting the fetal brain. The World Health Organization (WHO) and other organizations recommend its administration to pregnant women who are expected to have a preterm birth at less than 32 weeks gestation. In contrast, there is a lack of evidence that long-term use of ritodrine hydrochloride improves the neurological prognosis of infants. There is also a report that oral ritodrine hydrochloride administration increases the risk of CP associated with placental abruption [11]. Maternal steroid administration has been associated with improved pulmonary maturation and neurodevelopmental prognosis in infants.

After birth, high-quality systemic management that maintains cerebral blood flow and avoids hypoxemia, hypotension, and infection, while attempting to understand the characteristics of prematurity in preterm infants, will help prevent cerebral palsy associated with prematurity.

References

1. Kono Y. Hattatsuyogo no genjyou [Current status of developmental prognosis]. Perinat Med. 2017;47:859–62. Japanese.
2. Kono Y. Neonatal Research Network of Japan (NRNJ) database karamita kyokuteishusseitaijyuuji no yogo [Prognosis of extremely low birth weight infants from the Neonatal Research Network of Japan (NRNJ) database]. J Japan Soc Perinat Neonat Med. 2020;56:203–12. Japanese.

3. Ishii N, Kono Y, Yonemoto N, et al. Outcomes of infants born at 22 and 23 weeks' gestation. Pediatrics. 2013;132:62–71. https://doi.org/10.1542/peds.2012-2857.
4. Oskoui M, Coutinho F, Dykeman J, et al. An update on the prevalence of cerebral palsy: a systematic review and meta-analysis. Dev Med Child Neurol. 2013;55:509–19. https://doi.org/10.1111/dmcn.12080.
5. Marret S, Marchand-Martin L, Picaud JC, et al. Brain injury in very preterm children and neurosensory and cognitive disabilities during childhood: the EPIPAGE cohort study. PLoS One. 2013;8:e62683. https://doi.org/10.1371/journal.pone.0062683.
6. Synnes A, Luu TM, Moddemann D, et al. Determinants of developmental outcomes in a very preterm Canadian cohort. Arch Dis Child Fetal Neonatal Ed. 2017;102:F235–43. https://doi.org/10.1136/archdischild-2016-311228.
7. Serenius F, Källén K, Blennow M, et al. Neurodevelopmental outcome in extremely preterm infants at 2.5 years after active perinatal care in Sweden. JAMA. 2013;309:1810–20.
8. Pierrat V, Marchand-Martin L, Arnaud C, et al. Neurodevelopmental outcome at 2 years for preterm children born at 22 to 34 weeks' gestation in France in 2011: the EPIPAGE-2 cohort study. BMJ. 2017;358:j3448. https://doi.org/10.1136/bmj.j3448.
9. Kono Y, Yonemoto N, Nakanishi H, et al. Changes in survival and neurodevelopmental outcomes of infants born at <25 weeks' gestation: a retrospective observational study in tertiary centres in Japan. BMJ Paediatr Open. 2018;2:e000211. https://doi.org/10.1136/bmjpo-2017-000211.
10. Japan Society of Obstetrics and Gynecology/The Japan Association of Obstetricians and Gynecologists, editor. Sanfujinka shinryou Guideline [Guidelines for Obstetrics and Gynecology]. Tokyo: Japan Society of Obstetrics and Gynecology. 2020. Japanese.
11. Ichizuka K, Toyokawa S, Ikenoue T, et al. Risk factors for cerebral palsy in neonates due to placental abruption. J Obstet Gynaecol Res. 2021;47:159–66.

Intraventricular Hemorrhage, Periventricular Leukomalacia

Aiko Aoyama and Masahiro Hayakawa

Contents

Summary

- Intracranial hemorrhage (ICH) is estimated to occur in full-term infants with a frequency of 4.9/10,000 live births. In full-term infants, most of ICH are subdural hemorrhage. The incidence of intraventricular hemorrhage (IVH) in full-term infants is as low as 0.2%. On the other hand, in preterm infants, the incidence of IVH is 12.3% according to Neonatal Research Network Japan (August 2020). Especially, the incidence is high in very preterm infants of 24–27 weeks' gestation.
- Periventricular leukomalacia (PVL) is an ischemic necrotic lesion of cerebral white matter. The incidence of PVL is 3.0% in extremely low-birth-weight infants according to Neonatal Research Network Japan (August 2020), with a peak incidence in preterm infants of 25–29 weeks' gestation.

A. Aoyama · M. Hayakawa (✉)
Division of Neonatology, Center for Maternal-Neonatal Care, Nagoya University Hospital, Nagoya, Aichi, Japan
e-mail: masahaya@med.nagoya-u.ac.jp

Y. Matsuda (ed.), *Cerebral Palsy*, https://doi.org/10.1007/978-981-19-2217-6_28

1 Intracranial Hemorrhage/Intraventricular Hemorrhage

1.1 Pathophysiology

Intracranial hemorrhage (ICH) in full-term infants causes birth trauma, hemorrhagic infarction, coagulation abnormalities (including complications of extracorporeal circulation therapy), vascular malformations, neoplastic lesions, and infections. The sites of hemorrhage are choroid plexus (35%), thalamus (24%), germinal matrix (17%), parenchymal hemorrhage (14%), and unknown (10%).

In preterm infants, the blood vessels and connective tissue of the germinal matrix are fragile. The cerebral veins are also immature, delicate, and tortuous. Therefore, they are unable to compensate for the changes in cerebral circulation caused by changes in the systemic circulation, and the germinal matrix and thalamic striatal veins are easily destructed, resulting in intraventricular hemorrhage (IVH) and parenchymal hemorrhage. The systemic circulatory is fluctuated by acidosis, rapid administration of bicarbonate, pneumothorax, tracheal aspiration, neonatal seizures, and excessive handling.

Papile's classification by CT [1] and Volpe's classification by ultrasound [2] are used to classify the severity of IVH. Grade III and IV are severe IVH (Table 1).

1.2 Prognosis and Prevention

In Grade III/IV IVH, about 70% of infants develop posthemorrhagic hydrocephalus, and about 30% of infants are necessary for ventriculoperitoneal (VP) shunt. On the other hand, about 7% of infants with Grade I/II develop ventricular dilation, but only about 1% of infants are eligible for shunting [2].

Prevention of ICH in full-term infants is nothing less than prevention of birth trauma. In preterm infants, prevention of IVH includes avoiding preterm birth,

Table 1 Classification of intraventricular hemorrhage

Papile's classification (by CT scan)	
Grade I	Subependymal hemorrhage
Grade II	Intraventricular hemorrhage without ventricular dilation
Grade III	Intraventricular hemorrhage with ventricular dilation
Grade IV	Intraventricular hemorrhage with parenchymal hemorrhage
Classification of Volpe (by ultrasonography)	
Grade I	Germinal matrix hemorrhage with no or minimal intraventricular hemorrhage (<10% of ventricular area on parasagittal view)
Grade II	Intraventricular hemorrhage (10–50% of ventricular area on parasagittal view)
Grade III	Intraventricular hemorrhage (>50% of ventricular area on parasagittal view, usually distends lateral ventricle)

maternal transport (to avoid preterm birth in a not-perinatal center), prenatal maternal steroids, and delayed clamping of umbilical cord/umbilical cord milking. The risk of IVH decreases by 3.5% for each additional week of gestation by 32 weeks of gestation, In Japan, Grade IV IVH is remarkably common in infants born at the not-perinatal center at 23 weeks or less. Prenatal maternal steroid administration promotes fetal lung maturation and blood pressure elevation and stabilizes postnatal cerebral circulation. Delayed clamping of the umbilical cord and umbilical cord milking also reduce IVH. After birth, cerebral blood flow is affected not only by cardiac function but also by fluctuations in body temperature, inadequate ventilator care, and flighting in ventilator care. These factors may be seen as waveform variations on cerebral arterial Doppler ultrasound. Recently, catecholamines and vasodilators have been administered to evaluate the stress-velocity relationship, and fluctuations in the internal cerebral veins have been used as an index of increased venous pressure.

2 Periventricular Leukomalacia

2.1 Pathophysiology

Periventricular leukomalacia (PVL) is cell necrosis due to ischemia and inflammation and can occur both in utero and extra-utero (after birth). The causes of ischemia include premature placental abruption, placental insufficiency, asphyxia, twin-to-twin transfusion syndrome, hypotension, patent ductus arteriosus, and late circulatory collapse, while the causes of inflammation include chorioamnionitis, sepsis, and necrotizing enterocolitis. At the site of cellular necrosis in the white matter, microglia first infiltrate and become activated. Necrotic axons become swollen, astrocytes appear around 1 week, neovascularization begins, the center of the necrotic lesion gradually melts, and a cavity is formed around 2 weeks.

The characteristics of very preterm infants include (1) active myelination by oligodendrocytes around the ventricles, which may lead to myelination failure due to damage by inflammation, and (2) timing of injury coincides with axonal outgrowth, resulting in diffuse axonal degeneration with spongiform lesions and diffuse white matter volume loss. The MRI lesions seen in very preterm infants vary from punctate white matter lesions to cystic lesions, ventricular enlargement, and decreasing of white matter volume. Kidokoro et al. published cystic lesions were found in 7% and non-cystic lesions in 21% of infants less than 30 weeks of age, and 39% of infants had abnormal findings on MRI, including ventricular dilation and white matter volume loss [3].

2.2 *Prognosis and Prevention*

Because of the presence of corticospinal tracts around the ventricles, spastic paralysis occurs. Yoshida also classified 51 cases of PVL among 91 autopsied infants into four types based on the distribution of lesions: localized, extensive, diffuse, and spongiform [4] (Table 2).

Prenatal maternal steroids have been shown to decrease the incidence of PVL in infants 24 to 27 weeks of age, but no other circulatory management or anti-inflammatory therapy has been shown to be effective in preventing PVL. Late circulatory collapse, recurrent bradycardia attacks, IVH, necrotizing enterocolitis, and sepsis are a risk for PVL, so it is important to prevent or promptly treat these conditions when they occur.

3 Intraventricular Hemorrhage, Periventricular Leukomalacia, and Cerebral Palsy

IVH (Grade I/II) without white matter lesions has a relatively good prognosis (Table 3) [2]. However, oligodendrocyte progenitor cells are abundant in the germinal matrix, which is the site of hemorrhage, and their influence on future myelination is undeniable. Hemosiderin in the spinal fluid might be affected cerebellar maturation. Infants requiring VP shunt have a slightly higher rate of cerebral palsy

Table 2 Distribution and characteristics of periventricular leukomalacia in pathological tissues

Type of lesion	The most common gestational age	Characteristics of the clinical symptoms
Localized type	25–40 weeks of gestation	
Extensive type	27–29 weeks of gestation	Bilateral paralysis including the lower extremities, the upper extremities, and trunk Visual cognitive deficits when the optic radiation is involved
Diffuse type	Less than 26 weeks of gestation	In addition to tetraplegia, mental retardation and cognitive impairment
Spongiform	Less than 26 weeks of gestation	Nonspecific

Prepared based on reference [4]

Table 3 Long-term prognosis of intraventricular hemorrhage by grade

Severity	Cerebral palsy, mental retardation, or both (%)
Grade I	15
Grade II	25
Grade III	50
Grade III+ Parenchymal hemorrhage	75

(CP), and the prognosis is poor, with CP associated with parenchymal hemorrhage in 39–80% of patients with unilateral lesions and around 90% of patients with bilateral lesions [5].

In PVL, the rate of CP is high (about 60–70%), regardless of the severity of PVL and the presence or absence of IVH; spastic paraplegia is the most common, followed by ataxic paralysis and dyskinesia. It has also been reported that 39% of infants with PVL have developmental delays and half of the infants with PVL have learning disabilities. The incidence of visual impairment (7.9% vs. 24.6%), strabismus (15.5% vs. 40%), learning disability (31.6% vs. 53.5%), and epilepsy (10.5% vs. 31.6%) differs depending on whether the lesion is unilateral or bilateral [6]. In any case, long-term medical care and follow-up are necessary.

References

1. Papile LA, Burstein J, Burstein R, et al. Incidence and evolution of subependymal and intraventricular hemorrhage: a study of infants with birth weights less than 1,500gm. J Pediatr. 1978;92:529–34.
2. Volpe JJ. Volpe's neurology of the newborn. 6th ed. Amsterdam: Elsevier; 2018.
3. Kidokoro H, Neil JJ, Inder TE, et al. New MR imaging assessment tool to define brain abnormalities in very preterm infants at term. AJNR Am J Neuroradiol. 2013;34:2208–14.
4. Yoshida O, Takashima K, Morita S, et al. Chousouzanji—seikisan niokeru nouhattatsusyougai no tokuisei – noubyouri kara [Specificity of brain developmental disorders in very preterm to full-term infants: from brain pathology]. Rikuryo Kagaku. 2015;30:737–40. Japanese.
5. Gano D, Cowan FM, de Vries LS. Cerebral palsy after very preterm birth-an imaging perspective. Semin Fetal Neonatal Med. 2020;25:101106.
6. Resch B, Resch E, Maurer-Fellbaum U, et al. The whole spectrum of cystic periventricular leukomalacia in the preterm infant: results from a large consecutive case series. Childs Nerv Syst. 2015;31:1527–32.

Neonatal Stroke

Atsushi Uchiyama

Contents

Summary

- Neonatal stroke is a part of the perinatal stroke and refers to cases diagnosed after birth to less than 28 days of age. Neonatal stroke is a syndrome developing acute neurological impairment due to cerebral injury of vascular origins such as thrombus or embolus.
- Cerebral palsy caused by neonatal stroke is occurred by the damage of neurons controlling muscle tone, posture, and/or movement appropriately.
- It is very important for the prevention of developing neonatal stroke and reducing cerebral palsy or other neurological impairments by the disorder to clarify the cause and to treat appropriately.

A. Uchiyama (✉)
Department of Pediatrics, Tokai University School of Medicine, Isehara, Kanagawa, Japan
e-mail: uchiyama.atsushi@tsc.u-tokai.ac.jp

Y. Matsuda (ed.), *Cerebral Palsy*, https://doi.org/10.1007/978-981-19-2217-6_29

1 Overview of Neonatal Stroke

1.1 Definition

Neonatal stroke is considered under the umbrella of perinatal stroke diagnosed between at birth and less than 28 days of age [1, 2]. Perinatal stroke is a syndrome of acute neurological impairments caused by damage to the cerebral vasculature due to arterial or cerebral venous thrombus or embolus between 20 weeks of gestation and less than 28 days of age after birth [2, 3].

1.2 Classification

Perinatal stroke is classified into six subtypes by the onset time and the mechanism of cerebral vascular damage as follows [2, 3].

1. Presumed arterial presumed perinatal ischemic stroke
2. Periventricular venous infarction
3. Presumed perinatal hemorrhagic stroke
4. Neonatal arterial ischemic stroke (NAIS)
5. Neonatal cerebral sinus venous thrombosis (CSVT)
6. Neonatal hemorrhagic stroke (NHS)

Among these, NAIS, CSVT, and NHS are included in neonatal stroke: NAIS is speculated to result from emboli from the placenta passing through the patent foramen ovale into the aorta. CSVT is occurred due to impaired venous flow of at least one major cerebral sinus, and NHS is occurred due to an infarction related to the intracranial hemorrhage.

1.3 Etiology

The incidence of NAIS ranges from 6 to 17 per 100,000 live births [1], with a higher incidence of 7 per 1000 live births in preterm infants born at less than 34 weeks of gestational age [4]; the incidence of CSVT and NHS has been reported to range from 0.67 to 12 and 10.5 per 100,000 live births, respectively [5–7]. The actual incidence of neonatal stroke is estimated to be higher than these reports because some cases are asymptomatic.

1.4 Factors of the Development of Neonatal Stroke

Table 1 shows the main factors associated with the development of neonatal stroke. They can be divided into two major categories: maternal/fetal factors and neonatal factors. Many of these factors may contribute to the pathogenesis of NAIS, CSVT,

Table 1 Factors associated with the development of neonatal stroke

Clinical factors	Causes of developing neonatal stroke
Maternal and fetal factors	Chorioamnionitis Hypertensive disorders of pregnancy Premature rupture of membranes >24 h Non-reassuring fetal status Fetal growth restriction Twin-to-twin transfusion syndrome Thrombophilias in pregnancy Maternal autoimmune diseases Maternal inborn errors of metabolism
Neonatal factors	Male Birth asphyxia Hypoxic-ischemic encephalopathy Birth injury Hypoglycemia Polycythemia Dehydration Meningitis Disseminated intravascular coagulation Congenital heart disease Cerebrovascular anomalies
Iatrogenic factors	Use of an extracorporeal membrane oxygenation

and the NHS. However, some of these factors are associated with the development of specific subtypes, such as the use of extracorporeal membrane oxygenation is associated with the development of NAIS and NHS, dehydration is associated with CSVT, and cerebrovascular malformations are associated with NHS [3].

1.5 Clinical Characteristics

The typical clinical symptom of NAIS is a unilateral repetitive chronic seizure occurring between 1 and 3 days after birth due to infarction of the left, right, or bilateral middle cerebral artery [2]. The incidences of infarction in the left and right hemispheres are 66% and 27%, respectively. The incidence of it in bilateral hemispheres is only less than 10% [8].

Clinical symptoms of CSVT are seen within the first week of age. Seizures occur in 60–70% of the patients, and the rest shows nonspecific symptoms. Therefore, the diagnosis of CSVT is sometimes made incidentally on imaging studies performed for reasons such as suspect of central nervous infections or preterm birth [2].

NHS shows a variety of clinical symptoms, such as partial or generalized seizure, apnea, poor suckling, fever, and irritability [2].

1.6 Treatment and Management

Prophylactic antithrombotic therapy is not recommended, because the risk of recurrence is very low in NAIS [2].

The use of anticoagulants for neonatal CSVT is controversial, because the risk of recurrence is also low. However, the administration of anticoagulants such as low-molecular-weighted heparin should be considered on a case-by-case basis [2, 3].

In infants with NHS, the main focus is on supportive care to prevent the spread of bleeding.

When seizures are recognized due to NHS, anticonvulsants such as phenobarbital are used to treat them. However, this kind of medicine should be used for as short a time as possible, because neonatal seizures are often transient and there are concerns about the neurotoxic effects of anticonvulsants on the immature brains of newborn infants.

If the causes of neonatal stroke are clarified and treatable, it is very important to treat them concurrently.

2 Pathophysiology Associated with Cerebral Palsy

Neonatal stroke can cause a variety of neurological symptoms depending on the degree and location of the infarction. Among these, cerebral palsy (CP) develops when the infarction occurs in a central nervous system that is necessary for proper maintenance of movement and posture.

3 Current Status of Neonatal Stroke in CP

Neonatal stroke is a major cause of spastic hemiplegia, one of the subtypes of CP. A typical case is that a neonatal stroke is diagnosed on the basis of neurological imaging performed to clarify the cause of the seizure and subsequently diagnosed as CP based on the clinical symptoms.

However, there are some newborn infants in which a neonatal stroke is not diagnosed if they are asymptomatic during the neonatal period. In such cases, the presence of the infarction becomes apparent in infancy from symptoms such as hemiplegia.

Regarding the relationship between infarction and CP, it was reported that 76 of 111 patients (68%) with perinatal arterial ischemic stroke developed CP [9]. In another study based on differences in lesions of infarction, it was reported that all patients with infarction of the main branch of the middle cerebral artery (MCA) developed CP, whereas the incidence of the anterior, middle, and posterior MCA strokes were 12%, 19%, and 21%, respectively [10]. This report indicates that the incidence of CP differs depending on the infarction lesion even in the same blood vessel. It is also reported that some patients with infarction that were not diagnosed as CP were associated with learning disabilities and/or epilepsy. Therefore, long-term follow-up of such patients should be done.

4 Prevention and the Reduction of Incidence in Neonatal Stroke

The clinical factors developing neonatal stroke listed in Table 1 occur with a certain probability in newborn infants. Some of these factors are not preventable. However, there are preventable factors such as neonatal hypoglycemia and dehydration by careful management among of them.

For twin-to-twin transfusion syndrome, fetoscopic laser surgery of placental anastomotic vessels is now being performed. In addition, guidelines have been issued for the management of hereditary thrombophilia, such as deficiency of protein S or protein C, and autoimmune diseases, such as antiphospholipid antibody syndrome, during pregnancy.

Although various factors contribute to the development of neonatal stroke, there are also preventable and manageable factors among them. To prevent the onset of neonatal stroke and to reduce the incidences of developing CP or other neurological impairments induced by neonatal stroke, it is very important to clarify these factors and to perform appropriate treatment.

References

1. Rutherford MA, Ramenghi LA, Cowan FM. Neonatal stroke. Arch Dis Child Fetal Neonatal Ed. 2012;97:F377–84.
2. Fluss J, Dinomais M, Chabrier S. Perinatal stroke syndromes: similarities and diversities in aetiology, outcome and management. Eur J Paediatr Neurol. 2019;23:368–83.
3. Dunbar M, Kirton A. Perinatal stroke. Semin Pediatr Neurol. 2019;32:100767. https://doi.org/10.1016/j.spen.2019.08.003.
4. Benders MJ, Groenendaal F, Uiterwaal CS, et al. Perinatal arterial stroke in the preterm infant. Semin Perinatol. 2008;32:344–9.
5. Berfelo FJ, Kersbergen KJ, van Ommen CH, et al. Neonatal cerebral sinovenous thrombosis from symptom to outcome. Stroke. 2010;41:1382–8.
6. Ramenghi LA, Govaert P, Fumagalli M, et al. Neonatal cerebral sinovenous thrombosis. Semin Fetal Neonatal Med. 2009;14:278–83.
7. Cole L, Dewey D, Letourneau N, et al. Clinical characteristics, risk factors, and outcomes associated with neonatal hemorrhagic stroke: a population-based case-control study. JAMA Pediatr. 2017;171:230–8.
8. Miller V. Neonatal cerebral infarction. Semin Pediatr Neurol. 2000;7:278–88.
9. Golomb MR, Garg BP, Saha C, et al. Cerebral palsy after perinatal arterial ischemic stroke. J Child Neurol. 2008;23:279–86.
10. Wagenaar N, Martinez-Biarge M, van der Aa NE, et al. Neurodevelopment after perinatal arterial ischemic stroke. Pediatrics. 2018;142:e20174164.

Neonatal Hypoglycemia

Takeo Mukai and Naoto Takahashi

Contents

Summary

- In recent years, the association and prognosis of neonatal hypoglycemia and neurological sequelae have been reported successively.
- The risk factors for neonatal hypoglycemia include maternal diabetes mellitus, late preterm, SGA, and LGA infants, and neonatal hypoglycemia is thought to be particularly likely to damage the cerebral white matter.
- Regarding the relationship between neonatal hypoglycemia and neurological sequelae, it has been reported that neurodevelopmental and literacy deficits occur in mid-childhood, and the possibility of very long-term neurodevelopmental complications must be considered.
- The interventional glucose threshold is controversial. Currently, blood glucose should be kept at least 47 mg/dL (2.6 mmol/L).

T. Mukai (✉)
Department of Pediatrics, The University of Tokyo Hospital, Tokyo, Japan
e-mail: takeo-m@ims.u-tokyo.ac.jp

N. Takahashi
Department of Pediatric and Neonatal Intensive Care Unit, The University of Tokyo Hospital, Tokyo, Japan

Y. Matsuda (ed.), *Cerebral Palsy*, https://doi.org/10.1007/978-981-19-2217-6_30

Hypoglycemia in neonates has been reported for a long time [1], and subsequently, the association between neonatal hypoglycemia and neurological sequelae has been reported successively.

In this section, we define neonatal hypoglycemia and discuss about its relation to neurological disorders leading to cerebral palsy (CP).

1 What Is Neonatal Hypoglycemia?

Although specific uniform standards for neonatal hypoglycemia have not been established, European and American societies [American Academy of Pediatrics (AAP), Pediatric Endocrine Society (PES)] have issued guidelines for the management of blood glucose over time using limited observational data (Table 1) [2, 3].

In 1988, Lucas et al. conducted a multicenter study of 661 preterm infants, defining neonatal hypoglycemia as less than 47 mg/dL (2.6 mmol/L), and discussed the neurological prognosis with 47 mg/dL as the boundary [4]. This will be discussed later.

2 Risk Factors for Neonatal Hypoglycemia

Risk factors for neonatal hypoglycemia include maternal diabetes mellitus, late preterm infants, small-for-gestational-age (SGA) infants, and large-for-gestational-age (LGA) infants. All of these factors are risk factors that should be considered for postnatal hypoglycemia, and more severe hypoglycemia should be considered when multiple factors are present (Fig. 1) [5].

In addition, the use of ritodrine hydrochloride has been cited as a risk of neonatal hypoglycemia in the perinatal period that has recently been reported from Japan, and the possibility of neonatal hypoglycemia must be kept in mind, especially with the long-term use of ritodrine hydrochloride and its discontinuation immediately before delivery [6].

Table 1 Criteria for neonatal hypoglycemia over time

Less than 4 h after birth	<25–40 mg/dL (1.4–2.2 mmol/L)
From 4 h after birth to less than 24 h	<35–45 mg/dL (1.9–2.5 mmol/L)
After 24 h and less than 48 h of age	<45–50 mg/dL (2.5–2.8 mmol/L)
After 48 h of age	<60 mg/dL (3.3 mmol/L)

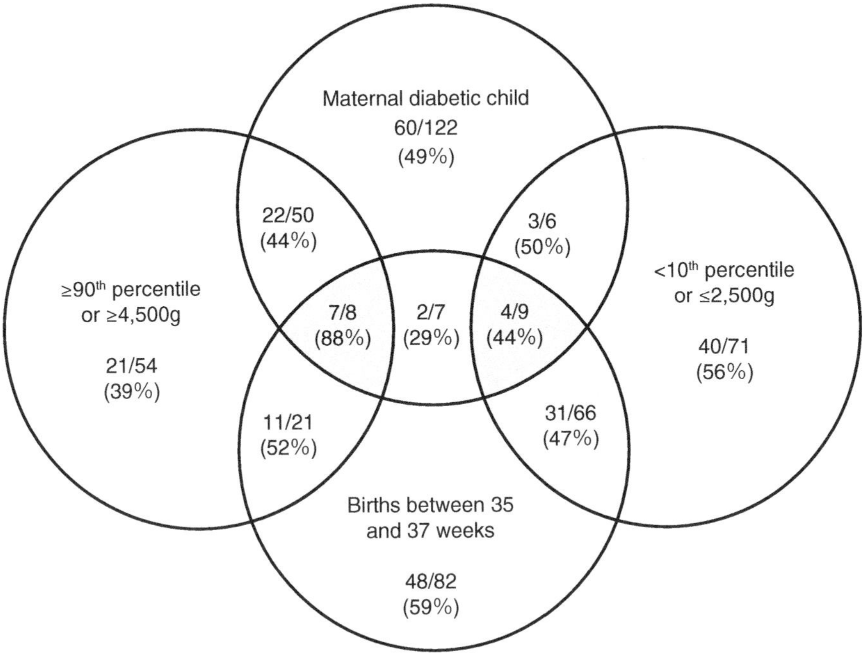

Fig. 1 Risk factors for neonatal hypoglycemia and incidence of neonatal hypoglycemia (47 mg/dL)

3 The Mechanism of Neonatal Hypoglycemia Causing Neurological Disorders

There are several theories on the mechanism by which neonatal hypoglycemia causes neurological disorders. It has been reported that under hypoglycemic conditions, excitatory neurotoxin is excessively secreted, stimulating N-methyl-D-aspartate (NMDA)-type glutamate receptors and producing free radicals, which induce neuronal apoptosis and alter brain energy metabolism [7, 8]. It is also reported to alter the energy metabolism of the brain [7, 8].

In addition, Charlotte et al. [9] reported that the MRI of 35 children with neonatal hypoglycemia showed white matter lesions in 94% of the children as a region susceptible to damage by neonatal hypoglycemia. In addition, 51% of the children had cortical lesions and 40% had basal ganglia and thalamus lesions (Table 2) [7].

Thus, the reason for the high incidence of white matter lesions in neonatal hypoglycemia has been reported in animal models, in which a significant decrease in cerebral blood flow was observed in the white matter due to an unbalanced redistribution of cerebral blood flow in hypoglycemic conditions [10]. This vulnerability in the white matter region of the brain is thought to be one of the reasons why neonates are more susceptible to damage during hypoglycemia.

Table 2 Sites of brain damage and their proportions in neonatal hypoglycemia

Site of a lesion		Proportion (%) among hypoglycemic children (35)
White matter	Mild	5 (14)
	Moderate	13 (37)
	Severe	15 (43)
Properties of white matter lesions	Bleeding	2 (13)
	Infarction of the middle cerebral artery territory	3 (20)
	Wide area infarction	10 (67)
Leukemic lesion area	The whole area	13 (39)
	Back of head	6 (18)
	Forehead	0 (0)
	One side	2 (6)
	Periventricular	12 (36)
Basal ganglia or thalamus		14 (40)
Endopod		4 (11)
Cerebellum		2 (6)
Cerebral cortex		18 (51)
Brain stem		2 (6)

4 The Association Between Neonatal Hypoglycemia and Cerebral Palsy

The relationship between neonatal hypoglycemia and neurological sequelae has been reported since the 1960s [11], and in 1988, Lucas et al. investigated neonatal hypoglycemia of less than 47 mg/dL (2.6 mmol/L) and the number of days of onset in 661 preterm infants (weight less than 1850 g). The longer the number of days of hypoglycemia, the worse the neurological prognosis at 18 months of correction [4].

In 1999, hypoglycemia of less than 47 mg/dL (2.6 mmol/L) occurred in 72.9% of 85 SGA children, and children with two or more episodes of hypoglycemia had significantly lower psychomotor development at 3.5 and 5 years of age than those with a single episode of hypoglycemia [12].

In a 2019 systematic review meta-analysis, neonatal hypoglycemia did not worsen neurodevelopmental outcomes in early childhood [n = 1657, odds ratio (OR) 1.16 [95% confidence interval (95% CI): 0.86–1.57]], but it did cause visuomotor dysfunction [n = 508, OR 3.46 (95% CI: 1.13–10.57)], visuomotor impairment [n = 508, OR 3.46 (95% CI: 1.13–10.57)], and executive function impairment [n = 463, OR 2.50 (95% CI: 1.20–5.22)]. In mid-childhood, neurodevelopmental deficits [n = 54, OR 3.62 (95% CI: 1.05–12.42)] and literacy deficits [n = 1395, OR 2.04 (95% CI: 1.20–3.47)] were observed. However, developmental assessment in adolescence has not yet been performed [13]. Based on these results, the possibility that neonatal hypoglycemia may lead to very long-term neurodevelopmental complications must be considered.

With regard to the hypoglycemic threshold for neurological impairment, a neurological outcomes cohort study was reported in 2015 in The New England Journal of Medicine (NEJM), in which blood glucose was kept at 47 mg/dL (2.6 mmol/L). A total of 404 hypoglycemic risk children [born <37 weeks, low birth weight (<10th percentile or <2500 g), high birth weight (>90th percentile or >4500 g)] were intermittently followed for blood glucose until 7 days after birth. Of these, 216 (53%) had hypoglycemia and were treated with additional feeding, dextrose gel, and intravenous fluids to maintain blood glucose levels above 47 mg/dL. At 2 years of age, developmental assessment by the Bayley scales of infant development III (BSID III) showed no significant difference compared with the control group without hypoglycemia. As a result, developmental evaluation of the Bayley scales of infant development III (BSID III) at 2 years of age showed no significant difference compared with the control group without hypoglycemia [14].

On the other hand, a paper on the therapeutic threshold for neonatal hypoglycemia was reported in the NEJM in 2020. According to the paper, the developmental assessment of BSID III at 18 months modified proved non-inferiority when the treatment threshold was 36 mg/dL (2.0 mmol/L), which is lower than the conventional treatment threshold of 47 mg/dL (2.6 mmol/L). In other words, a treatment threshold of 36 mg/dL (2.0 mmol/L) did not result in a worse developmental outcome than the conventional threshold of 47 mg/dL (2.6 mmol/L) [15]. A comparison of developmental outcomes over a longer period of time will be necessary in the future.

Neonatal hypoglycemia is frequent in infants at risk for maternal ritodrine hydrochloride use, preterm birth, maternal diabetes, SGA, and LGA. Studies have shown that neonatal hypoglycemia can cause cerebral cell damage, particularly in the cerebral white matter, and may pose a risk of long-term neurodevelopmental impairment. Although there are various theories on the interventional blood glucose threshold, at this stage, it should be managed so that the blood glucose level does not fall below 47 mg/dL (2.6 mmol/L) as shown in Table 1 over time and as a constant value.

References

1. Brown RJ, Wallis PG. Hypoglycaemia in the newborn infant. Lancet. 1963;1:1278–82.
2. Adamkin DH. Postnatal glucose homeostasis in late-preterm and term infants. Pediatrics. 2011;127:575–9.
3. UpToDate®: management and outcome of neonatal hypoglycemia.
4. Lucas A, Morley R, Cole TJ. Adverse neurodevelopmental outcome of moderate neonatal hypoglycaemia. BMJ. 1988;297:1304–8.
5. Stark J, Simma B, Blassnig-Ezeh A. Incidence of hypoglycemia in newborn infants identified as at risk. J Matern Fetal Neonatal Med. 2020;33(18):3091–6.
6. Yada Y, Ohkuchi A, Otsuki K, et al. Synergic interaction between ritodrine and magnesium sulfate on the occurrence of critical neonatal hyperkalemia: a Japanese nationwide retrospective cohort study. Sci Rep. 2020;10:7804.

7. Papagapiou MP, Auer RN. Regional neuroprotective effects of the NMDA receptor antagonist MK-801 (dizocilpine) in hypoglycemic brain damage. J Cereb Blood Flow Metab. 1990;10:270–6.
8. Wieloch T. Hypoglycemia-induced neuronal damage prevented by an N-methyl-D-aspartate antagonist. Science. 1985;230:681–3.
9. Burns CM, Rutherford MA, Boardman JP, et al. Patterns of cerebral injury and neurodevelopmental outcomes after symptomatic neonatal hypoglycemia. Pediatrics. 2008;122:65–74.
10. Mujsce DJ, Christensen MA, Vannucci RC. Regional cerebral blood flow and glucose utilization during hypoglycemia in newborn dogs. Am J Physiol. 1989;256(6 Pt 2):H1659–66.
11. Cornblath M, Reisner SH. Blood glucose in the neonate and its clinical significance. N Engl J Med. 1965;273:378–81.
12. Duvanel CB, Fawer CL, Cotting J, et al. Long-term effects of neonatal hypoglycemia on brain growth and psychomotor development in small-for gestational-age preterm infants. J Pediatr. 1999;134:492–8.
13. Shah R, Harding J, Brown J, et al. Neonatal glycaemia and neurodevelopmental outcomes: a systematic review and meta-analysis. Neonatology. 2019;115:116–26.
14. McKinlay CJ, Alsweiler JM, Ansell JM, et al. Neonatal Glycemia and neurodevelopmental outcomes at 2 years. N Engl J Med. 2015;373:1507–18.
15. van Kempen A, Eskes PF, Nuytemans D, et al. Lower versus traditional treatment threshold for neonatal hypoglycemia. N Engl J Med. 2020;382:534–44.

Bilirubin Encephalopathy

Akihisa Okumura

Contents

Summary

- Bilirubin encephalopathy results from selective central nervous system damage induced by neurotoxicity of unbound bilirubin. The primary sites of involvement include the globus pallidus, subthalamic nucleus, and brainstem auditory nucleus.
- Bilirubin encephalopathy in full-term infants is always associated with marked hyperbilirubinemia, whereas bilirubin encephalopathy in preterm infants often lacks marked hyperbilirubinemia. The manifestations of bilirubin encephalopathy during the remote period are characterized by athetotic cerebral palsy, auditory impairment, paresis of vertical upward gaze, and dental enamel dysplasia.
- In addition to neurological examination, head MRI and auditory brainstem responses are useful for diagnosis, and head MRI should be performed at 6–18 months of corrected age [1].
- A new method of neonatal jaundice management has been proposed [2], which is expected to reduce the occurrence of new cases.

A. Okumura (✉)
Department of Pediatrics, Aichi Medical University School of Medicine, Nagakute, Aichi, Japan
e-mail: okumura.akihisa.479@mail.aichi-med-u.ac.jp

Y. Matsuda (ed.), *Cerebral Palsy*, https://doi.org/10.1007/978-981-19-2217-6_31

1 Medical Examination

The "Diagnostic Criteria for Bilirubin Encephalopathy in Preterm Infants" developed by the Japan Agency for Medical Research and Development (AMED) Research Project for Practical Application of Intractable Diseases "Development of Comprehensive Clinical Guidelines for Kernicterus in Preterm Infants" group is shown in Table 1 [3]. The basis for the diagnosis of bilirubin encephalopathy is the neurological examination, which confirms the presence of athetotic cerebral palsy. It is not uncommon that typical athetotic cerebral palsy is misdiagnosed to be spastic cerebral palsy. Head MRI and auditory brain responses (ABR) are useful and should be performed when bilirubin encephalopathy is suspected.

The diagnostic criteria for bilirubin encephalopathy in preterm infants can be applied to the diagnosis of bilirubin encephalopathy in full-term infants except for gestational age.

2 Symptoms

Bilirubin encephalopathy in full-term infants is associated with marked hyperbilirubinemia and neurological symptoms known as Praagh's symptoms in the acute phase [3]. Bilirubin encephalopathy in preterm infants often lacks marked hyperbilirubinemia and rarely has distinct neurological symptoms in the acute phase. Therefore, bilirubin encephalopathy cannot be ruled out on the basis of the absence of marked hyperbilirubinemia in preterm infants.

The most characteristic neurological symptom in the remote phase of bilirubin encephalopathy is athetotic cerebral palsy [3]. Delay in motor development with asymmetrical posture and fluctuating muscle tone is evident from infancy. The child

Table 1 Provisional diagnostic criteria for chronic bilirubin encephalopathy (nuclear jaundice) in preterm infants. Modified from [3]

1. Cerebral palsy or delay in motor development characterized by asymmetrical posture, fluctuation of muscle tone due to emotional changes, and opisthotonus
2. Born before 37 weeks of gestational age
3. Abnormal signal intensity in bilateral globus pallidus on head MRI (T2-weighted image)*1
4. Auditory brainstem response is abnormal, but auditory response is preserved
5. Exclude other gross brain lesions, brain malformations, and progressive diseases*2
*1: It is desirable to confirm the abnormality by MRI between 6 months and 1.5 years of corrected age, when the rate of abnormality is high
*2: Nonspecific ventriculomegaly, thinning of the corpus callosum, and mild PVL should not be excluded. Patients with bilateral lesions in thalamus and putamen should be excluded
• Confirmed cases: 1, 2, 3, and 5 are satisfied
• Suspicious cases: 1, 2, 4, and 5 are satisfied

PVL periventricular leukomalacia

is difficult to hold due to neck instability and opisthotonus. The predominance of joint flexion results in an inverted triangle shape with elevated hips in the supine position. Muscle tone is easily affected by emotion and varies widely even in the same patient, from marked hypotonia to hypertonia, from dystonic posture (hypomobility) to athetotic dance (hyperactivity), and shifting laterality of asymmetrical posture. Physical or emotional stress may cause persistent severe hypertonia leading to rhabdomyolysis. On the other hand, verbal communication, language, and intellectual development are relatively good in many cases, and oral intake is often possible, although it takes time to have a meal.

Auditory disorders are also known to be a symptom of bilirubin encephalopathy. Auditory neuropathy is characteristic in patients with bilirubin encephalopathy, and it is not uncommon to maintain hearing in daily life even though ABR is severely abnormal [3]. In this case, the patient is able to speak sufficiently. Such a discrepancy between daily hearing and ABR findings is characteristic of bilirubin encephalopathy and provides a strong basis for diagnosis.

Head MRI is characterized by abnormal signal intensities in the globus pallidus and subthalamic nucleus (Fig. 1) [3]. High signal intensity of the globus pallidus on T1-weighted images has been reported in full-term infants in the acute phase. On the other hand, the time of onset is difficult to determine in preterm infants, and MRI is usually performed before discharge from the neonatal intensive care unit (NICU). MRI abnormalities are rarely found in preterm infants before discharge from NICU. In contrast, abnormal high signal intensity in the globus pallidus is frequently observed on T2-weighted images at 6–18 months of corrected age [1]. Lesions in the subthalamic nucleus are difficult to identify without clear high-resolution images. The lesions in the globus pallidus tends to be difficult to identify after

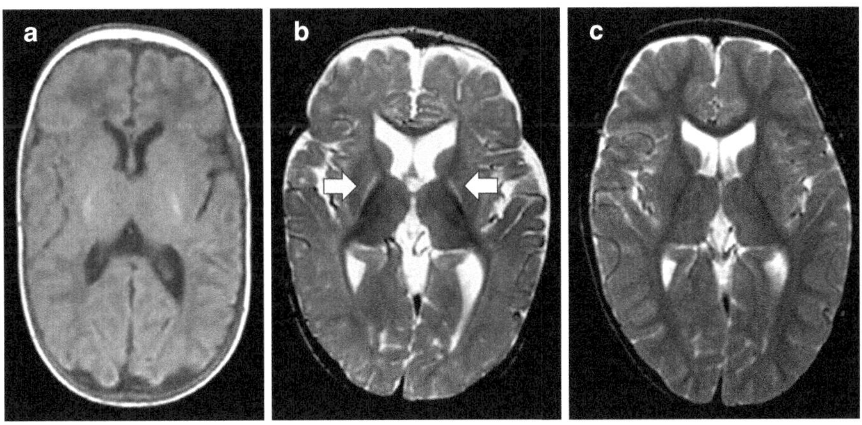

Fig. 1 Longitudinal changes of globus pallidus lesions in head MRI of bilirubin encephalopathy in preterm infants [1]. (**a**) T1-weighted image at 40 weeks (post menstrual age; PMA). MRI of the head at term equivalent age shows no obvious abnormality. (**b**) T2-weighted image at 8 months (corrected age; CA). High signal intensity is seen in bilateral globus pallidus. (**c**) T2-weighted image at 32 months of CA. No high signal intensity is present in the globus pallidus

2 years of corrected age. If preterm bilirubin encephalopathy is suspected, head MRI should be performed at 6–18 months of corrected age.

Paresis of vertical upward gaze and tooth enamel dysplasia are also known symptoms of bilirubin encephalopathy, but the symptoms are not always easy to identify and their actual situation is not fully understood.

3 Pathophysiology Associated with Cerebral Palsy

Bilirubin encephalopathy is a central nervous system disorder caused by the neurotoxicity of unbound bilirubin (UB). Histopathological studies have demonstrated that UB-induced neurotoxicity is selective, with histopathological changes occurring predominantly in the globus pallidus, subthalamic nucleus, hippocampus, oculomotor nucleus, ventral nucleus of the cochlear nerve, cerebellar Purkinje cells, and cerebellar dentate nucleus. It has been postulated that UB interacts with phospholipids in cell membranes, resulting in endoplasmic reticulum stress, oxidative stress, decreased enzyme activity, and impaired energy production, but the detailed mechanism of neuronal damage has not been fully elucidated. Excitotoxicity and inflammation are presumed to promote UB-induced neurological damage. These effects are thought to result in the influx of calcium ions into neurons, leading to apoptosis and cell cycle arrest.

No obstetric factors are known to be directly associated with bilirubin encephalopathy. Among genetic factors, a polymorphism in the UGT1A1 gene, UGT1A1*6 (p.G71R), which is involved in the glucuronidation of bilirubin, is known to be associated with the risk of bilirubin encephalopathy [4]. Hemolytic anemia due to genetic factors such as glucose-6-phosphate dehydrogenase (G6PD) deficiency is an important risk factor for bilirubin encephalopathy, although it is rare in Japanese.

4 Current Status in Cerebral Palsy

In Japan, bilirubin encephalopathy in full-term infants seems to be quite exceptional. On the other hand, in preterm infants, especially those born very preterm (<30 weeks), the number of cases has been increasing with the improvement of survival rate. Morioka et al. estimated the incidence to be 1.8 per 1000 live births in preterm infants of less than 30 weeks' gestation [5]. According to the results of a survey conducted by the "Development of Comprehensive Treatment Guidelines for Nuclear Jaundice in Preterm Infants" group of the Practical Application Research Project for Intractable Diseases of the Japan Agency for Medical Development (AMED), it is estimated that about 10 preterm infants develop bilirubin encephalopathy in Japan every year.

5 Toward Prevention

Bilirubin encephalopathy can be prevented by appropriate management of neonatal jaundice. The results of previous studies suggest that conventional jaundice management may not be able to prevent bilirubin encephalopathy completely in preterm infants. To overcome this problem, Morioka et al. [2] proposed a new method of neonatal jaundice management and are currently evaluating its efficacy and safety. The new method is characterized by the introduction of UB as a management criterion, the change of the criterion value according to the gestational age and the days after birth, and a longer period of jaundice management than the conventional method. For details of the new jaundice management method, please refer to "Guide to the treatment of bilirubin encephalopathy (nuclear jaundice) in preterm infants" [3].

References

1. Kitai Y, Hirai S, Okuyama N, et al. Diagnosis of bilirubin encephalopathy in preterm infants with dyskinetic cerebral palsy. Neonatology. 2020;117:73–9.
2. Morioka I. Hyperbilirubinemia in preterm infants in Japan: new treatment criteria. Pediatr Int. 2018;60:684–90.
3. Japan Medical Research and Development Organization Research Grant "Development of Comprehensive Treatment Guidelines for Nuclear Jaundice in Preterm Infants" Group, editor. Souzanji kakuoudan no houkatsuteki shinryou guideline no sakusei [Guide to the treatment of bilirubin encephalopathy (nuclear jaundice) in preterm infants]. 2020. Japanese.
4. Yanagi T, Nakahara S, Maruo Y. Bilirubin uridine diphosphate-glucuronosyltransferase polymorphism as a risk factor for prolonged hyperbilirubinemia in Japanese preterm infants. J Pediatr. 2017;190:159–162.e1.
5. Morioka I, Nakamura H, Koda T, et al. Current incidence of clinical kernicterus in preterm infants in Japan. Pediatr Int. 2015;57:494–7.

Apparent Life-Threatening Event (ALTE)

Ineko Kato

Contents

Summary

- The early neonatal period is a period of adaptation to life outside the womb immediately after birth, and even infants that appear to be normal may have some abnormalities, such as respiratory distress, cyanosis, and decreased muscle tone.
- Although some congenital anomalies may be present in apparent life-threatening event (ALTE), the cause of the disease may not be clear even after various tests.
- Careful observation by medical personnel is necessary for all newborns, especially in the early neonatal period, due to the possibility of serious sequelae.

I. Kato (✉)
Department of Medical Research and Development, Kinjo Gakuin University, Nagoya, Aichi, Japan
e-mail: ikato@kinjo-u.ac.jp

Y. Matsuda (ed.), *Cerebral Palsy*, https://doi.org/10.1007/978-981-19-2217-6_32

1 Concept

An ALTE is defined by the Japanese Ministry of Health, Labour, and Welfare (MHLW) Research Team as "an episode in which one or more of the following symptoms occur suddenly, leading the observer to believe that the child is about to die: abnormal breathing, change in skin color, abnormal muscle tone, or change in state of consciousness. It is not relevant to the means or strength of the stimulation for recovery, or with or without cause" [1]. In other words, ALTE is defined as a concept rather than a diagnosis. Therefore, the search for the cause is important.

The Japanese MHLW research team prepared the "Guide to the Procedure for Searching for the Causes of an Apparent Life-Threatening Event (ALTE)" in fiscal year (FY) 2016 [2]. A search for the cause of the disease is performed based on the patient's history, onset status, examination findings, and laboratory findings; however, if the cause cannot be identified by various tests, the patient is diagnosed with an unknown cause of ALTE (idiopathic ALTE).

2 Sudden Infant Death Syndrome

Sudden infant death syndrome (SIDS) is defined by the Japanese MHLW research team as "a syndrome of sudden death in a child younger than 1 year of age in which death is unpredictable on the basis of previous health status and history, and in which the cause cannot be identified by death scene investigation or autopsy." Autopsy and death scene investigation are essential for the diagnosis of SIDS. The onset of SIDS occurs primarily in the first 2–5 months of life, and the frequency of the disease in the neonatal period is thought to be low.

3 SUPC (Sudden Unexpected Postnatal Collapse)

Although cases of ALTE or SIDS in the neonatal period have been reported for some time, sudden neonatal death or sudden cardiopulmonary insufficiency or collapse without death has been defined as SUPC. SUPC is considered an unpredictable condition that occurs in the early neonatal period and could have serious consequences.

In 2010, the British Association of Perinatal Medicine (BAPM) developed a guideline to review the incidence and pathogenesis of sudden unexpected postnatal collapse (SUPC) [3]. According to this guideline, SUPC is defined as a term or near-term (>35 weeks) infant who (1) was well at birth (normal 5-min Apgar score and received usual postnatal care), (2) developed an unexpected sudden change that required resuscitation with positive pressure breathing within 7 days of birth, and (3) died, required intensive care, or developed encephalopathy or other disabilities.

SUPC does not include neonatal death and ALTE which have risk factors, such as preterm birth (<35 weeks), perinatal asphyxia, or congenital abnormalities. Since SUPC includes both deaths and surviving cases, some cases of death are considered sudden unexpected early neonatal death (SUEND), and some cases of surviving cases are considered ALTE.

4 Epidemiology of ALTE/SUPC

In 1994, Yamanami [4] reported on early neonatal onset of SIDS and ALTE using a nationwide questionnaire survey of obstetric facilities. A total of 57 cases of SIDS and 69 cases of ALTE were reported over a 5-year period from 1989 to 1993, and the incidence rates were SIDS = 0.040 per 1000 live births and ALTE = 0.048 per 1000 live births. The mean onset time of ALTE was 40 h after birth.

Ohki et al. [5] conducted a nationwide questionnaire survey on early neonatal sudden unexpected changes in 2008 and 2009 in perinatal facilities. A total of 118 cases (56 inborns and 62 outborns) responded to the survey over 2 years, and 32 cases developed within 2 h after birth, 74 within 24 h, and 84 within 48 h. The incidence rate was 0.176–0.233 for all sudden unexpected changes per 1000 births, 0.013–0.017 for deaths, and 0.031–0.042 for serious sequelae, according to the report.

5 Causes and Prognosis of ALTE/SUPC

According to Yamanami's study, 15 patients were rescued but later died, 5 patients had cerebral palsy (CP), 1 patient had epilepsy, and the other 18 patients survived without sequelae.

Ohki et al. reported that the most common causes of sudden unexpected change in newborns up to 2 h after birth were transient tachypnea, hemorrhagic pulmonary edema, respiratory distress syndrome, respiratory leakage syndrome, respiratory failure and paraplegia, persistent pulmonary hypertension, meconium aspiration syndrome, and congenital anomalies. After 48 h, ductal shock due to congenital heart disease and abnormalities of the central nervous system abnormalities were reported to be more common. The investigation in cases within the first hour of life was also reported to have revealed that early skin-to-skin contact (early SSC) had no effect on the incidence of sudden unexpected change. The outcome of the sudden unexpected change in newborns was 15 deaths, 28 were with sequelae, 73 improved, and 2 were unknown. Among the 28 patients with sequelae, 23 patients required tube feeding and artificial ventilation, 1 patient had mild athetosis after cerebral hypothermia treatment, 1 patient was able to walk after grade IV intraventricular hemorrhage, and the prognosis of 3 patients was unknown.

Suzuki [6] reported in 2016 on the clinical characteristics of cases whose causes were analyzed on the basis of the obstetric medical compensation system, in which he analyzed 26 cases that were evaluated as normal newborns immediately after birth without any problems in the delivery process but later developed sudden unexpected changes and remained with severe CP. The 26 cases included 15 cases of ALTE (unexplained ALTE), 12 cases of group B streptococcus (GBS) infection, 6 cases of herpes infection, 6 cases of hypoglycemia, 3 cases of hyperkalemia, 3 cases of cerebral infarction, and 6 cases with other diagnoses. In a review of 15 of these cases diagnosed with ALTE, 33% of the onset was within 2 h of birth and 80% within 1 day.

It is important to provide intensive care to newborns who develop sudden unexpected postnatal changes and to perform a thorough examination for possible causes. Guidelines for the investigations of SUPC or ALTE from the UK and Italy stated that examinations for congenital infections, congenital anomalies, respiratory disorders, anemia, hypoglycemia, congenital adrenal hyperplasia, nervous system or neuromuscular diseases, and metabolic diseases are required (Table 1) [3, 7]. When the cause of the disease is unclear even after various investigations, idiopathic ALTE or idiopathic SUPC is diagnosed.

Table 1 Relevant investigations for cases of sudden unexpected neonatal change (ALTE/SUPC)

1. Histopathological investigations of the placenta and umbilical cord
2. Maternal blood test: Kleihauer method, virus test (acute phase serum cryopreservation), toxicology test
3. Maternal vaginal secretion test
4. Neonatal blood tests: blood count, coagulation system, blood gases, renal function, liver function, blood glucose, lactic acid, magnesium, ammonia, β-hydroxybutyrate, amino acids, free fatty acids, acylcarnitine profile, cortisol (at three different points in time), viral tests, DNA and chromosome tests, filter paper blood storage If unexplained hypoventilation/apnea is suspected: collect a DNA sample to search for abnormalities in the PHOX2B gene associated with congenital central hypoventilation syndrome
5. Cerebrospinal fluid: biochemical, sugar, culture, virus test, lactic acid, glycine, specimen preservation
6. Bacterial culture of various surface swabs
7. Urine: bacteriological test, viral test, poison, orotic acid, preservation of amino acid, urine specimen preservation
8. Imaging: head ultrasound, magnetic resonance imaging, renal/adrenal ultrasound, electrocardiography, cardiac ECHO
9. Fundus examination/RetCam®
10. Skin biopsy for fibroblast culture
11. Muscle biopsy if neuromuscular disease or mitochondrial disorders cannot be excluded
12. Electroencephalography

6 Reducing the Risk of Sudden Unexpected Neonatal Change

The neonatal period is a time for extrauterine adaptation, during which the newborn should adapt to changes in the environment. To reduce the risk of sudden unexpected life threatening events, especially in the early neonatal period, careful observation of all newborns and their mothers is necessary. Attention should be paid to the safe sleep environment, skin color, respiratory status, respiratory rate, oxygen saturation, and body temperature for newborns.

References

1. Togari H, et al. Heisei 24 nendo kouseiroudoukagakukenkyuu nyuuyouji totsuzensi syoukougun (SIDS) oyobi nyuuyouji toppatsusei kikyuujitai (ALTE) no byoutaikaimei oyobi yobouhou kaihatsu nimuketa fukusuuryouiki senmonka niyoru tougouteki kenkyu [2012 Health and Labor Sciences Research: an integrated study by multi-disciplinary experts for elucidation of the pathogenesis and development of prevention methods for Sudden Infant Death Syndrome (SIDS) and Sudden Infant Death Emergency (ALTE)]. 2012. Japanese.
2. Kato I et al. Heisei 28 nendo kouseiroudoukagakukenkyu nyuuyouji totsuzensi syoukougun (SIDS) oyobi nyuuyouji toppatsusei kikyuujitai (ALTE) no byoutaikaimei to shibousuu genshou notameno kenkyu [2016 Health and Labor Sciences Research on the pathogenesis of Sudden Infant Death Syndrome (SIDS) and sudden unexpected critical incident in infants (ALTE) and reduction of deaths]. 2016. Japanese.
3. Guidelines for the investigation of newborn infants who suffer a sudden and unexpected postnatal collapse in the first week of life. Recommendations from a professional group on sudden unexpected postnatal collapse. 2010. [Internet]. https://www.cpsig.org.uk/documents/InvestigationsinSUPC.draftguideline.pdf. Accessed 25 Nov 2020.
4. Yamaminami S. Neonatal SIDS. Pediatrics. 1997;29:498–502. Japanese.
5. Ohki S, Kajiwara M, Amizuka T, et al. Shusseigobunbenshisetsu deno shinseiji kyuhen nikansuru zenkokuchousa [Nationwide survey on sudden neonatal changes in postnatal delivery facilities]. J Japan Soc Premature Infants Newborns. 2012;24:73–81. Japanese.
6. Suzuki S. Shusseigo no shinseijikyuhen ni taiousuru [Dealing with sudden neonatal changes after birth]. J Nissan Womens Assoc. 2016;68:3133–6. Japanese.
7. Piumelli R, Davanzo R, Nassi N, et al. Apparent life-threatening events (ALTE): Italian guidelines. Ital J Pediatr. 2017;43:111. [Internet]. https://www.ncbi.nlm.nih.gov/pmc/articles/PMC5728046/pdf/13052_2017_Article_429.pdf. Accessed 26 Nov 2020.

Part III
Prevention

Neonatal Hypothermia

Masaki Shimizu

Contents

Summary

- Neonatal hypothermia is the only currently available evidence-based treatment for neonatal paresis and associated neonatal hypoxic-ischemic encephalopathy.
- Although moderate or severe neonatal hypoxic-ischemic encephalopathy is a major cause of cerebral palsy due to permanent brain damage in the central nervous system, neonatal hypothermia after injury provides effective brain protection.
- Hypothermia therapy is strictly regulated by the International Guidelines on Resuscitation, including the indication criteria, cooling period, and temperature rewarming.
- In recent years, however, it has become clear that the long-term prognosis at school age is not sufficiently improved.

M. Shimizu (✉)
Department of Neonatology, Saitama Children's Medical Center Perinatal and Child Health Care Center, Saitama, Japan
e-mail: shimizu.masaki@saitama-pho.jp

Y. Matsuda (ed.), *Cerebral Palsy*, https://doi.org/10.1007/978-981-19-2217-6_33

The incidence of neonatal hypoxic-ischemic encephalopathy (HIE) following neonatal paralysis has decreased with the widespread use of neonatal resuscitation programs, and the associated incidence of cerebral palsy (CP) has also decreased. However, moderate or severe HIE is still a major cause of CP, and neonatal therapeutic hypothermia (TH) has been introduced in perinatal care facilities nationwide. However, in recent years, long-term outcomes around school age have been reported, and although the rate of CP has decreased, developmental and cognitive impairments have relatively increased. In this section, we describe the basics of TH for the prevention of CP, its short- and long-term prognosis, and cognitive dysfunction without CP.

1 What Is Neonatal TH?

Neonatal TH is a treatment that is initiated to prevent or reduce permanent brain damage caused by neonatal hypoxic-ischemic encephalopathy. It is the current standard of care for postnatal HIE and was demonstrated to be cerebroprotective by reducing the brain metabolism and inhibiting intracellular metabolic activities. The number of CP cases due to polycystic encephalomalacia, which was frequently observed before the introduction of TH for moderate or severe HIE, has decreased, and the brain protective effects on the cerebral cortex are considered to be high. However, there are still severe CP cases with deep white matter and basal ganglia necrosis. In recent years, studies on the long-term prognosis of CP before and after school age revealed that developmental disorders due to higher-order dysfunction occur in school-aged children.

2 Basics of Neonatal TH

TH is effective for improving the survival rate and neurological developmental prognosis of HIE infants at 18–24 months, and reducing the risk of CP to one-third if the 72-h brain core's temperature (e.g., rectal temperature) is maintained at 33–34 °C within 6 h after injury for moderate or severe HIE in full-term or preterm infants. There is no difference in effects between selective head cooling and whole-body cooling.

HIE is caused by a severe anaerobic metabolic disorder that leads to adenosine triphosphate (ATP) depletion, accumulation of excitatory amino acids (EAAs) caused by Na/K^{++} ATP-dependent pump failure in the neuronal cell membrane, cytotoxic oxidation, and an increase in free radicals and nitric oxide (NO), which damage the cell membrane and intracellular organelles. Accumulation of these metabolites causes neurological depolarization and neuronal edema, and cerebral edema is induced by disruption of the blood-brain barrier. TH suppresses these brain metabolites, reduces the accumulation of EAAs, suppresses NO release, and reduces leakage at the blood-brain barrier. These neuroprotective effects inhibit inflammatory responses and cell apoptosis induced by ischemic injury [1–3].

3 Indication Criteria for Neonatal TH (Table 1)

Neonatal TH for HIE is performed according to the guidelines set by the International Liaison Committee on Resuscitation (ILCOR), with indication and exclusion criteria. HIE patients must be selected based on these exclusion and indication criteria.

Table 1 Guidelines for neonatal therapeutic hypothermia (TH) for neonatal hypoxic-ischemic encephalopathy (HIE)

Exclusion criteria
• If the child is more than 6 h old at the time of the start of cooling
• Those with less than 36 weeks of gestation
• Those whose birth weight is less than 1800 g
• Conditions with potential complications during cooling or major malformations
• When it is judged that the benefits of TH cannot be obtained due to the general condition or complications or when the risk of TH exceeds the benefits
• When the necessary system as an organization cannot be established
If none of the above applies, the next step is to determine if the adaptation criteria apply.
Adaptation criteria
• The child was born at 36 weeks or more of gestation and meets at least one of the following conditions:
– Apgar score of 5 or less at 10 min after birth
– Continuous neonatal resuscitation (tracheal intubation, bag ventilation) for more than 10 min is required
– Blood gas (cord blood, arterial, venous, peripheral capillary) within 60 min of birth with pH less than 7
– Blood gas (cord blood, arterial, venous, peripheral capillary) within 60 min of birth with a base deficit of 16 mmol/L or greater
The next step is to determine the presence of encephalopathy in HIE. Moderate to severe encephalopathy (equivalent to Sarnat class 2 or higher), i.e., impaired consciousness (somnolence, dullness, coma) and at least one of the following (preferably examined by a neonatologist or pediatric neurologist with expertise in neonatal encephalopathy):
• Decreased muscle tone
• Abnormal reflexes, including loss of the "doll's eye" reflex or abnormal pupillary reflex
• Decreased or absent sucking
• Clinical convulsions
aEEG (amplitude EEG) findings were previously included in the indication criteria, but as they do not always correspond to the neurological prognosis, they are now considered reference criteria. Patients must have at least a 30-min aEEG recording with moderate or greater abnormalities in the underlying rhythm or seizures. Classical electroencephalographic evaluation is not used as a criterion.
– Moderately abnormal = upper margin >10 μV and lower margin <5 μV or highly abnormal = upper margin <10 μV
– Sudden increase in potential and narrowing of amplitude, followed by a short burst of suppression

EEG electroencephalography
Adapted from the International Liaison Committee on Resuscitation (ILCOR)

4 Neonatal TH in Practice

There are three cooling methods for TH: selective head cooling with a cooling cap on the head, whole-body cooling with a cooling blanket, and intravascular cooling with a special intravascular catheter or extracorporeal circulation. The guidelines do not specify a specific cooling method but state that the deep body temperature (rectal temperature and esophageal temperature) should be cooled to a target temperature of 34 °C within 6 h after birth. In practice, when a child with HIE is admitted to the hospital, it is first necessary to confirm that none of the exclusion criteria are met, including systemic complications, and then to determine whether the child meets the criteria for TH within 6 h of birth. If TH is indicated, the patient should be immediately placed on a cooling pad and cooled to a target temperature of 33–34 °C. TH is a treatment to protect the brain by reducing the brain temperature to 33–34 °C. However, other organs are also exposed to low temperature, and strict systemic temporary management is required, including cerebral oxygen metabolism, cerebral activity, circulation, respiration, blood coagulation, electrolytes, infusion, infection, and seizure. Therefore, neonatal TH for HIE should be performed in a neonatal intensive care unit (NICU) under the guidance of a neonatologist who is skilled in the systemic management of neonates. According to the guidelines, the cooling period should be 72 h, and the temperature should be rewarmed to 37 °C at a rate of 0.5 °C/h after cooling.

5 Short-Term Outcomes of Neonatal TH

RCTs of TH in children with moderate or severe neonatal HIE reported outcomes at 18–24 months. Shankaran et al. [4] reported from the National Institute of Child Health and Human Development (NICHD) that whole-body cooling is a safe and effective treatment. The Cochrane review group conducted a meta-analysis of the effects of TH on death or neurological developmental outcomes in 1505 full-term or late preterm infants. They found that TH resulted in a statistically significant and clinically important reduction in the combined outcome of mortality or major neurodevelopmental disability to 18 months of age (typical RR 0.75 (95% CI 0.68 to 0.83); number needed to treat for an additional beneficial outcome (NNTB) 7 (95% CI 5 to 10) [5]. In addition, a recent meta-analysis of 13 articles including 1805 neonates concluded that TH for HIE is safe but associated with a risk of thrombocytopenia [RR, 1.08 (95% CI: 1.02–1.37), $p = 0.03$] and arrhythmia [RR, 2.52 (95% CI: 1.62–3.93), $p < 0.0001$].

As described above, TH was demonstrated to be an effective treatment for moderate or severe HIE, but it is not effective at improving the neurological prognosis. There are also cases of abnormal findings in the deep white matter and basal ganglia due to TH even if there is no abnormality in the cerebral cortex on head MRI, and children with mental impairment but no motor impairment due to the so-called CP have been reported.

6 Long-Term Outcomes of Neonatal TH

In recent years, large clinical trials of TH for HIE have reported neuroprotective effects around school age and in late childhood. According to the Cool Cap study, which assessed the prognosis at 6–7 years of age based on interviews with parents, 62 of 135 surviving children were disabled at 18 months, and there was no benefit of TH [6]. The NICHD group investigated the long-term prognosis of 190 neonatal encephalopathy patients at 6–7 years of age, with the primary outcome being death or intelligence quotient (IQ) of <70 and the secondary outcome being the presence of disability [7]. The prospective TH study investigated motor skills, cognitive function, growth, and functional disability as reported by parents. The primary outcome of death or IQ of less than 70 was observed in 46 (47%) of 97 subjects in the TH group and in 58 (62%) of 93 subjects in the control group [RR, 0.78 (95% CI: 0.61–1.01), $p = 0.06$], mortality was 28% vs. 44% ($p = 0.04$), and death or severe neurological impairment was 41% vs. 60% ($p = 0.03$). Other outcome data were available for 70 patients in the TH group and 52 in the control group. Moderate to severe disability was noted in 24 of 69 (35%) and 19 of 50 (38%) patients, respectively ($P = 0.87$). Attention and executive functions were impaired in 4% and 13% of children who received TH and standard care, respectively ($P = 0.19$), and visuospatial dysfunction was observed in 4% and 3% of children who received TH and standard care, respectively ($P = 0.80$). As a result, cognitive dysfunction and substandard IQ were observed in more than 25% of the children at the age of 6–7 years. Most children surviving CP (96%) had an IQ lower than 70, 9% of children without CP had an IQ below 70, and 31% had an IQ between 70. Of children with an IQ below 70, 23% were able to walk normally, 16% had complex motor functions, and 10% had normal fine motor development and motor coordination assessments. Twenty percent of the children with a normal IQ and 28% of those with an IQ of 70–84 received special education support and were retained for one or more years, revealing that all neonatal HIE children remain cognitively impaired [7].

In the TOBY trial using whole-body cooling, a survey of 145 school-aged children demonstrated that 75 of 145 (52%) had IQ scores of 85 or higher, which was greater than the 52 of 132 (39%) in the target group [RR, 1.31 (95% CI: 1.01–1.71), $p = 0.04$]. The motor function score was significantly lower in the TH group (21% vs. 36%, $p = 0.03$), with moderate or severe disability (22% vs. 37%, $p = 0.03$) [8].

Although there have been no RCTs of TH in Japan, the long-term prognosis of the 42 patients who received TH for HIE (autologous cases) was as follows: 33% (14/42) had an IQ of ≥85, 2% had an IQ of ≥85 with CP only, 12% (5/42) had an IQ of 71–84, and 33% (14/42) had an IQ of <70. Of the 33% (14/42) with an IQ of <70, 14% were ambulatory and 86% had CP. Overall, 31% (13/42) had CP. The mortality rate was 17%.

The median (range) scores on the Wechsler test of intelligence in children without CP [15 self-tested cases, mean age at test 6 years 0 months (5:0–7:3)] were as follows: total test IQ (FIQ) = 93.2 (67–150), verbal IQ (VIQ) = 90.8 (60–140),

Table 2 Results of the Wechsler system intelligence test in children without cerebral palsy

[15 patients, mean age at test 6 years 0 months (5:0–7:3)]			
IQ	Mean (SD)	WISC-III	WPPSI
Total test IQ (FIQ)	93.2 (±20.9) (67–150)	98.3 (±22.7)	84.3 (±15.0)
Verbal IQ (VIQ)	90.8 (±20.1) (60–140)	96.3 (±20.7)	81.3 (±15.9)
Motor IQ (PIQ)	96.7 (±17.2) (69–125)	98.8 (±18.3)	93.1 (±15.9)

Difference between VIQ and PIQ	
Mean (SD)	14.8 (±9.5) (WISC-III 12.6 (±7.2)/WPPSI 18.7 (±12.2))
15 points or more	9 patients (47%) (WISC-III 5/WPPSI 4)
VIQ < PIQ	7 patients (WISC-III 3/WPPSI 4)
Less than 10–15 points	6 patients (32%) (WISC-III 4/WPPSI 2)
VIQ < PIQ	2 patients (WISC-III 2/WPPSI 0)
Less than 9 points	4 patients (22%) (WISC-III 3/WPPSI 1)

WISC-III Wechsler intelligence scale for Children-III, *WPPSI* Wechsler Preschool and Primary Scale of Intelligence, *VIQ* Verbal IQ, *PIQ* Performance IQ

motor IQ (PIQ) = 96.7 (69–125); 47% (7/15) had a difference of 15 points or more between VIQ and PIQ, and 86% (6/7) were characterized by a predominance of motor skills (Table 2). Thus, children with a large discrepancy between verbal and motor skills may have a high risk of developing learning disabilities and developmental disorders and should be carefully followed up when they start school.

7 Neonatal TH for HIE in Preterm Infants

HIE associated with neonatal asphyxia also develops in preterm infants, and at our institution, TH has been used with great care in preterm infants with HIE of 33–35 weeks of gestation. Although the current TH guidelines exclude patients who are younger than 36 weeks of age, studies are underway to improve the neurological outcome of preterm HIE. TH as a treatment for HIE in preterm infants has not been examined on a large scale, but a recent study of preterm infants at 34–35 weeks of gestation reported increased mortality and morbidity compared with TH for HIE in full-term infants. However, this report did not compare preterm infants with those who did not receive TH for HIE (control group) [9].

In December 2020, the NICHD Neonatal Research Network Preemie Hypothermia for Neonatal Encephalopathy started NCT01793129, an RCT to evaluate the safety and efficacy of 72-h TH for preterm infants at 33–35 weeks of age with moderate to severe HIE encephalopathy who survive at 6 h after birth. The primary outcome is death or severe disability at 18–22 months of age.

8 Expanded Options for Neonatal TH

Whether a lower temperature setting or longer cooling period improves the prognosis of TH for HIE has been investigated. Neither a longer cooling time (>72–120 h), a lower temperature setting (32–33.5 °C or lower), nor their combination reduced mortality or moderate/severe disability at 18 months compared with the standard cooling method (33.5 °C for 72 h) [10]. On the other hand, a 76% reduction in death or disability was reported for TH after 6–24 h of life [11].

The use of neonatal TH for HIE reduced the incidence of CP. Children who undergo neonatal TH should be followed up after discharge from the NICU for evaluation of motor neural development and cognitive dysfunction around school age.

References

1. Gunn AJ, Gunn TR, Gunning MI, et al. Neuroprotection with prolonged head cooling started before postischemic seizures in fetal sheep. Pediatrics. 1998;102:1098–106.
2. Edwards AD, Yue X, Squier MV, et al. Specific inhibition of apoptosis after cerebral hypoxia-ischaemia by moderate post-insult hypothermia. Biochem Biophys Res Commun. 1995;217:1193–9.
3. Globus MY, Alonso O, Dietrich WD, et al. Glutamate release and free radical production following brain injury: effects of posttraumatic hypothermia. J Neurochem. 1995;65:1704–11.
4. Shankaran S. Hypoxic-ischemic encephalopathy and novel strategies for neuroprotection. Clin Perinatol. 2012;39:919–29.
5. Jacobs SE, Berg M, Hunt R, et al. Cooling for newborns with hypoxic ischaemic encephalopathy. Cochrane Database Syst Rev. 2013.
6. Guillet R, Edwards AD, Thoresen M, et al. Seven- to eight-year follow-up of the Cool Cap trial of head cooling for neonatal encephalopathy. Pediatr Res. 2011;71:205–9.
7. Shankaran S, Pappas A, McDonald SA, et al. Childhood outcomes after hypothermia for neonatal encephalopathy. N Engl J Med. 2012;366:2085–92.
8. Azzopardi D, Strohm B, Fau-Marlow N, et al. Effects of hypothermia for perinatal asphyxia on childhood outcomes. N Engl J Med. 2014;371:140–9.
9. Rao R, Trivedi S, Vesoulis Z, et al. Safety and short-term outcomes of therapeutic hypothermia in preterm neonates 34–35 weeks gestational age with hypoxic-ischemic encephalopathy. J Pediatr. 2017;183:37–42.
10. Shankaran S, Laptook AR, Pappas A, et al. Effect of depth and duration of cooling on death or disability at age 18 months among neonates with hypoxic- ischemic encephalopathy: a randomized clinical trial. JAMA. 2017;318:57–67.
11. Laptook AR, Shankaran S, Tyson JE, et al. Effect of therapeutic hypothermia initiated after 6 hours of age on death or disability among newborns with hypoxic-ischemic encephalopathy: a randomized clinical trial. JAMA. 2017;318:1550–60.

Recent Findings on the Perinatal Brain Protective Effects of Magnesium

Hiroshi Sameshima

Contents

Summary

- Magnesium administered transmaternally reduces brain damage. This has been proven in animal studies and in clinical studies. In a Cochrane review, it reduced cerebral palsy by 1/3 without changing mortality in preterm infants.
- The number needed to treat to prevent one cerebral palsy is calculated to be 42–46 individuals. Recent animal studies have shown a preconditioning effect of this mechanism. If so, prophylactic administration during pregnancy may also have a cerebral palsy-preventive effect, and forward-looking studies are awaited.

1 Current Status of the Neuroprotective Effect of Magnesium on the Brain

There are two types of drugs validated in brain protection for preterm infants that can be administered during pregnancy.

H. Sameshima (✉)
University of Miyazaki Hospital, Miyazaki, Japan
e-mail: hsameshima@med.miyazaki-u.ac.jp

Y. Matsuda (ed.), *Cerebral Palsy*, https://doi.org/10.1007/978-981-19-2217-6_34

One is corticosteroid, which has a protective effect on the brain such as prevention of intraventricular hemorrhage as well as lung maturation in preterm infants. The other is magnesium sulfate hydrate (Mg), which is described in this section.

Mg is transmissible through the human placenta. Based on clinical data from 111 pregnant women, the fetal/maternal blood concentration ratio was reported to be 0.94 [1]. Therefore, transmaternal administration can maintain the fetal blood concentration and is expected to have a brain protective effect.

A recommendation for the use of Mg in obstetrics was issued by the American College of Obstetricians and Gynecologists (ACOG) in 2016 [2]. According to this, the indications for Mg use were narrowed down to three: (1) eclampsia prevention and treatment, (2) prolongation of pregnancy up to 48 h for preterm birth, and (3) fetal brain protection (for preterm births less than 32 weeks). All of these are for short-term use up to 48–72 h.

Many papers have been reported on the brain protective effects of Mg on preterm infants. Historically, several relatively large randomized controlled trials (RCTs) were subsequently conducted because of the controversy that erupted in observational studies regarding the brain protective effects [3–7]. Among them, meta-analyses on the brain protective effects in preterm infants have been repeatedly reported using five RCTs that met certain selection criteria [8–10]: four studies used Mg for brain protection in preterm infants [3–6], and the remaining one was administered for eclampsia prevention.

Although analyses using summary data have been widely used for meta-analyses [8, 9], the usefulness of meta-analyses of individual data has recently become apparent [10]. Table 1 shows the results of the meta-analysis based on individual participant data [10]. The results were similar to those of previous analyses using summary data. The upper part of the table shows the results of the meta-analysis using all five studies, and the lower part shows the results of the meta-analysis using only four studies for the purpose of brain protection (Table 1).

Table 1 Results of the meta-analysis 1: effect of transmaternal magnesium administration on infant brain protection

Primary endpoint	Risk ratio (RR)	95% confidence interval (CI)	Number of children	Number of RCTs
1. Death or cerebral palsy	0.94	0.85–1.05	6131	All 5 studies
	0.86	0.75–0.99	4448	4 studies, only RCTs for neuroprotection, NNT = 41
2. Death	1.03	0.91–1.17	6131	All 5 studies
	0.95	0.80–1.13	4448	Four studies, examining only RCTs for neuroprotection
3. Cerebral palsy in survivors	0.68	0.54–0.87	4601	All 5 studies, survivors only, NNT = 46
	0.68	0.53–0.87	3988	4 studies, RCTs only for neuroprotection, survivors only, NNT = 42

NNT number needed to treat

First, for the primary endpoint of reducing death or cerebral palsy, a meta-analysis of all five studies found no significant difference. On the other hand, the four studies for brain protection showed a significant reduction with a relative risk (RR) of 0.86. Therefore, it cannot be said to reduce "death or cerebral palsy."

Next, we focused only on the deaths in the "death or cerebral palsy" category and found that Mg was not involved in the mortality of the children. This clearly indicates that the maternal administration of Mg does not increase infant mortality, which may answer a possible concern that Mg may rescue the frequency of cerebral palsy in the surviving infants by increasing infant mortality.

Finally, an analysis of the incidence of cerebral palsy (CP) in survivors showed that Mg significantly reduced the incidence of CP by RR 0.68 or 32% compared with the control group.

Based on the results of these analyses, it is concluded that transmaternal Mg administration during pregnancy can reduce brain damage in preterm infants by about two-thirds without increasing infant mortality. The number needed to treat (NNT) to prevent the development of cerebral palsy in one person was calculated to be 42–46.

This cerebroprotective effect of Mg was found to be similar regardless of the cause of preterm birth and regardless of the timing of Mg administration (weeks of gestation), total dose, or whether Mg was administered as maintenance therapy, according to the current meta-analysis [10]. However, the number of cases is insufficient for such a secondary analysis, and further RCTs are required.

Table 2 summarizes the results of the meta-analysis based on individual data for the child's secondary endpoints for brain protection [10]. The results of the meta-analysis showed that neonatal acute complications such as neonatal seizures, severe intraventricular hemorrhage of grade 3 or higher, and periventricular leukomalacia (PVL) were not affected by Mg administration. In addition, no significant effect of Mg on long-term prognosis, such as blindness and developmental delay, was observed.

Table 2 Results of the meta-analysis 2: secondary effects of transmaternal magnesium administration on the child

Binomial factor	Risk ratio (RR)	95% confidence interval (CI)
Apgar score <7.5 quantile	1.01	0.89–1.14
Chronic lung disease	1.08	0.96–1.22
Neonatal convulsions	0.75	0.54–1.03
Intraventricular hemorrhage, grade 3 or 4	0.83	0.63–1.09
Periventricular leukomalacia (leukomalacia)	0.91	0.66–1.25
Necrotizing enterocolitis	1.22	0.97–1.53
Cavernous arteriopathy of prematurity requiring treatment	1.03	0.91–1.16
Loss of eyesight	0.88	0.65–1.06

The five studies used in this meta-analysis are, in order of citation, referred to as the MAGNET, ACTOMgSO4, PREMAG, BEAM, and MAGPIE studies [3–7]. In addition, the MAGENTA study, an RCT of 1676 patients at 30–34 weeks, is also well known [11]. Furthermore, in April 2020, the MASP study, an RCT of 560 preterm births (<32 weeks' gestation), was newly reported from Denmark [12]. The frequency of moderate to severe CP was 2% in the Mg group, compared with 3.3% in the control group, an overall decrease of 39%. A meta-analysis incorporating these data as individual participant data (Cochrane review) is awaited.

2 Methods of Administration of Magnesium for Cerebral Neuroprotective Purposes

Most of the RCTs are administered to women with a fetal age of less than 32 or 34 weeks, with a lower limit of 24 weeks or later, and in whom preterm labor is judged to be imminent within 24 h. The method of administration is to load 4 g of Mg over 20–30 min, followed by intravenous administration of 1 g per hour to the mother.

It has been shown that the Mg concentration in fetal blood increases in about 1 h and in amniotic fluid increases in about 3 h. It is thought that a protective effect is observed more than 4 h after the loading dose, but the basis for this is not clear, and some suggest 6–12 h.

Mg administration should be continued until the end of labor or after 24 h of continuous administration according to the method used in the RCTs. On the other hand, if the steroid effect is expected in the case of imminent preterm labor, 48–72 h should be used.

The efficacy and safety of multiple doses of Mg have not yet been established.

The method of administering Mg for cerebroprotection is the same as that widely used for eclampsia prophylaxis and imminent preterm labor, and the side effects should be treated accordingly.

Thus, the cerebroprotective effect of Mg has been studied only for short-term administration. The reason for this is that in Europe and the United States, Mg is only administered for a short period of time, even when used as a countermeasure against imminent preterm labor. Therefore, there is still no clear scientific evidence for the brain protective effect of long-term administration of Mg, which has been used in Japan. In addition, there is no clear scientific evidence for the effect of combination therapy of Mg with other uterine contraction inhibitors on brain protection.

3 Mechanism of Neuroprotective Effect of Magnesium on the Brain

The mechanism of the cerebroprotective effect of Mg has not been clearly elucidated, but since Mg ions have a competitive antagonism with calcium ions, many possible mechanisms have been postulated.

In vivo studies on the mechanism of action have been verified in animal experiments on sheep, goats, and rats. The results suggest that Mg stabilizes cerebral blood flow, inhibits intracellular calcium influx, stabilizes neuronal cell membranes, and has antioxidant, anti-inflammatory, anti-apoptotic, and mitochondria-mediated tolerance effects.

Among them, the study by Hagberg et al. published in 2019 is interesting from the viewpoint of preconditioning [13, 14]. In general, it is known that tolerance to strong stress can be obtained by adding a mild stimulus or another stimulus before applying a strong stress load, which is called preconditioning (tolerance).

Therefore, Hagberg et al. examined whether administering a small amount of Mg before hypoxic-ischemic loading (preconditioning), which would normally cause brain damage, could reduce hypoxic-ischemic brain damage (tolerance effect) in a rat brain damage model [13, 14]. As a result, they reported that a single preadministration of Mg from a minimum of 12 h to a maximum of 6 days before hypoxic-ischemic stress improved subsequent brain damage. In particular, 24-h preadministration showed the greatest preconditioning effect [14]. Hagberg et al. concluded that this was not a direct effect of Mg but a preconditioning effect, because the Mg blood concentration recovered to within the normal range after hypoxic-ischemic stress. This effect was demonstrated not only in 7-day-old rats, which are close to full term in terms of human brain development, but also in more immature brains. That is, hypoxic-ischemic brain damage was significantly suppressed by preloading Mg 24 h before hypoxia-ischemia even in 4- and 5-day-old rats [13]. Based on these results and those of other studies, we hypothesize that Mg alters mitochondrial function and metabolism and induces tolerance to subsequent hypoxic-ischemic challenge.

There are still many research issues to be addressed, such as whether there is a preconditioning effect in humans, when the preconditioning effect should be observed (at what week of pregnancy), and whether it is better to administer Mg immediately before pregnancy, as has been proposed, or to administer Mg in advance with the expectation of a preconditioning effect. If there is a preconditioning effect, it may be possible to prevent brain damage in preterm infants by preadministering Mg during pregnancy.

4 A Multicenter, Retrospective Study from Japan

As mentioned above, the efficacy of long-term Mg administration for brain protection, which has been used in Japan, is unknown. Therefore, we conducted a collaborative study among four institutions in Japan to retrospectively examine whether long-term Mg administration improves the frequency of brain damage in preterm infants, the effect of concomitant administration of β-stimulants, and the optimal timing and duration of Mg administration [15]. The subjects were 1083 preterm births between 28 and 36 weeks of gestation, 39% without uterine contraction inhibitors, 47% with Mg, 41% with β-stimulants, and 27% with both drugs.

Multivariate and multiple comparisons were made using the following confounding factors: uterine contraction inhibitors, weeks of pregnancy, sex, presence of asphyxia, and prenatal steroids. The results showed that Mg significantly reduced the incidence of poor prognosis (infant death or brain damage) compared with the group without uterine contraction inhibitors, even after adjusting for confounding factors [odds ratio (OR), 0.27 [95% confidence interval (95% CI), 0.10–0.72]]. In contrast, beta-stimulants did not change the frequency of poor outcome (OR, 1.28). Interestingly, the cerebroprotective effect of Mg disappeared when the two drugs were combined. The cerebroprotective effect of Mg was also observed when the drug was used for 1 week or less, but not when it was administered for longer periods. Cerebroprotection was observed in preterm infants between 28 and 32 weeks of gestation but not in preterm infants over 32 weeks.

Although the number of cases was too small to draw any conclusions, there was no difference between the duration of Mg withdrawal before delivery and the frequency of brain damage, indicating the possibility of a preconditioning effect of Mg.

These results indicate that the brain protective effect of Mg was observed in preterm infants born between 28 and 32 weeks of gestation within 1 week of use and that the brain protective effect disappeared when Mg was combined with beta-stimulants. The efficacy within 1 week was similar to that of short-term administration in Western countries. Further studies are needed to investigate the effect of the combination of beta-stimulants, the preconditioning effect, and the effect on very preterm infants born between 22 and 28 weeks of gestation.

References

1. Brookfield KF, Su F, Elkomy MH, et al. Pharmacokinetics and placental transfer of magnesium sulfate in pregnant women. Am J Obstet Gynecol. 2016;214:737.e1–9.
2. ACOG. Committee opinion number 652: magnesium sulfate use in obstetrics. Obstet Gynecol. 2016;127:239–51.
3. Mittendorf R, Covert R, Boman J, et al. Is tocolytic magnesium sulphate associated with increased total paediatric mortality? Lancet. 1997;330:1517–8.
4. Crowther CA, Hiller JE, Doyle LW, et al.; Australasian Collaborative Trial of Magnesium Sulphate (ACTOMgSO4) Collaborative Group. Effect of magnesium sulfate given for neuroprotection before preterm birth: a randomized controlled trial. JAMA. 2003;290:2669–76.
5. Marret S, Marpeau L, Zupan-Simunek V, et al.; PREMAG Trial Group. Magnesium sulphate given before very preterm birth to protect infant brain: the randomised controlled PREMAG trial. BJOG. 2007;114:310–8.
6. Rouse DJ, Hirtz DG, Thom E, et al. A randomized, controlled trial of magnesium sulfate for the prevention of cerebral palsy. N Engl J Med. 2008;359:895–905.
7. Altman D, Carroli G, Duley L, et al.; MAGPIE Trial Collaboration Group. Do women with pre-eclampsia, and their babies, benefit from magnesium sulphate? The Magpie trial: a randomised placebo-controlled trial. Lancet. 2002;359:1877–90.
8. Doyle LW, Crowther CA, Middleton P, et al. Magnesium sulphate for women at risk of preterm birth for neuroprotection of the fetus. Cochrane Database Syst Rev. 2009;CD004661.

9. Shepherd E, Salam RA, Middleton P, et al. Antenatal and intrapartum interventions for preventing cerebral palsy: an overview of the Cochrane systematic review. Cochrane Database Syst Rev. 2017;8:CD012077.
10. Crowther CA, Middleton PF, Voysay M, et al. Assessing the neuroprotective benefits for babies of antenatal magnesium sulphate: an individual participant data mete-analysis. PLoS Med. 2017;14:e1002398.
11. Crowther CA, Middleton P, Wilkinson D, et al. Magnesium sulphate at 30 to 34 weeks' gestational age: neuroprotection trial (MAGENTA)—study protocol. BMC Pregnancy Childbirth. 2013;13:91.
12. Wolf HT, Brok J, Henriksen TB, et al. Antenatal magnesium sulphate for the prevention of cerebral palsy in infants born preterm: a double-blind, randomized, placebo-controlled, multicenter trial. BJOG. 2020;127(10):1217–25. https://doi.org/10.1111/1471-0528.16239. [Epub ahead of print].
13. Koning G, Lyngfelt E, Svedin P, et al. Magnesium sulphate induces preconditioning in preterm rodent models of cerebral hypoxia-ischemia. Int J Dev Neurosci. 2018;70:56–66.
14. Koning G, Leverin AL, Nair S, et al. Magnesium induces preconditioning of the neonatal brain via profound mitochondrial protection. J Cereb Blood Flow Metab. 2019;39:1038–55.
15. Kino E, Ohhashi M, Kawagoe Y, et al. Impact of tocolysis-intent magnesium sulfate and beta-adrenergic agonists on perinatal brain damage in infants. J Obstet Gynecol Res. 2020;46:2027–35.

Mechanism and Current Status of Umbilical Cord Blood Stem Cell Transplantation

Haruo Shintaku

Contents

Summary

- In 1982, Nakahata et al. in Japan were the first in the world to discover that umbilical cord blood contains stem cells, and in 1989, Gluchman et al. began to use it to treat Fanconi anemia. This led to the establishment of umbilical cord blood banks, and cord blood stem cell transplantation became a popular practice throughout the world and has been widely applied to the treatment of leukemia for the purpose of reconstructing hematopoietic tissue.
- In 2014, Cotten et al. in the United States reported the potential of cord blood stem cell transplantation for the treatment of hypoxic-ischemic encephalopathy in neonates, which is a regenerative medicine that aims to regenerate brain tissue rather than reconstruct hematopoietic tissue.

In general, the human brain tissue has a low regenerative capacity and does not recover spontaneously after injury. Once brain damage is complete and cerebral palsy (CP) develops, there is no effective treatment. It is important to develop treatment methods in the neonatal period, before brain damage is complete. Therapeutic hypothermia (TH) for perinatal hypoxic ischemic encephalopathy (HIE), which is

H. Shintaku (✉)
Endowed Department of Disability Medicine and Regenerative Medicine, Osaka Metropolitan University Graduate School of Medicine, Osaka, Japan
e-mail: shintakuh@omu.ac.jp

Y. Matsuda (ed.), *Cerebral Palsy*, https://doi.org/10.1007/978-981-19-2217-6_35

the main cause of cerebral palsy, has already been widely used as an effective treatment under the guidelines; although the mortality rate was reduced in severe HIE, half of the patients with TH alone were found to have some residual disease [1, 2]. In 2014, it was reported in the United States that the combination of TH and cord blood transfusion (CBT) for the treatment of HIE improved the prognosis [3]. In Japan, a clinical trial of autologous umbilical cord blood stem cell therapy for HIE was started at the end of 2014 by the Japan Agency for Medical Research and Development (AMED) as one of the projects for practical application of regenerative medicine. In Japan, a clinical trial of autologous umbilical cord blood stem cell therapy for HIE was started by the Japan Agency for Medical Research and Development (AMED) at the end of 2014.

1 Umbilical Cord Blood Stem Cells and Regenerative Medicine (Fig. 1)

Hematopoietic stem cells (HSCs) and mesenchymal stem cells (MSCs), which exist everywhere in our body, have long played play a role in tissue maintenance and regeneration. These cells, called somatic stem cells, are safer and less ethically

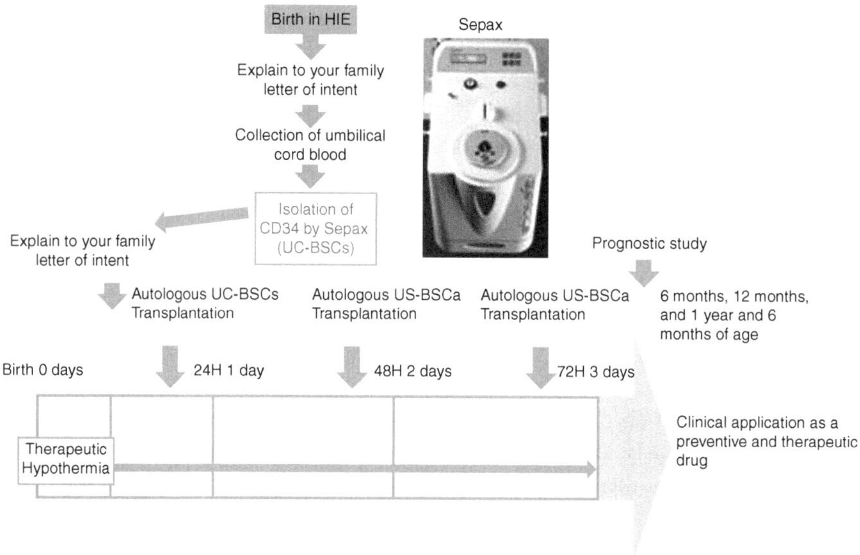

Fig. 1 Autologous cord blood stem cell therapy protocol. In neonates born with moderate or severe hypoxic-ischemic encephalopathy (HIE), cord blood is collected with the consent of the family, aseptically isolated using Sepax, and administered intravenously for 3 days with hypothermia in three divided doses. *HIE* hypoxic-ischemic encephalopathy

problematic than ES cells (embryonic stem cells) and iPS cells (pluripotent stem cells), which have been the focus of attention recently, and their clinical application is advancing. In the neonatal field, umbilical cord blood stem cells (UC-BSCs) and umbilical cord-derived mesenchymal stem cells (UC-MSCs) are obtained from the umbilical cord blood and the umbilical cord, which are normally discarded after birth, and they are attracting attention as a source of supply.

In 1982, Nakahata et al. in Japan [4] were the first in the world to discover that the umbilical cord blood contained stem cells (UC-BSCs), and CBT was subsequently performed for the treatment of Fanconi anemia. Such CBT is the same as conventional transplantation in that it reconstructs hematopoietic tissue using hematopoietic stem cells. However, CBT as a treatment for HIE described here is not homologous use but type 2 regenerative medicine technology because UC-BSCs are administered for the purpose of treating brain tissue rather than reconstructing hematopoietic tissue, although they are not cultured. In this sense, CBT as a treatment for HIE should be correctly described as UC-BSCs therapy rather than transplantation based on the "Act on Securing the Safety of Regenerative Medicine" (New Regenerative Medicine Act) enacted in 2014.

2 Treatment of Hypoxic-Ischemic Encephalopathy with UC-BSCs

In 2014, Cotten et al. [3] from Duke University, USA, isolated and administered stem cells from an autologous umbilical cord blood to moderately to severely ill neonates with HIE and found no safety issues and no difference in survival between TH alone and TH plus autologous CBT. The normal survival rate of developmental quotient (DQ) of 85 or higher was 72% in the TH plus autologous CBT group compared with 41% in the TH alone group.

Japan has started a phase I trial of autologous umbilical cord blood stem cell therapy for HIE based on the new regenerative medicine law in accordance with the treatment method of Cotten et al. Based on the guidelines of TH for HIE, this clinical trial was conducted on newborns with moderate or severe HIE who were born at 36 weeks or more of gestation and weighed 1800 g or more at birth. UC-BSCs were aseptically isolated using Sepax (Global Life Sciences Technologies Japan Co., Ltd.) and were administered intravenously for 3 days in triplicate (Fig. 1) [5]. We have already conducted the six cases necessary to confirm the safety of this treatment, and all patients were able to be weaned from the ventilator and were discharged from the hospital without any deaths, which is almost equivalent to the results reported by Cotten et al. [6]. Since the phase I study was completed and the safety was confirmed, the phase II study has been started.

3 Treatment Mechanism of UC-BSCs

Basic research on the application of UC-BSCs and UC-MSCs to brain regenerative medicine has been conducted, and UC-BSCs and UC-MSCs have been shown to have the pluripotency to transform into neurons in vitro, and their therapeutic effects on the central nervous system have been demonstrated in in vivo experimental systems such as animal experiments. However, recent studies have shown that these stem cells do not directly replace damaged nerve cells in the brain tissue but that UC-BSCs promote repair mainly by improving energy metabolism and promoting angiogenesis in the damaged area, and UC-MSCs promote regeneration of brain nerve cells mainly by suppressing tissue damage by suppressing inflammatory reactions in the acute phase. In addition, UC-MSCs have been shown to promote the regeneration of brain neurons by inhibiting tissue damage, mainly by suppressing acute inflammatory reactions.

4 From Prevention to Treatment of Cerebral Palsy

Until now, direct treatment of CP has been difficult, and treatment of the causative disease has been focused on preventing CP as a sequela. Recently, however, clinical trials have been conducted in Japan and overseas to treat CP directly by administering self-UC-BSC to children diagnosed with CP, rather than to prevent CP. Overseas, Kurtzberg et al. at Duke University conducted a randomized placebo-controlled trial of self-administered UC-BSCs in children with cerebral palsy aged 1–7 years and reported that motor function improved significantly after 1 year in the group that received 2×10^7or more self-administered UC-BSCs [7]. In Japan, Kochi University has started a phase I clinical trial of self-administered UC-BSCs in CP children aged 2–7 years, and safety has already been confirmed in the six cases conducted.

Thus, the treatment of CP, which was considered to be impossible in the past, has become a reality with the progress of regenerative medicine using autologous cord blood stem cells, and further development is expected.

References

1. Shankaran S, Pappas A, McDonald SA, et al. Childhood outcomes after hypothermia for neonatal encephalopathy. N Engl J Med. 2012;366:2085–92.

2. Tsuda K, Mukai T, Iwata S, et al. Therapeutic hypothermia for neonatal encephalopathy: a report from the first 3 years of the Baby Cooling Registry of Japan. Sci Rep. 2017;7:39508.
3. Cotten CM, Murtha AP, Goldberg RN, et al. Feasibility of autologous cord blood cells for infants with hypoxic-ischemic encephalopathy. J Pediatr. 2014;164:973–979.e1.
4. Nakahara T, Ogawa M. Hemopoietic colony-forming cells in umbilical cord blood with extensive capability to generate mono- and multipotential hemopoietic progenitors. J Clin Invest. 1982;70:1324–8.
5. Nabetani M, Shintaku H, Hamazaki T. Future perspectives of cell therapy for neonatal hypoxic-ischemic encephalopathy. Pediatr Res. 2018;83:356–63.
6. Tsuji M, Sawada M, Watabe S, et al. Autologous cord blood cell therapy for neonatal hypoxic-ischaemic encephalopathy: a pilot study for feasibility and safety. Sci Rep. 2020;10:4603.
7. Sun JM, Song AW, Case LE, et al. Effect of autologous cord blood infusion on motor function and brain connectivity in young children with cerebral palsy: a randomized, placebo-controlled trial. Cells Transl Med. 2017;6:2071–8.

GPSR Compliance

The European Union's (EU) General Product Safety Regulation (GPSR) is a set of rules that requires consumer products to be safe and our obligations to ensure this.

If you have any concerns about our products, you can contact us on ProductSafety@springernature.com

In case Publisher is established outside the EU, the EU authorized representative is:

Springer Nature Customer Service Center GmbH
Europaplatz 3
69115 Heidelberg, Germany

Batch number: 10732090

Printed by Printforce, the Netherlands